Yearbook of Anesthesiology-10

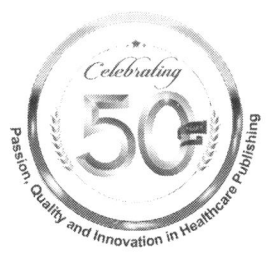

Editorial Board

1. **VP Kumra** MD DAc FICA
   Past President and Advisor
   Indian College of Anaesthesiologists
   Former Vice President
   Indian Society of Anaesthesiologists (National)
   Emeritus Consultant and Advisor
   Institute of Anesthesiology, Pain and Perioperative Medicine
   Sir Ganga Ram Hospital, New Delhi, India
   ved_kumra@yahoo.com

2. **B Radhakrishnan** MD MPhil FICA
   President
   Indian College of Anaesthesiologists
   Past President
   Indian Society of Anaesthesiologists (National)
   Senior Professor and Consultant
   Gokulam Medical College and GG Hospital
   Thiruvananthapuram, Kerala, India
   brktvm@yahoo.com

3. **Jayashree Sood** MD FFARCS PGDHHM FICA
   CEO, Indian College of Anaesthesiologists
   Professor and Chairperson
   Institute of Anesthesiology, Pain and Perioperative Medicine
   Honorary Jt Secretary, Board of Management
   Sir Ganga Ram Hospital, New Delhi, India
   drjayashreesood@gmail.com

4. **Baljit Singh** MD FICA
   CEO, Indian College of Anaesthesiologists
   Past President
   Indian Society of Anaesthesiologists (National)
   Former Director Professor
   GB Pant Institute of Postgraduate Medical Education and Research, New Delhi
   Professor and Head
   Department of Anesthesiology and Critical Care
   Faculty of Medicine and Health Sciences
   SGT University, Gurugram, Haryana, India
   drbaljitsingh@gmail.com

Yearbook of Anesthesiology-10

Editors
Raminder Sehgal MD DA FICA
Former Director Professor
Department of Anesthesiology
Maulana Azad Medical College, New Delhi
Former Senior Consultant
Institute of Anesthesiology, Pain and Perioperative Medicine
Sir Ganga Ram Hospital, New Delhi, India
ramindersehgal@hotmail.com

Anjan Trikha MD DA FICA FAMS FAOA
Professor
Department of Anesthesiology, Pain Medicine
and Critical Care
All India Institute of Medical Sciences
New Delhi, India
anjantrikha@gmail.com

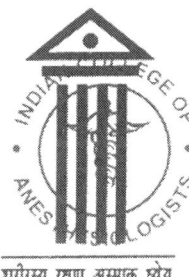

शरीरस्य खलु अस्माकं ध्येय
Indian College of Anaesthesiologists

Foreword
Muralidhar K

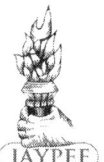

JAYPEE BROTHERS MEDICAL PUBLISHERS
The Health Sciences Publisher
New Delhi | London

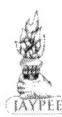 **Jaypee Brothers Medical Publishers (P) Ltd**

Headquarters
Jaypee Brothers Medical Publishers (P) Ltd
EMCA House, 23/23-B
Ansari Road, Daryaganj
New Delhi 110 002, India
Landline: +91-11-23272143, +91-11-23272703
+91-11-23282021, +91-11-23245672
Head Office: 011-43574357
Email: jaypee@jaypeebrothers.com

Corporate Office
Jaypee Brothers Medical Publishers (P) Ltd
4838/24, Ansari Road, Daryaganj
New Delhi 110 002, India
Phone: +91-11-43574357
Fax: +91-11-43574314
Email: jaypee@jaypeebrothers.com

Overseas Office
JP Medical Ltd
83 Victoria Street, London
SW1H 0HW (UK)
Phone: +44 20 3170 8910
Fax: +44 (0)20 3008 6180
Email: info@jpmedpub.com

Website: www.jaypeebrothers.com
Website: www.jaypeedigital.com

© 2021, Jaypee Brothers Medical Publishers

The views and opinions expressed in this book are solely those of the original contributor(s)/author(s) and do not necessarily represent those of editor(s) of the book.

All rights reserved. No part of this publication may be reproduced, stored or transmitted in any form or by any means, electronic, mechanical, photocopying, recording or otherwise, without the prior permission in writing of the publishers.

All brand names and product names used in this book are trade names, service marks, trademarks or registered trademarks of their respective owners. The publisher is not associated with any product or vendor mentioned in this book.

Medical knowledge and practice change constantly. This book is designed to provide accurate, authoritative information about the subject matter in question. However, readers are advised to check the most current information available on procedures included and check information from the manufacturer of each product to be administered, to verify the recommended dose, formula, method and duration of administration, adverse effects and contraindications. It is the responsibility of the practitioner to take all appropriate safety precautions. Neither the publisher nor the author(s)/editor(s) assume any liability for any injury and/or damage to persons or property arising from or related to use of material in this book.

This book is sold on the understanding that the publisher is not engaged in providing professional medical services. If such advice or services are required, the services of a competent medical professional should be sought.

Every effort has been made where necessary to contact holders of copyright to obtain permission to reproduce copyright material. If any have been inadvertently overlooked, the publisher will be pleased to make the necessary arrangements at the first opportunity. The **CD/DVD-ROM** (if any) provided in the sealed envelope with this book is complimentary and free of cost. **Not meant for sale.**

Inquiries for bulk sales may be solicited at: jaypee@jaypeebrothers.com

Yearbook of Anesthesiology-10

First Edition: **2021**

ISBN: 978-93-90595-01-3

Printed at: Replika Press Pvt. Ltd.

Contributors

Amita Gupta MD
Consultant and Professor
Department of Anesthesiology and Intensive Care
Vardhman Mahavir Medical College (VMMC) and Safdarjung Hospital
New Delhi, India
amitaguptadr@gmail.com

Anjan Trikha MD DA FICA FAMS FAOA
Professor
Department of Anesthesiology, Pain Medicine and Critical Care
All India Institute of Medical Sciences
New Delhi, India
anjantrikha@gmail.com

Anju Gupta
MBBS MD DNB IDRA MNAMS PGCCHM
Assistant Professor
Department of Anesthesiology, Pain and Critical Care
All India Institute of Medical Sciences
New Delhi, India
dranjugupta09@gmail.com

Anoop Raj Gogia MD
Consultant and Professor
Department of Anesthesiology and Intensive Care
Vardhman Mahavir Medical College (VMMC) and Safdarjung Hospital
New Delhi, India
gogiaanoop@gmail.com

Anudeep Jafra MD
Assistant Professor
Department of Anesthesiology and Intensive Care
Postgraduate Institute of Medical Education and Research
Chandigarh, India
anu_gmch@yahoo.co.in

Arunthevaraja Karuppiah MBBS MD
Obstetric Anesthesiology
Clinical Fellow
Department of Anesthesiology
University of Maryland
School of Medicine
Baltimore, MD, USA
arunks8401@gmail.com

Bharti Wadhwa MD
Professor
Department of Anesthesiology
Maulana Azad Medical College
New Delhi, India
drbhartitaneja@gmail.com

Bhavani Shankar Kodali MBBS MD
Professor
Department of Anesthesiology
University of Maryland
School of Medicine, Baltimore
Division Chief
Obstetric Anesthesiology
Chief Safety Officer, Anesthesiology
University of Maryland Medical Center
Baltimore, MD, USA
bkodali@som.umaryland.edu

Chhavi Sawhney DNB
Professor
Department of Anesthesiology
Jai Prakash Narayan Apex Trauma Center (JPNATC)
All India Institute of Medical Sciences
New Delhi, India
drchhavisawhney@gmail.com

Girija Prasad Rath MD DM FICA
Professor
Department of Neuroanesthesiology and Critical Care
Neurosciences Center
All India Institute of Medical Sciences
New Delhi, India
girijarath@yahoo.co.in

Contributors

Gunchan Paul MD IDCCM
Associate Professor
Department of Critical Care Medicine
Dayanand Medical College and Hospital
Ludhiana, Punjab, India
gunchan@gmail.com

Jayashree Sood MD FFRCA PGDHHM FICA
Senior Consultant and Chairperson
Institute of Anesthesiology, Pain and Perioperative Medicine
Sir Ganga Ram Hospital
New Delhi, India
drjayashreesood@gmail.com

Jyotsna Goswami MD
Senior Consultant and Head
Department of Onco-Anesthesia, Critical Care and Pain
Tata Medical Center
Kolkata, West Bengal, India
jyotsnagoswami@gmail.com

Kamakshi Garg MD MAMS
Associate Professor
Department of Anesthesiology
Dayanand Medical College and Hospital
Ludhiana, Punjab, India
drkamakshigarg@gmail.com

Lt Col Shyam Madabhushi
MD DNB DM (Critical Care Medicine)
Classified Specialist and Intensivist
Department of Anesthesiology
Army Hospital (Research and Referral)
New Delhi, India
drmshyam@yahoo.com

Manjula Sarkar MD
Professor In-charge
Department of Cardiac Anesthesia
Dr DY Patil Medical College, Pune
Former Head
Department of Cardiac Anesthesia
King Edward Memorial (KEM) Medical College
Mumbai, Maharashtra, India
drmanjusarkar@gmail.com

Manpreet Kaur MD
Assistant Professor
Department of Anesthesiology, Pain Medicine and Critical Care
All India Institute of Medical Sciences
New Delhi, India
manpreetkaurrajpal@yahoo.com

Medha Mohta MD MAMS
Director Professor
Department of Anesthesiology and Critical Care
University College of Medical Sciences and Guru Teg Bahadur Hospital
New Delhi, India
medhamohta@gmail.com

Neerja Bhardwaj MD
Professor
Department of Anesthesiology and Intensive Care
Postgraduate Institute of Medical Education and Research
Chandigarh, India
neerja.bhardwaj@gmail.com

Neeru Luthra MD
Associate Professor
Department of Anesthesiology
Dayanand Medical College and Hospital
Ludhiana, Punjab, India
drneeru1977@yahoo.co.in

Neeti Makhija MD
Professor
Department of Cardiac Anesthesia, Cardiothoracic Center
All India Institute of Medical Sciences
New Delhi, India
neetimakhija@hotmail.com

Neha Aeron MD DNB MNAMS
Assistant Professor
Department of Anesthesiology
Sardar Patel Medical College
Bikaner, Rajasthan, India
nga6016@gmail.com

Nitin Sethi DNB
Consultant
Institute of Anesthesiology, Pain and Perioperative Medicine
Sir Ganga Ram Hospital
New Delhi, India
nitinsethi77@yahoo.co.in

PL Gautam MD DNB FICCM MNAMS
Professor and Head
Department of Critical Care Medicine
Liver Transplant Anesthesiologist
Dayanand Medical College and Hospital
Ludhiana, Punjab, India
drplgautam@gmail.com

PN Jain MD MNAMS FICA FIAPM
Professor and Head
Division of Pain
Department of Anesthesiology, Critical Care and Pain
Tata Memorial Center, Mumbai
Homi Bhabha National Institute (HBNI)
Mumbai, Maharashtra, India
Pnj5@hotmail.com

Prakash Srinivas Shastri
MD FRCA FICCM
Senior Consultant and Vice Chairman
Institute of Critical Care Medicine
Sir Ganga Ram Hospital
New Delhi, India
prakashshastri@live.in

Pratibha Jain Shah MD
Professor and Former Head
Department of Anesthesiology and Critical Care
Pt Jawahar Lal Nehru Memorial Medical College
Raipur, Chhattisgarh
Faculty, Academy of Traumatology
Ahmedabad, Gujarat, India
prati_jain@rediffmail.com

Raj Tobin MD EDRA FICA PGDHHM
Director and Head
Department of Anesthesiology
Max Super Speciality Hospital
Saket, New Delhi, India
rajtobin@gmail.com

Rohan Magoon MD
Assistant Professor
Department of Anesthesiology
Dr Ram Manohar Lohia Hospital
New Delhi, India
rohanmagoon21@gmail.com

RS Thota
MD MNAMS Fellowship in Pain Management (Singapore)
Professor
Department of Anesthesiology, Critical Care and Pain
Tata Memorial Center, Mumbai
Homi Bhabha National Institute (HBNI)
Mumbai, Maharashtra, India
Ragstho24@gmail.com

Rudranil Nandi MD DM (Oncoanesthesia)
Consultant
Department of Onco-Anesthesia, Critical Care and Pain
Tata Medical Center
Kolkata, West Bengal, India
drrudranilnandi@gmail.com

Sadik Mohammed MD
Associate Professor
Department of Anesthesiology and Critical Care
All India Institute of Medical Sciences
Jodhpur, Rajasthan, India
drmsadik@gmail.com

Sanjay Agrawal
MD PDCC (Neuroanesthesia)
Professor and Head
Department of Anesthesiology
All India Institute of Medical Sciences
Rishikesh, Uttarakhand, India
sanjay.anaesth@aiimsrishikesh.edu.in

Contributors

Senthil Kumar DA DNB
Assistant Professor
Department of Anesthesiology and Pain Medicine
Sri Ramachandra Medical College and Research Institute
Chennai, Tamil Nadu, India
drsenthilkumar17@gmail.com

Shashi Kiran
DA DNB MD FICA
Senior Professor
Department of Anesthesiology
Pt Bhagwat Dayal Sharma Post Graduate Institute of Medical Sciences
Rohtak, Haryana, India
drshashi64@rediffmail.com

Shobana Bharadwaj MBBS
Assistant Professor
Department of Anesthesiology
Director, Obstetric Anesthesiology Fellowship Program
University of Maryland School of Medicine
Baltimore, MD, USA
sbharadwaj@som.umaryland.edu

Soma Ganesh Raja
MD FIPM
Assistant Professor
Department of Anesthesiology and Pain Medicine
Sri Ramachandra Medical College and Research Institute
Chennai, Tamil Nadu, India
drsoms@gmail.com

Subodh Kumar MD
Assistant Professor
Department of Anesthesiology and Intensive Care
Government Medical College and Hospital
Chandigarh, India
subodh.kgmc@gmail.com

Sukanya Mitra MD MAMS
Professor and Head
Department of Anesthesiology and Intensive Care
Government Medical College and Hospital
Chandigarh, India
drsmitra12@yahoo.com

Swati Chhabra MD DNB
Associate Professor
Department of Anesthesiology and Critical Care
All India Institute of Medical Sciences
Jodhpur, Rajasthan, India
swati_virgo83@yahoo.co.in

Vanitha Rajagopalan MD DM
Assistant Professor
Department of Neuroanesthesiology and Critical Care
Neurosciences Center
All India Institute of Medical Sciences
New Delhi, India
vanitharajagopalan@gmail.com

Veena Asthana MD
Professor and Head
Department of Anesthesiology
Himalayan Institute of Medical Sciences
Swami Ram Himalayan University
Dehradun, Uttarakhand, India
drvasthana@gmail.com

Venkata Ganesh MBBS MD
Assistant Professor
Department of Anesthesiology, Pain Medicine and Critical Care
All India Institute of Medical Sciences
New Delhi, India
bjfiero@gmail.com

Yudhyavir Singh MD
Assistant Professor
Department of Anesthesiology
Jai Prakash Narayan Apex Trauma Center (JPNATC)
All India Institute of Medical Sciences
New Delhi, India
yudhyavir@gmail.com

Foreword

I am delighted to write foreword for the 10th volume of *Yearbook of Anesthesiology*, which is being published annually under the auspices of Indian College of Anaesthesiologists (ICA), India. ICA is an academic body which was established to promote education, improve anesthesia standards and bring about equity in training nationwide. The college has come a long way from the time of its inception in 2008. It has taken long strides by collaborating with American Society of Anesthesiology, Society of Ambulatory Medicine and other international organizations. These steps will help to turn its goals into reality.

With great pleasure I would like to acknowledge the contributions of editors, Dr Raminder Sehgal and Dr Anjan Trikha, who have taken up the onus of publishing the Yearbook on a regular basis. The Yearbook is a highly acclaimed publication with the authors carefully chosen to include experts as well brilliant youngsters to provide the best and up-to-date knowledge to its readers. It is heartening to know that the *Yearbook of Anesthesiology-10* has a wide variety of subjects relating to the contemporary practice of anesthesia and intensive care. The contributors have put in a huge effort to provide us the current information on topics such as anesthesia for laser surgery, vasodilatory shock, blood conservation strategy, new anticoagulants, opioid-free anesthesia, nonoperation room anesthesia, carbon footprint and cardiac drugs. I know that this is going to be a boost to the youngsters and the practitioners of anesthesia in this country. The contents are of immense value aimed to provide evidence-based patient care, safety and benefit the humanity at large.

Muralidhar K MD FIACTA FICA MBA FASE
Dean, Indian College of Anaesthesiologists
Director (Academic), Senior Consultant and Professor
Department of Anesthesiology and Intensive Care
Narayana Institute of Cardiac Sciences
Narayana Health City, Bengaluru, Karnataka
Professor of International Health
University of Minnesota, Minneapolis, MN, USA
Principal
Narayana Hrudayalaya Institute of Allied Health Sciences
Bengaluru, Karnataka, India
*muralidhar.kanchi.dr@narayanahealth.org/
kanchirulestheworld@gmail.com*

Preface

The present *Yearbook of Anesthesiology* is the 10th volume in the series of yearly updates, published under the auspices of the Indian College of Anaesthesiologists, India, an academic body focused on improving anesthesia education. It was in 2011 that the idea of yearly updates was envisaged and the first edition was published in 2012 by the college, with Dr Umesh Chandra as its editor. At that time there were many apprehensions regarding the book's acceptability among anesthesiologists in the country as it was for the first time that such a volume was being published from India. The members of the college and the editorial board were surprised at the overwhelming response that the first volume received, thus the saga of the *Yearbook of Anesthesiology* continued and the 10th volume is being released.

As in all previous volumes, this year too, the contents can be divided into three subgroups—anesthesiology, pain and critical care medicine. The contents of the present volume have a mix both classical anesthesia topics like capnography, blood-brain barrier and anesthesia circuits and those that are being hotly discussed and are likely to gain popularity in the coming years such as carbon footprint analysis of perioperative care and opioid-free anesthesia. Opioids are not freely available in India, especially in smaller cities and towns, therefore practicing and administration of opioid-free anesthesia would be a boon for the anesthesiologists. Similarly, extracorporeal therapies like use of CytoSorb for management of sepsis have been found to be helpful for abdominal sepsis and other similar therapies are likely to be used in future. Other important topics relate to maternal and child health and include analysis of maternal morbidity and mortality, difficult pediatric airway and management of children with congenital cardiac disease.

The chapters on postdural puncture headache, colloids, perioperative thromboembolism, blood conservation strategies, peripheral effects of opioids, management of head and neck neuralgias and cancer pain would be very useful for practicing anesthesiologists. The postgraduate students in anesthesia are likely to find the chapters on newer anticoagulants, latest modes of ventilation, trauma care, anesthesia for laser surgery and non-operating room anesthesia very helpful. Issues related to newer cardiac drugs and vasodilatory shock have been discussed extensively. Regional anesthesia is an integral part of the practice of anesthesia, and understandably we included a chapter on the controversies which surround it. Last but not the least, this book would have been incomplete without a chapter on COVID in this year of the pandemic. To accommodate it, we had to forgo the much appreciated section related to "Journal Scan" which had been a regular feature of the Yearbook ever since we took over as editors.

Like always, the specialty chapters have been written by experts in their fields and the topics that have been chosen are the ones that have seen newer concepts being used for patient care. It was a challenge to bring out the

10th edition due to the COVID pandemic that has derailed academic programs all over the world, especially the anesthesiology programs because most of the anesthesiologists are at the helm of COVID Task Forces. We would like to express our gratitude to all contributors for sparing their precious time for contributing to this Yearbook without any kind of financial rewards. Our special thanks are also due for the staff of M/s Jaypee Brothers Medical Publishers (P) Ltd, New Delhi, India, for their cooperation and support, as they too had to work with limited staff under trying circumstances due to the pandemic.

As editors, we would welcome opinions, suggestions and criticism regarding our efforts in bringing out the Yearbook so that we can improve the content of the future volumes.

Raminder Sehgal
Anjan Trikha

Contents

1. **Capnography: An Indispensable Noninvasive Tool** 1
   Bhavani Shankar Kodali, Arunthevaraja Karuppiah, Shobana Bharadwaj
   - Physics *1*
   - Colorimetric Device *3*
   - Physiological Overview *4*
   - Limitations *12*
   - Future Trends and Conclusion *13*

2. **Recent Trends in Trauma Care** 16
   Chhavi Sawhney, Yudhyavir Singh
   - Prehospital Phase *16*
   - Trauma Damage Control *18*
   - REBOA and Resuscitative Thoracotomy *19*
   - Trauma Critical Care *19*
   - Hybrid Operating Rooms *20*
   - Trauma Training *20*
   - Specific Injuries *21*

3. **Anesthesia for Laser Surgery** 26
   Soma Ganesh Raja, Senthil Kumar
   - Laser Physics *26*
   - Components of Laser *26*
   - Laser Effectiveness *27*
   - Clinical Effects of Laser *28*
   - Laser Classification *28*
   - Laser Hazards *28*
   - Anesthetic Considerations for Laser Airway Surgery *35*

4. **Anesthesia Circuits: Bain and Closed** 45
   Swati Chhabra, Sadik Mohammed
   - Bain Circuit *46*
   - Circle System *51*

5. **What's New in the Management of Vasodilatory Shock?** 67
   Shyam Madabhushi
   - Vasopressors *67*
   - Intravenous Fluid Administration and Timing of Vasopressors *69*
   - Adjunctive Therapies: Steroids and Vitamins *70*
   - Mechanical Circulatory Support for Distributive Shock *71*

6. **Controversies and Gray Zones in Regional Anesthesia** 74
   Raj Tobin
   - Neuraxial Anesthesia in Thrombocytopathy and Thrombocytopenia *75*
   - Neuraxial Anesthesia in Patients under General Anesthesia/Deep Sedation *75*
   - Epidural Blood Patch *76*

- Epidural Test Dose *76*
- Regional Anesthesia and Acute Compartment Syndrome *77*
- Adjuvants in Nerve Blocks *78*
- Regional Anesthesia and Peripheral Nerve Injury *81*
- Regional Anesthesia and Rebound Pain *81*
- Regional Anesthesia in Diabetics *82*

7. Intraoperative Blood Conservation Strategies 88
Jyotsna Goswami, Rudranil Nandi
- Preoperative Assessment and Optimization to Reduce Intraoperative Blood Loss *89*
- Intraoperative Strategies *92*
- Intraoperative Monitoring *97*
- Biological and Clinical Consequences of Perioperative Allogenic Blood Transfusion *98*

8. Newer Anticoagulants and Anesthesia 102
Bharti Wadhwa
- Understanding the Coagulation Pathway *102*
- Physiology of Therapeutic Anticoagulation *103*
- Limitations of Traditionally used Anticoagulants *103*
- Direct Acting Oral Anticoagulants *104*
- Pharmacokinetics of Newer Oral Anticoagulants *104*
- Practical Concerns with Perioperative Management of Anticoagulation *106*
- Perioperative Management of Newer Oral Anticoagulant *108*
- Emergency Surgery *110*
- Administration of Antidote *111*
- Neuraxial Block and Newer Oral Anticoagulant *113*

9. The Blood-Brain Barrier 118
Girija Prasad Rath, Vanitha Rajagopalan
- Historical Perspective *118*
- Anatomy and Physiology *118*
- Development of Blood-Brain Barrier *121*
- Regulation and Homeostasis *121*
- Transport across Blood-Brain Barrier *121*
- Blood-Brain Barrier and Disease *124*
- Imaging the Blood-Brain Barrier *127*
- Markers of Damaged Blood-Brain Barrier *127*
- Future Perspectives *128*

10. Pediatric Difficult Airway 132
Neerja Bhardwaj, Anudeep Jafra
- Principle Approach to a Difficult Pediatric Airway *132*
- Predictors of Difficult Airway in Children *133*
- Preoperative Assessment of the Airway *134*
- Investigations *135*
- Anesthetic Management *136*
- Unexpected Difficult Intubation *140*
- Difficult Airway Algorithms *141*
- Extubation *141*
- Role of Ultrasound in Airway Management in Children *141*

11. **Peripheral Analgesic Effect of Opioids** 145
    Manpreet Kaur
    - Need for Peripheral Administration of Opioids   145
    - Peripheral Opioid Receptors   145
    - Inflammation and Peripheral Opioid Receptor   146
    - Routes of Administration   147
    - Recent Advances   149

12. **Maternal Morbidity and Mortality: An Anesthesiologist's Role and Perspective** 152
    Medha Mohta
    - Definitions   152
    - The Current Situation   152
    - Causes of Maternal Morbidity and Mortality   153
    - Role of Anesthesiologist in Management of Parturients   154
    - Anesthesia-related Complications   154
    - Nonanesthetic Perioperative Complications   159
    - Measures to be taken to Reduce Severe Maternal Morbidity and Mortality   162
    - Anesthesiologists as Peridelivery Physicians   163

13. **Opioid-free Anesthesia and Analgesia** 169
    Sukanya Mitra, Subodh Kumar
    - Definition   169
    - Why is Opioid-free Anesthesia Necessary?   169
    - Components   171
    - Goal   171
    - Indications   171
    - Advantages and Disadvantages   171
    - Nonopioid Adjuncts   172
    - Measurement of Nociception   176
    - Opioid-free Anesthesia for Different Surgeries   177
    - Controversies, Questions, and the Way Ahead   179

14. **Nonoperating Room Anesthesia: Challenges and Safety** 187
    Kamakshi Garg, Neeru Luthra
    - Novel Characteristics of NORA Cases and Challenges to the Anesthesia Provider   187
    - Safety during Anesthesia Practice   188
    - Preprocedural Assessment for Outpatient Anesthesia Procedures   190
    - Monitoring in Nonoperating Room Anesthesia Locations   190
    - Specific Procedures-related Issues   190
    - Anesthesia for Image-guided Interventions: Evolution of a New Interface   192
    - Anesthesiologists in the Catheterization Laboratory   197

15. **Anesthetic Management in Pediatric Patients with a Congenital Heart Disease Undergoing Noncardiac Surgery** 201
    Manjula Sarkar, Anju Gupta
    - Classification of Congenital Heart Disease   201
    - Pathophysiology   201

- Signs and Symptoms *203*
- Risk Categorization *203*
- Anesthetic Management *203*
- Recommendation for Management of Congenital Heart Disease Children Posted for Elective Procedures *207*
- Recommendation for Management of Congenital Heart Disease Children Posted for Emergency Surgeries *207*
- General Principles of Anesthetic Management *208*
- Regional Anesthesia *210*
- Anesthetic Considerations of Management of Specific Cardiac Lesions *212*
- Limitations in Managing Congenital Heart Disease Patients *214*

16. Panorama of Postdural Puncture Headache: Current Evidence 218
Pratibha Jain Shah
- History *218*
- Pathophysiology *219*
- Risk Factors *221*
- Associated Problems *225*
- Prevention *225*
- Diagnostic Evaluation *227*
- Treatment *228*

17. Perioperative Venous Thromboembolism: A Review 236
Nitin Sethi, Jayashree Sood
- Pathophysiology *236*
- Diagnosis of Venous Thromboembolism *237*
- Treatment of Pulmonary Embolism *240*
- Guidelines for Perioperative Venous Thromboembolism Prophylaxis *241*
- Pharmacological Prophylaxis Drugs *248*

18. Carbon Footprint Analysis in Perioperative Care 255
Shashi Kiran, Neha Aeron
- Technique of Estimation of Carbon Footprint *255*
- Role of Perioperative Care in CO_2 Footprint *256*
- Adverse Effects of Carbon Footprint *259*
- Reduction of Perioperative CO_2 Footprint: Strategies *259*
- Role of Anesthesiologist *261*

19. Colloids: An Overview.. 265
Sanjay Agrawal, Veena Asthana
- Albumin *265*
- Semisynthetic Colloids *266*
- Crystalloids versus Colloids *270*
- Clinical Efficacy of Various Colloids *270*

20. Newer Modes of Ventilation 273
PL Gautam, Gunchan Paul
- Dual Control within a Breath *277*
- Dual Control in Subsequent Breaths *278*
- Smart Modes (Closed-loop Systems) *283*
- Physiological Closed-loop Ventilation and Highly Automated Systems— NeoGanesh SmartCare *290*

21. **New Cardiac Drugs Anesthesia Implications**.. 295
    Neeti Makhija, Rohan Magoon
    - Antiarrhythmics *295*
    - Anticoagulants *297*
    - Reversal Agents against New Oral Anticoagulants *300*
    - Antiplatelet Agents *300*
    - Metabolic Modulators *302*
    - Antihypertensives *303*
    - Antiheart Failure Drugs *304*
    - Therapeutics in Pulmonary Arterial Hypertension *305*
    - Anesthetic Implications *308*
    - Recommendations *309*

22. **Role of Extracorporeal Therapy in Sepsis**... 314
    Prakash Shastri
    - Blood Purification Devices used in the Treatment of Septic Shock *314*

23. **Recent Advances in the Management of Cancer Pain**................................ 318
    PN Jain, RS Thota
    - Pharmacological Treatment *320*
    - World Health Organization three-step Analgesic Ladder *324*
    - Bone Pain *325*
    - Interventional Treatment *325*

24. **Management of Head and Neck Neuralgia** 330
    Anoop Raj Gogia, Amita Gupta
    - Trigeminal Neuralgia *330*
    - Glossopharyngeal Neuralgia *333*
    - Herpes Zoster and Postherpetic Neuralgia *335*
    - Occipital Neuralgia *339*
    - Other Facial Pains *339*

25. **Anesthesia Implications in COVID Positive Patients**...................... 344
    Anjan Trikha, Venkata Ganesh
    - Infection Control for Anesthesia *345*
    - Protection of Anesthesia Equipment *346*
    - Operating Room Decontamination *347*
    - Management of Anesthesia *348*
    - Obstetric Anesthesia *353*
    - Pediatric Anesthesia *354*
    - Anesthesia and Bronchoscopy *354*
    - Postoperative Management *355*

Index *363*

Plate 1

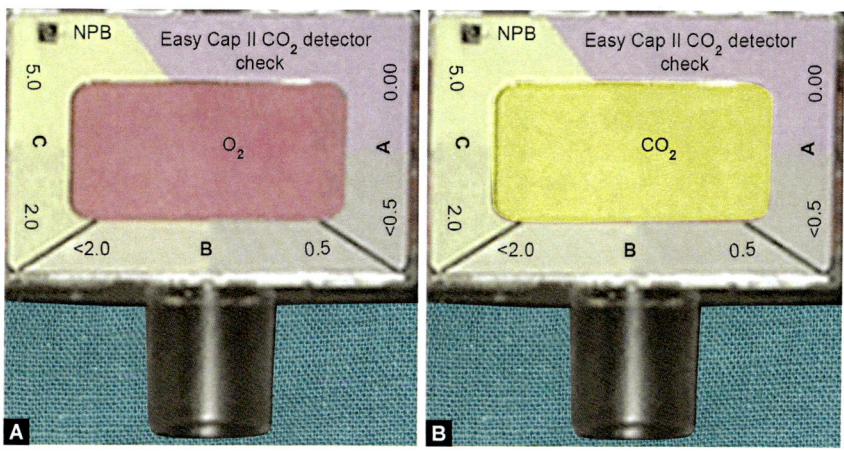

Figs. 4A and B: Calorimetric capnometer. The pH sensitive paper changes from purple to yellow when CO_2 is detected. *(Chapter 1)*

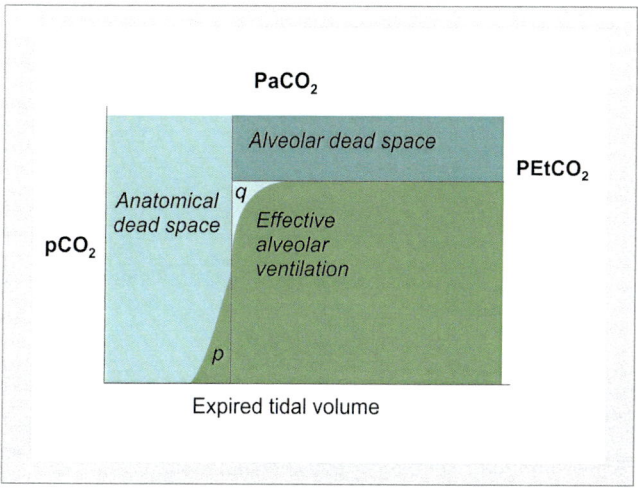

Fig. 6: Volume capnogram. *(Chapter 1)*

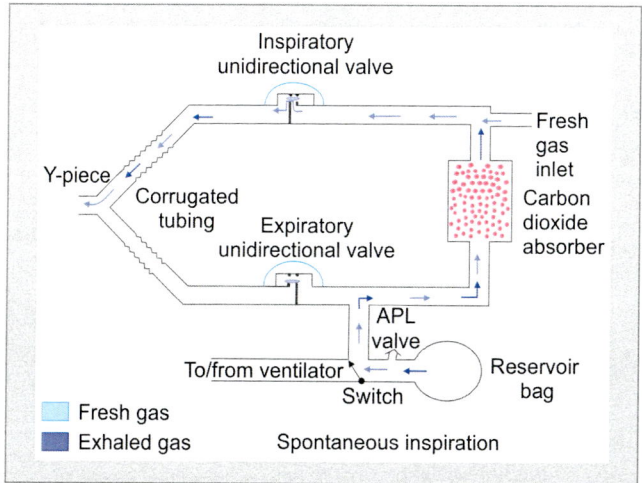

Fig. 17: Diagrammatic representation of flow mechanics of a circle system during inspiratory phase of spontaneous ventilation. *(Chapter 4)*

Plate 2

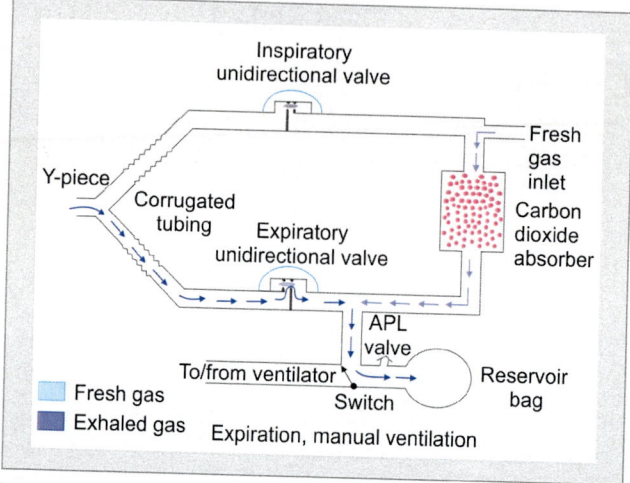

Fig. 18: Diagrammatic representation of flow mechanics of a circle system during expiratory phase of spontaneous ventilation. *(Chapter 4)*

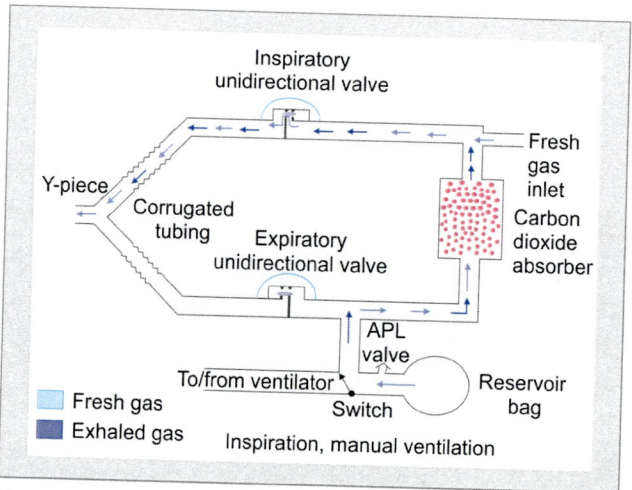

Fig. 19: Diagrammatic representation of flow mechanics of a circle system during inspiratory phase of manual ventilation. *(Chapter 4)*

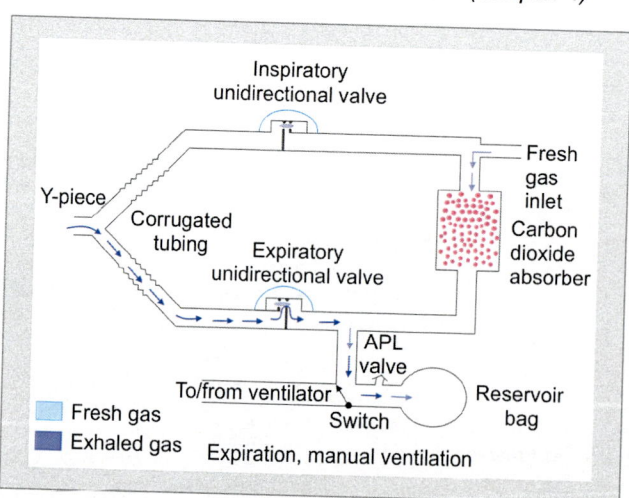

Fig. 20: Diagrammatic representation of flow mechanics of a circle system during expiratory phase of manual ventilation. *(Chapter 4)*

CHAPTER 1

Capnography: An Indispensable Noninvasive Tool

Bhavani Shankar Kodali, Arunthevaraja Karuppiah, Shobana Bharadwaj

INTRODUCTION

Capnography is the measurement of the partial pressure of exhaled carbon dioxide (CO_2) and display of CO_2 waveform. The graphic representation is expressed as expired CO_2 concentration over time, or volume and is known as time, or volume capnogram. Capnography became a standard of monitoring during anesthesia practice in Europe in the late 1970s and the United States in mid-1980s. Since then, it has evolved as an essential component of standard anesthesia monitoring armamentarium.[1] Capnography has also expanded beyond the operating room into the emergency department, radiology, gastroenterology procedures, adult, and pediatric sedation sites. Furthermore, capnography has also made its impact in intensive care units (ICUs) across the world for monitoring ventilation and assuring correct location of endotracheal tube (ETT) continuously. Capnometry is a numeric measurement and display of the level of CO_2 concentration without waveform. The waveform of capnography is more valuable and reliable than capnometry for clinical interpretation.[2,3]

PHYSICS

There are two types of capnography devices **(Figs. 1, 2 and Table 1)**: (1) "sidestream" and (2) "mainstream"[4] depending upon where the CO_2 analyzer is located in relation to the ventilator circuit. In a "mainstream" analyzer, sampling window is in the ventilator circuit (near the hub of ETT) and measures CO_2, while in a "sidestream", the gas is located out of the ventilator circuit and gas sample is aspirated via 6 feet sampling tube. In both types, the gas analyzers work mostly using the principle of infra-red (IR) absorption spectroscopy **(Fig. 3)**. An IR diode emits the light that traverses the chamber containing airway sample. The CO_2 molecules absorb IR light and unabsorbed IR light is detected by an IR detector. Molecules of CO_2 absorb IR radiation at a very specific wavelength (4.26 µm), with the amount of radiation absorbed having a nearly exponential relation to the CO_2 concentration (Beer-Lambert Law) present in the breath sample. The difference between the source light and absorbed light is transformed into CO_2 concentration and displayed as

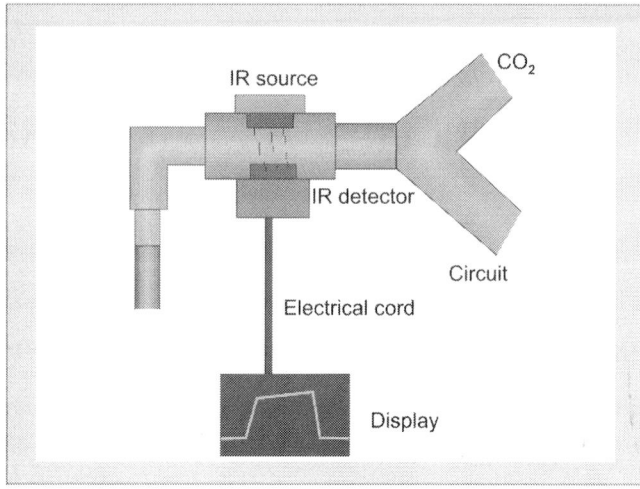

Fig. 1: Mainstream capnography: Infra-red (IR) light sensor is positioned in the airway circuit.

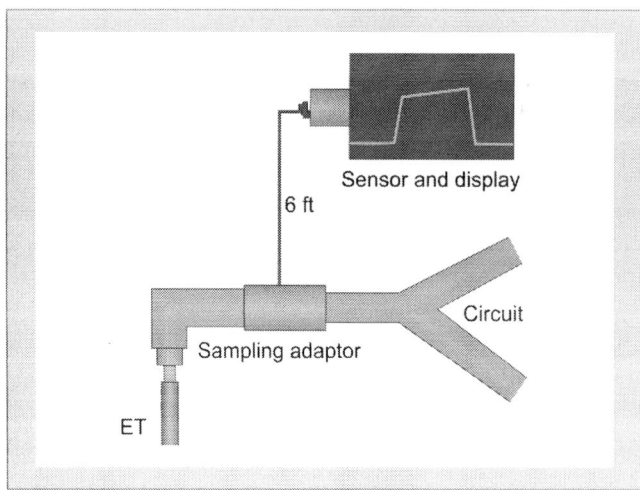

Fig. 2: Sidestream capnography: Infra-red (IR) light sensor is positioned outside the airway circuit. A T-piece adapter with a 6 feet disposable tubing is inserted between the breathing tube and airway circuit. (ET: endotracheal tube)

a capnography waveform. Water vapor, nitrous oxide, and anesthetic agents absorb IR light, but at a different wavelength. There are other techniques of measuring CO_2 using photoacoustic spectroscopy, Raman scattering, and mass spectrometry, which are not commonly used.

In the majority of capnographs, the exhaled concentration is plotted against the time (time capnography) and is the common method in practice. In volume capnography, the exhaled CO_2 is serially plotted against expired lung volume. Volume capnography is not routinely used. However, this may be a preferred technique in near future, as it enables indirect estimation of physiological dead space.[5]

TABLE 1: Types of capnography and their characteristics

Sidestream capnography	Mainstream capnography
Used both for intubated and nonintubated patients	Predominantly used for intubated patients
Most widely used method	The sensor contains an infra-red (IR) measurement device with an electrical cord. The newer versions are extremely light
The gas sampling tube is inserted in between the breathing circuit and endotracheal tube. Only manufacturer recommended tubing material and length must be used	Adaptor containing IR sensor is interposed between the patient's breathing circuit and endotracheal tube. Sensor emits IR light to a photodetector on the other side of the adapter
Slight delay in the display of the CO_2 waveform	CO_2 waveform is measured immediately
Main advantage of sidestream capnography is that, it can be used in nonintubated patients, for instance, patients with oxygen facemask	Need special smaller lighter weight adapters for use in the nonintubated patients
A drawback is that the tubing may become blocked from water vapor or secretions	The mainstream sensor is heated above body temperature, which prevents water vapor condensation and allows the sensor to function in high moisture environments

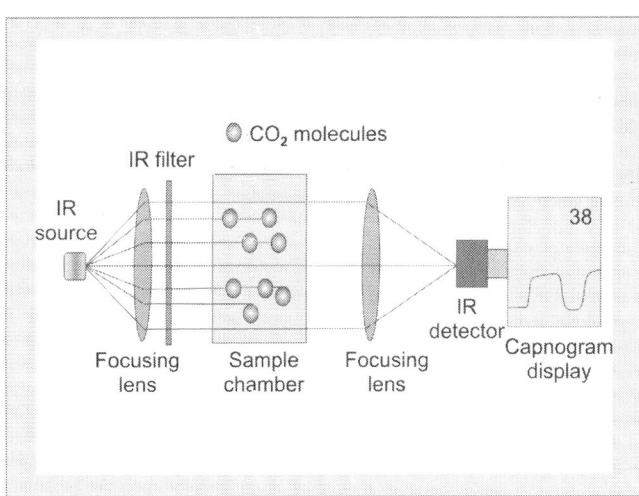

Fig. 3: Measurement of carbon dioxide (CO_2) by infra-red (IR) technology.

COLORIMETRIC DEVICE

The colorimetric CO_2 detector **(Figs. 4A and B)** can be used for verification of correct placement of an ETT in the trachea. It has especially treated litmus paper, which changes color from purple to yellow. The device is not

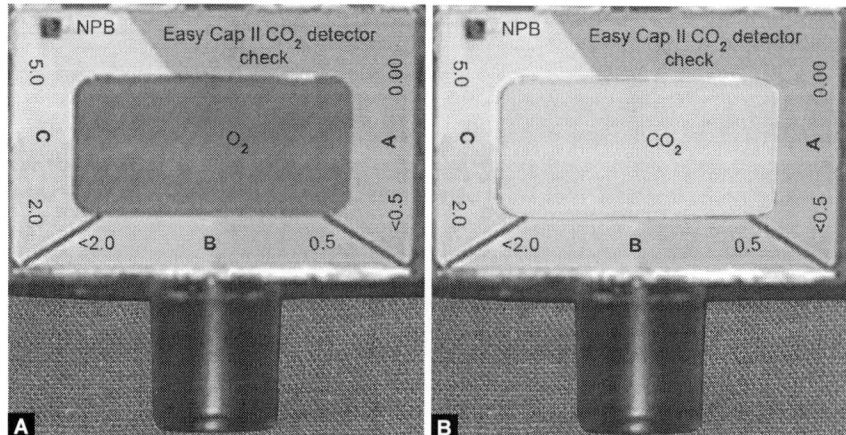

Figs. 4A and B: Calorimetric capnometer. The pH sensitive paper changes from purple to yellow when CO_2 is detected. *(For color version see Plate 1)*

very accurate, particularly when CO_2 output is low during CPR. Waveform capnography is the preferred approach currently. Nonetheless, the colorimetric device is a reasonable option to check placement of an ETT for emergency intubations.

PHYSIOLOGICAL OVERVIEW

A good understanding of time capnogram **(Fig. 5)** and volume capnogram **(Fig. 6)** will help clinicians to avail of full benefit of capnography in clinical practice.

Time Capnography

Time capnogram **(Fig. 5)** is usually interpreted as two segments—(1) an inspiratory segment and (2) an expiratory segment, and two angles— alpha and beta.[6] Capnograms may be evaluated breath by breath, or trends may be assessed as valuable clues to a patient's physiologic status. Expiratory segment is divided into three phases, I to III. Inspiratory segment is designated as phase 0 **(Table 2)**.

The angle between phase II and III is called alpha angle, which increases as slope of phase III increases. Normally, it is about 100–110°. Airway obstruction increases the angle due to increase in the slope phase II and phase III. The response time of the capnograph, sweep speed, and the respiratory cycle time also affect the angle. On the other hand, the angle between phase III and phase 0 is called beta angle, which is normally about 90°. During rebreathing, this angle increases. Occasionally, an upward blip or spike, known as phase IV, can occur towards the end of phase III. This terminal elevation represents emptying of alveoli with long time constants containing higher CO_2 concentration. The maximal CO_2 level, the best reflection of alveolar CO_2, is known as end-tidal CO_2 ($EtCO_2$). This is generally depicted in concentration as $EtCO_2$ or if in partial pressure of CO_2, $PEtCO_2$. This is the number that is displayed on the monitor. $PEtCO_2$ is the best reflection of alveolar CO_2 (P_ACO_2)

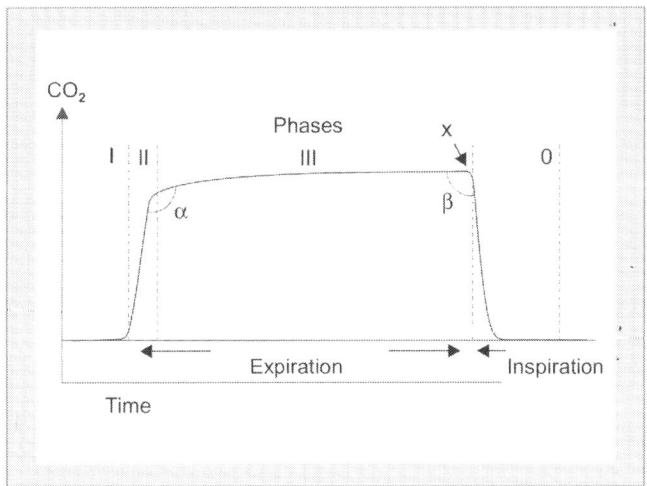

Fig. 5: Normal time capnogram: *Phase I:* End of inhalation and beginning of exhalation (dead space ventilation). *Phase II:* Rapid rise of CO_2 due to mixing of the dead space gas with alveolar CO_2. *Phase III:* Alveolar plateau. The exhalation of the CO_2 from the alveoli. It reaches a peak where the partial pressure of CO_2 is the highest. *Phase 0:* Partial pressure of CO_2 decreases rapidly at the beginning of the inspiration.

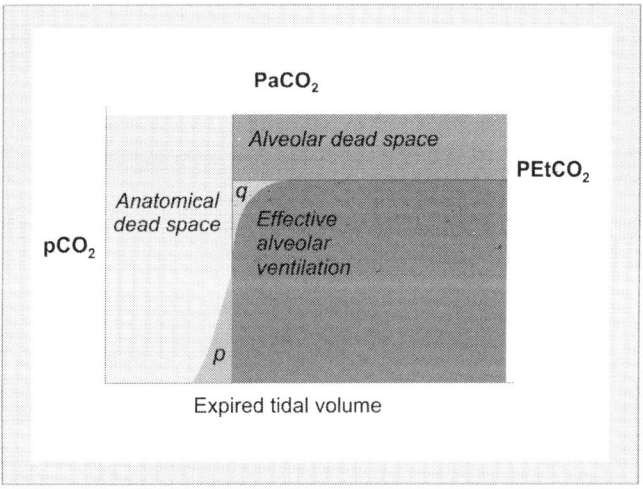

Fig. 6: Volume capnogram. *(For color version see Plate 1)*

and, normally the arterial CO_2 ($PaCO_2$)–$PEtCO_2$ difference is about 5 mm Hg due to the alveolar dead space. There are several clinical possibilities where abnormal capnograms can occur; the most common to anesthesia practice are depicted in **Figures 7A to F**.

Applications of Time Capnography

In the operating rooms, capnography plays a vital role in detecting breathing circuit disconnection instantly when the capnograph no longer detects

TABLE 2: Segments of time capnography

Segment	Phase	
Expiratory segment	Phase I	Initial stage of exhalation, in which the gas sampled is anatomical dead space and apparatus dead space gas, free of CO_2 (dead space ventilation)
	Phase II	Expiratory upstroke—combination of dead space and alveolar gas
	Phase III	Alveolar plateau phase—exhalation of mostly alveolar gas. It is important to note that the expiratory plateau is not an isocapnic trace but rather it progresses with a very slight and steady increase in the pCO_2 as the alveolar fraction is expelled from the lungs
Inspiratory segment	Phase 0	Inspiratory downstroke—inhalation of CO_2 free gas; patient inspiring fresh gas

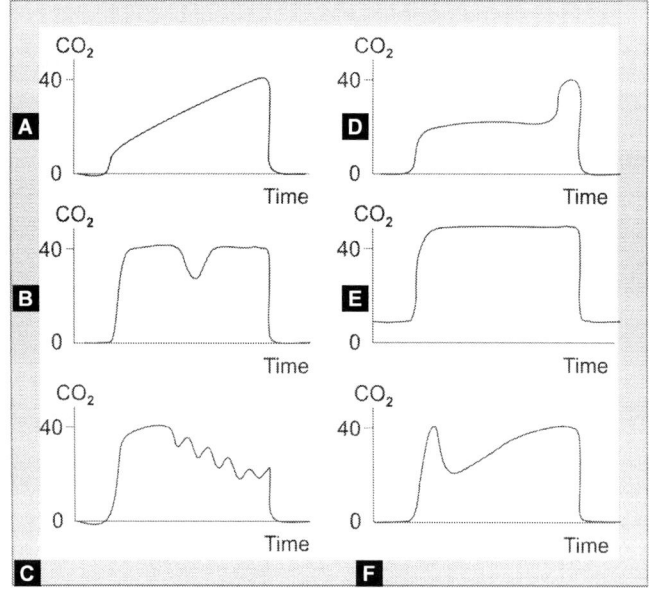

Figs. 7A to F: Examples of several abnormal capnograms. (A) Capnogram of a patient with severe chronic obstructive pulmonary disease (COPD), or other causes leading to the increased airway resistance, such as asthma, endobronchial intubation, endotracheal tube kinking. No plateau is reached before the next inspiration. The gradient between $PEtCO_2$ and arterial CO_2 is increased; (B) Downward wave during plateau phase indicates spontaneous respiratory effort; (C) Cardiogenic oscillations appear as small, regular, tooth like humps at the latter part of the expiratory phase. The rate of the "humps" is identical to the patient's heart rate; (D) A leak in the sampling line during positive pressure ventilation; (E) Failure of inspired CO_2 to return to zero due to an incompetent expiratory valve or exhausted CO_2 absorbent; (F) Bifid waveform of expired CO_2 in patient with emphysema undergoing elective surgery after unilateral lung transplantation. The initial upstroke represents gas from the normal (transplanted) lung, which is followed by gas exhaled from the remaining (emphysematous) lung.

the $EtCO_2$. This is followed by drop-in oxygen saturation. $EtCO_2$ is probably the best method to detect disconnections; a decrease or absence of $EtCO_2$ is highly sensitive but not specific for anesthesia circuit disconnections. Beyond this important and vital application, capnography serves to provide the clinician with enormous data information about the patient's overall physiology that can help clinicians to identify cardiac, ventilatory, and metabolic abnormalities and they are outlined below:

- *Confirmation of tracheal intubation:* 2015 American Heart Association Guidelines on Advanced Adult Cardiac Life Support endorsed continuous waveform capnography in addition to clinical assessment for confirming the ETT placement.[7] To note, a normal waveform can occur when the tube has been placed in the right mainstem bronchus too. A flatline waveform immediately after ETT placement usually indicates esophageal placement. Other common scenarios with a flatline waveform include:
  - Anesthesia circuit disconnections.
  - Technical malfunction of the monitor or sampling tube.
  - Endotracheal tube complete obstruction (e.g., clotted blood).
  - Prolonged cardiac arrest with cellular death (no CO_2 production at a cellular level).

  Unrecognized misplaced endotracheal intubation by healthcare providers was widespread in the past[8,9] and has been significantly reduced by the use of $EtCO_2$ monitoring. Confirmation of correct tube placement using clinical signs has shown to be unreliable. The "Fourth National Audit Project" by Royal College of Anesthetists (RCoA) and Difficult Airway Society stressed the importance of capnography in confirming tracheal intubation in all clinical settings through "No Trace = Wrong Place" campaign. Capnography also provides reliable information on the correct placement of supraglottic airway devices.

- *Assessing tracheal tube and tracheostomy patency and position:* Capnography for the duration the patient remains on artificial airway was cited as the most effective way of reducing morbidity and mortality.[10] Capnography monitoring gives real-time information on the patient's airway patency. A change in waveform is usually seen before a decrease in oxygen saturation and should be immediately assessed.[11]

- *Guide adequacy of ventilation:* Capnography is commonly used to detect hypercapnia due to hypoventilation and hypocapnia due to hyperventilation.[11] In general, the $PaCO_2$ levels are higher by about 5 mm Hg. In patients with essentially normal lungs and cardiac output, $EtCO_2$ can be used to noninvasively monitor $PaCO_2$. An initial arterial blood gas can be performed to determine the gradient (Arterial-$EtCO_2$), further ventilatory adjustments can be made just using $EtCO_2$ as a guide. If the patient has chronic obstructive pulmonary disease (COPD) or unstable cardiac output, $EtCO_2$ may not be a perfect guide. It can also be used for weaning patients from mechanical ventilation. Arterial to $EtCO_2$ difference gives a fair idea about physiological dead space. If the gradient stabilizes or it decreases over time from initially a large gradient, this demonstrates indirectly that the patient's V/Q status is improving.[12]

- *Procedural sedation:* Capnography has been widely used as a respiratory monitor in addition to pulse oximeter during surgical procedures requiring sedation. Capnography will identify hypoventilation long before the pulse oximeter detects hypoxemia, this is especially true in patients receiving supplemental oxygen during sedation **(Figs. 8A and B)**. A comprehensive meta-analysis of 13 randomized clinical trials provides clear evidence that capnography monitoring is more sensitive to identify respiration related adverse events used during procedural sedation. In addition, there is a statistically significant and clinically meaningful reduction in episodes of desaturation as well as requirement of assisted ventilation.[13] During sedation, expired gases are diluted by oxygen administration, and the CO_2 waveforms may not appear in normal shape. Under these circumstances, a change from baseline is an important criterion of excessive sedation resulting in hypoventilation or airway obstruction. A systematic approach to changes in CO_2 waveforms can troubleshoot respiratory events during sedation **(Flowchart 1)**.

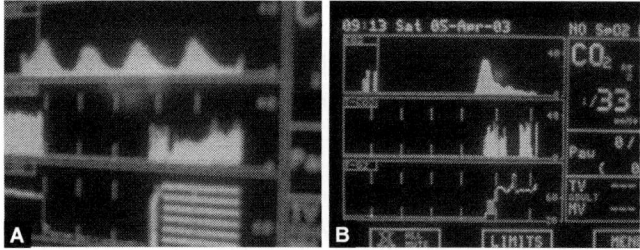

Figs. 8A and B: A drop in respiratory rate or height noticed in capnography during procedural sedation.

Flowchart 1: Algorithm for differential diagnosis of respiratory adverse events during sedation with capnography.

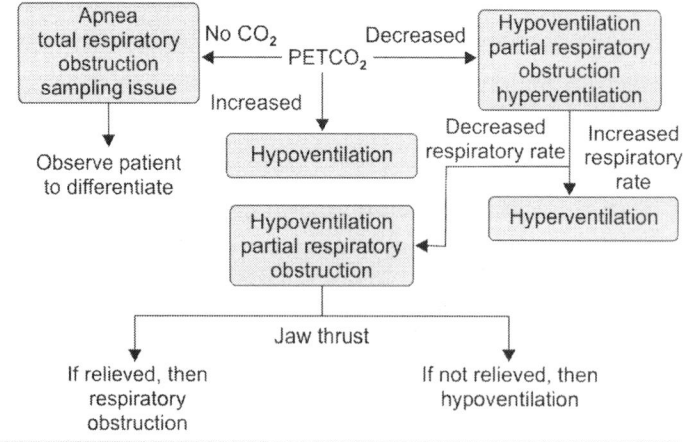

- *During percutaneous tracheostomy placement:* Percutaneous tracheostomy is an invasive procedure and may rarely result in significant patient harm due to incorrect placement. Capnography improves safety by confirming that the tracheostomy tube is correctly placed in the trachea at the end of the procedure. Capnography can be also used as an alternative to fiberoptic bronchoscopy, if unavailable or contraindicated, to detect correct tracheal needle placement before performing percutaneous tracheostomy.[14]
- *Monitoring patients with raised intracranial pressure:* Capnography is an essential tool for management of patients with raised intracranial pressure (ICP), both in the operating room and critical care setting. $PaCO_2$ has a profound and reversible effect on cerebral blood flow. Cerebral blood flow is linearly responsive to $PaCO_2$ level.[15] Capnography can be used as a continuous monitor of $EtCO_2$ which is the best reflective of $PaCO_2$ level during ICP management.
- *Monitoring response to treatment of bronchospasm:* A patient with bronchospasm usually has a capnogram with an exaggerated up-sloping plateau phase, with a prolonged phase II representing slow expiration of respiratory gases. In addition to conventional methods, capnography can be used to assess response to bronchodilators.[11] Capnography is advantageous when compared to peak flow meter because it is independent of efforts and provides continuous monitoring.
- *Estimation of cardiac output:* An increase in cardiac output and pulmonary blood flow results in better perfusion of the alveoli and a rise in $EtCO_2$. Provided the ventilation remains constant, the $EtCO_2$ provides a continuous trend of pulmonary blood flow and therefore, an estimation of cardiac output. During constant minute ventilation and tissue CO_2 production, an abrupt reduction in blood flow reduces $EtCO_2$ via two mechanisms. First, a reduction in venous return causes a decrease in delivered CO_2 to the alveoli, resulting in a decrease in alveolar $_pCO_2$ ($PaCO_2$) and, consequently, $EtCO_2$. Second, reduced pulmonary vascular flow will result in an increase in alveolar dead space, which will dilute the CO_2 from normally perfused alveolar spaces, thus decreasing $EtCO_2$ below $PaCO_2$.[16] A number of studies have shown that $EtCO_2$ can be useful in estimating a change in cardiac output in a variety of clinical scenarios like cardiac arrest, circulatory shock, and major surgeries.[17,18]
- *Assessment of efficacy of cardiopulmonary resuscitation (CPR) and prediction of survivability:* Utilization of capnography in the following ways during CPR improves the survival outcomes in cardiac arrest.[19,20]
    - Confirms the correct placement and patency of the airway device.
    - Monitor ventilation, avoiding hyper and hypoventilation.
    - Assess the adequacy of chest compression during CPR.
    - Early assessment of return of spontaneous circulation (ROSC) during CPR.
    - Used in decision making for prognostication during CPR. In intubated patients, failure to achieve an $EtCO_2$ of >10 mm Hg by waveform capnography after 20 minutes of CPR may be considered as one component of a multimodal approach to decide when to terminate resuscitative efforts but should not be as a sole criterion[7] **(Fig. 9)**.

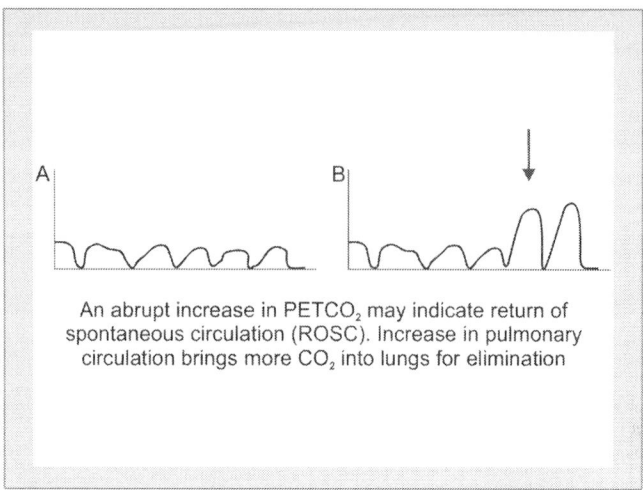

Fig. 9: Waveform capnography showing changes in the end-tidal carbon dioxide during cardiopulmonary resuscitation (CPR) and after ROSC.

- *Detection of inadvertently placed nasogastric tube:* In a meta-analysis of nine clinical trials of mechanically ventilated patients, the use of capnography for inadvertent tracheal placement of the nasogastric tube had a sensitivity ranging from 0.88 to 1.00, specificity 0.95–1.00, positive likelihood ratio 15.22–283.35, negative likelihood ratio 0.01–0.25.[21]
- *Monitoring during patient transport:* Monitoring capnography waveforms with pulse oximetry during transport assures the integrity of airway and prevents mishaps during interhospital or intrahospital transfers. If ventilation is kept constant, an abrupt decrease in $EtCO_2$ values must be immediately investigated; it may be due to decreased cardiac output.[22]
- *Sepsis:* Capnography has potential prognostic value in sepsis to gauge lactate levels. $EtCO_2$ demonstrates an inverse relationship with lactate levels.[23,24] $EtCO_2$ levels <25 mm Hg demonstrate a 0.93 sensitivity for mortality in these studies. In another study, a significant correlation was noted between $EtCO_2$ and sequential organ failure assessment (SOFA) score ($r = -0.35$, $p < 0.01$), and $EtCO_2$ and lactate level ($r = -0.35$, $p < 0.01$). A receiver operator curve for $EtCO_2$ and SOFA > 2 had an area under curve (AUC) of 0.69. $EtCO_2$ of <35 has a sensitivity of 0.73 (95% CI 0.56–0.85) and specificity 0.50 (0.38–0.62) in predicting SOFA scores >2. $EtCO_2$ < 35 mm Hg had a sensitivity of 0.60 (0.22–0.88) and specificity 0.42 (0.32–0.52) in predicting lactate >4 with an AUC of 0.62. There was a statistically significant correlation between $EtCO_2$ and SOFA scores, but association was not strong enough for clinical decision making.[25]
- *Trauma resuscitation:* In blunt trauma prehospital patients who underwent intubation, $EtCO_2$ were greater in survivors (30.8 mm Hg in survivors and 26.3 mm Hg in nonsurvivors). $EtCO_2$ also demonstrates a strong inverse relationship with lactate in patients with penetrating trauma.[26] A recent

study released in injury finds capnography levels <35 mm Hg had an association with indicators of shock and need for blood transfusion in the first 6 hours of admission.[27]
- *Fluid responsiveness:* In a recent study, capnography outperformed other indices such as, pulse pressure variation, systolic blood pressure, heart rate, and mean blood pressure during fluid challenge in patients undergoing mechanical ventilation.[28] Further studies are required to assess the efficacy of $EtCO_2$ for fluid management.
- *Seizures:* $EtCO_2$ can provide an assessment of the ventilatory status of a patient who is actively seizing or in a postictal state.[26]
- *Postoperative care:* Capnography use in the postoperative period can identify early respiratory depression before oxygen desaturation occurs, especially in patients receiving supplemental oxygen.[29] This can significantly improve patient outcomes and avoid the need for costly interventions.[30]

Volume Capnography

Volume capnography is the graphical representation of partial pressure of CO_2 versus exhaled volume. This measurement is made noninvasively at every breath by a combination of flow and CO_2 sensors, which are positioned together at the Y piece of ventilator circuit. Under normal circumstances there is a difference of 2–5 mm Hg between arterial and alveolar CO_2 ($PaCO_2$-$PEtCO_2$ gradient) but this can differ considerably with ventilation perfusion (V/Q) mismatch in the lungs. Volume capnography can provide much more information than time capnography in situations where there is an alteration in V/Q ratio. A volume capnogram can be divided into various components as defined here **(Fig. 6)**. A horizontal line representing $PaCO_2$ (arterial blood sampled during the $PEtCO_2$ recordings) is drawn on the CO_2 trace. The area under the curve (green area), is the volume of CO_2 in the breath and represents effective alveolar ventilation. The remaining area represents wasted ventilation (physiological dead space). A vertical line is drawn through phase II so that the two areas p and q are equal. Area under light blue represents anatomical dead space and area under dark blue represents alveolar dead space.[22]

Applications of Volume Capnography

- *Assessing adequacy of ventilation.*
  - Volume capnography can assess the adequacy of ventilation. However, in mechanically ventilated ICU patients, there is often a large difference between simultaneous measurements of $PaCO_2$ and $PEtCO_2$. Once the difference between $PEtCO_2$ and $PaCO_2$ is established volume capnography can be used as a guide of $PaCO_2$.
- *Estimation of optimal positive end-expiratory pressure (PEEP).*
  - Volume capnometry can help estimate optimal PEEP and response to PEEP can be used to guide therapy in patients with acute respiratory distress syndrome (ARDS). It can also be used to determine prognosis in patients with ARDS.

- *Exclusion of pulmonary embolism.*
  - Pulmonary embolism can be excluded by volume capnography when D-dimers are positive and track the efficacy of thrombolysis in patients with major thromboembolism.
- *Noninvasive estimation of cardiac output and volume responsiveness.*
  - The accuracy of estimation with volume capnography is similar to esophageal Doppler ultrasound, pulse contour analysis, and thoracic bioimpedance.
- *Estimation of dead space.*
  - Volume capnography can be used to determine breath by breath physiological dead space (Bohr Dead space).[5]

LIMITATIONS

Even more than 40 years after the introduction of capnography, patients are still dying because of unrecognized esophageal intubation or tracheal tube displacement. These deaths are occurring either through failure to use this reliable technology, or failure to interpret an abnormal capnograph waveform.[31] In some countries, capnography units are not used even when available due to lack of knowledge to interpret capnography.[31] Despite valuable information provided by capnography, there are few limitations like any other monitoring modality and hence requires caution in the interpretation of the data. Capnography is more reliable in patients where there is isolated ventilation, perfusion, or metabolism issue. However, patients with mixed pathophysiology pose challenges for interpretation.

False-positive CO_2 detection could occur in esophageal intubations if the patient ingested carbonated beverages. Acidic solution exposure, such as stomach content fluid or vinegar, can result in qualitative color change in colorimetric method. Waveform capnography is much more reliable under these circumstances.

Mainstream devices are near ETT and face, and hence caution must be exercised to avoid facial burns due to IR assembly. Sidestream devices may result in time delay, but this is of less clinical significance in clinical practice. The sampling lines and IR window are prone to obstructions by secretions. The sampling tube must be positioned antigravity (vertically upward) and a small filter between the sampling line and the ETT minimizes the blockade with secretions.

It is common to use $EtCO_2$ monitoring during transfer of patients by aircraft and in high altitude locations. In order to provide safe patient transport care, a knowledge about ambient pressure effect on gas analysis is essential. Gas analyzers are calibrated to measure partial pressure of the gas at sea level. Reduction of atmospheric pressure at high altitude will affect capnography in the following ways:[32]

- Pumping of gas through the sample chamber—more powerful pump may be required to maintain flow rates.
- Calibration inaccuracies may occur—this can be corrected by recalibration at high altitude.

- Fall in barometric pressure may be electronically sensed as a gas leak within the monitor. However, the clinical significance of these variations can be minimized, or must be considered while interpreting $EtCO_2$ values.

FUTURE TRENDS AND CONCLUSION

With growing understanding of capnography, and increasing litigations outside of the operating rooms, it is inevitable that many procedural sedation facilities, ICU, and emergency departments will use capnography in future. In the emergency medicine environment, capnography has expanded from CPR and ventilated patients, to use in spontaneously breathing patients in every clinical application, across the continuum of care. The use of capnography could soon become a standard of care in all critically ill on mechanical ventilation during interhospital or intrahospital transfer. The addition of algorithms and technology like integrated pulmonary index (IPI) has also helped clinicians to recognize and intervene in any respiratory compromise. Capnography can facilitate airway management in a neonate as an indicator of gas exchange, lung aeration, early identification of obstruction, early recognition of ROSC, and probably the quality of the administered chest compressions.[33] Volumetric capnography can make a profound impact on the respiratory weaning protocol and shorten the duration of respiratory life support on patients requiring mechanical ventilation. There is growing trend of utilization of this technology in the ICU to measure physiological dead space, oxygen consumption, and CO_2 production.

KEY POINTS

- Capnography is a standard of care monitoring during anesthesia procedures.
- Capnography has also become a standard of care to monitor ventilation during sedation procedures.
- American Heart Association has endorsed capnography to be used during cardiopulmonary resuscitation (CPR).
- Volume capnography can provide physiological dead space estimations breath by breath.
- A knowledge of physics, physiology and clinical interpretations of capnography are essential to avail full benefit of capnography in clinical practice.

REFERENCES

1. Gelb AW, Morriss WW, Johnson W, Merry AF, International Standards for a Safe Practice of Anesthesia Workgroup. World Health Organization-World Federation of Societies of Anaesthesiologists (WHO-WFSA) International Standards for a Safe Practice of Anaesthesia. Can J Anaesth. 2018;65(6):698-708.
2. Bhavani-Shankar K, Moseley H, Kumar AY, Delph Y. Capnometry and anaesthesia. Can J Anaesth. 1992;39(6):617-32.
3. Bhavani-Shankar K, Kumar AY, Moseley HS, Ahyee-Hallsworth R. Terminology and the current limitations of time capnography: a brief review. J Clin Monit. 1995;11(3):175-82.
4. Block FE Jr, McDonald JS. Sidestream versus mainstream carbon dioxide analyzers. J Clin Monit. 1992;8(2):139-41.

5. Verscheure S, Massion PB, Verschuren F, Damas P, Magder S. Volumetric capnography: lessons from the past and current clinical applications. Crit Care. 2016;20(1):184.
6. Bhavani-Shankar K, Philip JH. Defining segments and phases of a time capnogram. Anesth Analg. 2000;91(4):973-7.
7. Link MS, Berkow LC, Kudenchuk PJ, Halperin HR, Hess EP, Moitra VK, et al. Part 7: Adult Advanced Cardiovascular Life Support: 2015 American Heart Association Guidelines Update for Cardiopulmonary Resuscitation and Emergency Cardiovascular Care. Circulation. 2015;132(18 Suppl 2):S444-64.
8. Jones JH, Murphy MP, Dickson RL, Somerville GG, Brizendine EJ. Emergency physician-verified out-of-hospital intubation: miss rates by paramedics. Acad Emerg Med. 2004;11(6):707-9.
9. Katz SH, Falk JL. Misplaced endotracheal tubes by paramedics in an urban emergency medical services system. Ann Emerg Med. 2001;37(1):32-7.
10. Cook TM, Woodall N, Harper J, Benger J, Fourth National Audit P. Major complications of airway management in the UK: results of the Fourth National Audit Project of the Royal College of Anaesthetists and the Difficult Airway Society. Part 2: intensive care and emergency departments. Br J Anaesth. 2011;106(5):632-42.
11. Kerslake I, Kelly F. Uses of capnography in the critical care unit. BJA Education. 2016;17(5):178-83.
12. Lucangelo U, Bernabe F, Vatua S, Degrassi G, Villagra A, Fernandez R, et al. Prognostic value of different dead space indices in mechanically ventilated patients with acute lung injury and ARDS. Chest. 2008;133(1):62-71.
13. Saunders R, Struys M, Pollock RF, Mestek M, Lightdale JR. Patient safety during procedural sedation using capnography monitoring: a systematic review and meta-analysis. BMJ Open. 2017;7(6):e013402.
14. Mallick A, Venkatanath D, Elliot SC, Hollins T, Nanda Kumar CG. A prospective randomised controlled trial of capnography vs. bronchoscopy for Blue Rhino percutaneous tracheostomy. Anesthesia. 2003;58(9):864-8.
15. Carney N, Totten AM, O'Reilly C, Ullman JS, Hawryluk GW, Bell MJ, et al. Guidelines for the Management of Severe Traumatic Brain Injury, Fourth edition. Neurosurgery. 2017;80(1):6-15.
16. Isserles SA, Breen PH. Can changes in end-tidal $_pCO_2$ measure changes in cardiac output? Anesth Analg. 1991;73(6):808-14.
17. Matsumoto A, Itoh H, Eto Y, Kobayashi T, Kato M, Omata M, et al. End-tidal CO_2 pressure decreases during exercise in cardiac patients: association with severity of heart failure and cardiac output reserve. J Am Coll Cardiol. 2000;36(1):242-9.
18. Jin X, Weil MH, Tang W, Povoas H, Pernat A, Xie J, et al. End-tidal carbon dioxide as a noninvasive indicator of cardiac index during circulatory shock. Crit Care Med. 2000;28(7):2415-9.
19. Soar J, Nolan JP, Bottiger BW, Perkins GD, Lott C, Carli P, et al. European Resuscitation Council Guidelines for Resuscitation 2015: Section 3. Adult advanced life support. Resuscitation. 2015;95:100-47.
20. Kodali BS, Urman RD. Capnography during cardiopulmonary resuscitation: current evidence and future directions. J Emerg Trauma Shock. 2014;7(4):332-40.
21. Chau JP, Lo SH, Thompson DR, Fernandez R, Griffiths R. Use of end-tidal carbon dioxide detection to determine correct placement of nasogastric tube: a meta-analysis. Int J Nurs Stud. 2011;48(4):513-21.
22. Kodali BS. Capnography outside the operating rooms. Anesthesiology. 2013;118(1):192-201.
23. Guirgis FW, Williams DJ, Kalynych CJ, Hardy ME, Jones AE, Dodani S, et al. End-tidal carbon dioxide as a goal of early sepsis therapy. Am J Emerg Med. 2014;32(11):1351-6.

24. Hunter CL, Silvestri S, Ralls G, Bright S, Papa L. The sixth vital sign: prehospital end-tidal carbon dioxide predicts in-hospital mortality and metabolic disturbances. Am J Emerg Med. 2014;32(2):160-5.
25. McGillicuddy DC, Tang A, Cataldo L, Gusev J, Shapiro NI. Evaluation of end-tidal carbon dioxide role in predicting elevated SOFA scores and lactic acidosis. Intern Emerg Med. 2009;4(1):41-4.
26. Long B, Koyfman A, Vivirito MA. Capnography in the Emergency Department: a review of uses, waveforms, and limitations. J Emerg Med. 2017;53(6):829-42.
27. Stone ME, Jr., Kalata S, Liveris A, Adorno Z, Yellin S, Chao E, et al. End-tidal CO_2 on admission is associated with hemorrhagic shock and predicts the need for massive transfusion as defined by the critical administration threshold: a pilot study. Injury. 2017;48(1):51-7.
28. Lakhal K, Nay MA, Kamel T, Lortat-Jacob B, Ehrmann S, Rozec B, et al. Change in end-tidal carbon dioxide outperforms other surrogates for change in cardiac output during fluid challenge. Br J Anaesth. 2017;118(3):355-62.
29. Lam T, Nagappa M, Wong J, Singh M, Wong D, Chung F. Continuous pulse oximetry and capnography monitoring for postoperative respiratory depression and adverse events: A systematic review and meta-analysis. Anesth Analg. 2017;125(6):2019-29.
30. Whitaker DK. Time for capnography - everywhere. Anaesthesia. 2011;66(7):544-9.
31. Cook TM, Harrop-Griffiths W. Capnography prevents avoidable deaths. BMJ. 2019;364:l439.
32. Pattinson K, Myers S, Gardner-Thorpe C. Problems with capnography at high altitude. Anaesthesia. 2004;59(1):69-72.
33. Cereceda-Sanchez FJ, Molina-Mula J. Systematic review of capnography with mask ventilation during cardiopulmonary resuscitation maneuvers. J Clin Med. 2019;8(3):358.

CHAPTER 2

Recent Trends in Trauma Care

Chhavi Sawhney, Yudhyavir Singh

INTRODUCTION

Historically, trauma care dates back to 800–700 bc, when during the Trojan War many warriors possessed the knowledge of wound care and Machaon acted as the chief trauma surgeon. His techniques and skills can be considered as the origin of trauma management.[1] Most of the experience in trauma management was derived from the combat and then adapted to civilian trauma. The experience during the two world wars laid the foundations of current trauma care system and continues to improve with new innovations and techniques.

PREHOSPITAL PHASE

Most of the preventable deaths occur within minutes to few hours after trauma. There are two approaches regarding the extent of care provided to the trauma victims in the prehospital setting. The "scoop and run" approach mainly focuses on minimizing the prehospital time. The prehospital care is limited to cervical spine stabilization and splinting of long bone fractures which can be managed by the personnel trained in providing basic life support.[2]

Aeromedical Transport

Integration of aeromedical transport with the emergency medical services (EMS) is an asset to the prehospital care of trauma victims.[3] As a result of air evacuation, the 1-hour radii of hospitals has increased from 45 miles by ground to 150 miles. It is seen that airlifting a critical trauma patient decreases mortality, if ground transport is not possible or the distance is more than 45 miles.[4] However, the advantages of air transport in urban areas have been diluted by the cost and overtriage of patients with minor trauma. Bledsoe reported that 60% of the patients air transported had minor trauma and 25% required less than 24 hours of hospital stay. The operational cost of aeromedical services per hour is huge, hence overutilization of the service should be avoided. It is risky for the aeromedical personnel and there are instances of several deaths or injuries every year. Development of protocols to identify the candidates who would benefit from air transport would be helpful in conservation of resources.

Hemostatic Dressings

The other model for trauma care is the "stay and play" approach where, prehospital management is done by the physicians on the basis of clinical presentation, anatomical and physiological scoring system. Initial airway management and bleeding control is provided and depending upon the response, the patient is shifted to the designated facility.

Prehospital torso and junctional areas bleeding control is challenging but has the potential to improve survival. Previously, the strategies included minimal handling, direct pressure on wounds and fracture splinting. Now, devices such as junctional tourniquets, pelvic circumferential binders and ITClamp® have been developed to improve prehospital resuscitation.[5] There are reports which support the use of hemostatic dressings in situations where pressure dressings are unable to control the bleeding. Topical hemostatic compounds like zeolite and kaolin have been used for junctional zones such as neck, axilla, and groin which are problematic areas for hemorrhage control.[6] A variety of chitosan-based dressings (ChitoFlex, ChitoGauze, and CeloxGauze) which create a physical barrier and aid gauze adherence to the wound are also available.[7] As the systemic absorption is limited, there is no risk of inappropriate coagulation distant from the site of application. These dressings decrease prehospital blood loss and hence, reduce mortality. Large varieties of products are available but more robust data is required to compare these options.

Telemedicine

The advances in telecommunication technology have been associated with the simultaneous emergence of telemedicine. The electronic medical records and focused assessment with sonography for trauma (FAST) images are transmitted from rural or primary centers to tertiary care facilities using a satellite network.[8-10] These are a few examples of transferring real-time data from remote locations to expedite management. The "concept" of telemedicine is currently being employed in trauma emergency department (ED). Using bidirectional audiovisual equipment, level 1 trauma centers extend their expertise to guide resuscitation at community hospitals. Latifi et al. described their experience with five rural hospitals attached to a level 1 trauma hospital. The authors observed that the teleconsultation with a trauma surgeon helped in improving outcome by aiding in initial assessment and was cost-effective.[11] But, unreliable communication system and lack of prospective evidence are some of the limitations to the widespread use of telecommunication.[12]

In the present coronavirus disease (COVID-19) pandemic and even in the post COVID era, telemedicine will have an immense role such as scheduling postoperative follow up, managing recovery issues and even, wound care management. It works as "virtual personal protective equipment (PPE)" and helps in saving travel time, cost and conserving resources. Teleconsultation is also being used for new outpatient appointments, reviewing history and imaging.[13]

Telerehabilitation which includes home-based rehabilitation programs and video-based rather than direct physical training will also decrease in-hospital stay and expedite safe home discharge especially for trauma victims.[14]

TRAUMA DAMAGE CONTROL

Hemorrhage and neurologic injuries are the two most frequent causes of trauma-related mortality. Standard parameters for assessing shock severity included monitoring vital signs, urine output, and organ perfusion parameters such as base deficit and lactate levels. Recent techniques such as noninvasive cardiac output monitoring, near infrared spectrometry, and sublingual videomicroscopy have been recommended for continuous monitoring. All these techniques have their benefits and drawbacks and further studies are required.

High-volume fluid resuscitation after hemorrhagic shock may aggravate injury-related bleeding, acute traumatic coagulopathy (ATC), organ failure and even, mortality. Damage control resuscitation involves rapid hemorrhage control, permissive hypotension, early use of blood products and minimal crystalloids use.[15] Targeting the systolic blood pressure (SBP) at 80–85 mm Hg helps to maintain coronary perfusion and avoid exsanguination and clot disruption. But the patients with traumatic brain injury (TBI) require a higher SBP to maintain cerebral perfusion pressure.

There has been a significant change over the last 30 years in the resuscitation fluid for trauma patients. A balanced transfusion regimen with minimum crystalloids and resembling whole blood is recommended.[16] The transfusion of red blood cell (RBC), fresh frozen plasma (FFP) and platelets in ratio of 1:1:1 prevents early death from exsanguination by achieving hemostasis.[17,18] However, the timing and ratio of platelets to FFP and RBCs is still debatable. Although, component therapy is still in place, the use of whole blood has also made a resurgence. With the recent use of platelet sparing leukoreduction filters, platelet containing whole blood is readily available.[19] Based on the encouraging results and easy availability, whole blood transfusion has been suggested for prehospital transfusion protocol as well. However, severe hemorrhage and resuscitation can lead to a lethal triad of coagulopathy, metabolic acidosis and hypothermia. To prevent ATC, tranexamic acid administration within 3 hours of injury is recommended for patients who are in shock or likely to develop shock. The parameters used for coagulation monitoring like platelet count, prothrombin time and activated partial thromboplastin time are of limited value in trauma. The viscoelastic hemostatic assays (VHA) such as thromboelastography (TEG) and rotational thromboelastography (ROTEG) provide rapid and specific information about clot formation and lysis and hence, allow for a more targeted therapy.[20]

Recent guidelines suggest that dynamic parameters such as focused ultrasound and arterial pressure waveform analysis could be used for predicting volume responsiveness and adequacy of resuscitation.[21]

Damage control surgery is based on the principle of minimal manipulation in a short duration to control hemorrhage in high-risk or severely injured patients. Temporary closure techniques, vacuum assisted closure and negative pressure wound therapy have brought a paradigm shift in trauma resuscitation and critical care.[22]

REBOA AND RESUSCITATIVE THORACOTOMY

The use of resuscitative endovascular balloon occlusion of the aorta (REBOA) has gained momentum as endovascular approach to control noncompressible torso hemorrhage. Although the technique was originally described in 1950s, the increased availability and familiarity with the endovascular technique has led to a resurgence of REBOA. Intra-aortic balloon occlusion helps to augment mean arterial pressure to the proximal organs maintaining myocardial and cerebral perfusion. The circulating blood volume can be preserved till definitive surgical management is undertaken. Depending upon the suspected origin of bleeding, the intra-aortic occlusion is performed at different levels. Zone 1 is akin to thoracic aorta clamping that is performed during resuscitative thoracotomy (RT). In acute trauma patient with massive hemopericardium, RT is performed as a last resort. The technique is highly invasive with low survival rates.[23,24] As RT allows for direct access to thoracic vasculature for direct clamping or release of cardiac tamponade, it is indicated in suspected or confirmed major intrathoracic injury and cardiovascular collapse. The use of REBOA should be restricted to patients with exsanguinating hemorrhage arising from below the diaphragm. Moore et al. compared REBOA and RT for noncompressible truncal hemorrhage. The authors concluded that early deaths were fewer in patients undergoing REBOA and survival was equivalent when compared with RT.[25] Future multicenter studies are needed to expand on this approach.

TRAUMA CRITICAL CARE

Trauma resuscitation initiated in the ED may continue in the ICU. Hence, trauma ICU frequently works as an extension of ED for ongoing resuscitation. ATC is seen in 10–25% patients with severe trauma and is associated with increased mortality. The transfusion of packed red blood cells (PRBCs), FFP and platelets in a fixed ratio (1:1:1) focuses on balancing RBCs, platelets and FFP but it does not improve the fibrinogen level.[23] There is an increase in 28-day mortality with fibrinogen level less than 229 mg/dL and less than 100 mg/dL is another risk factor for mortality. So, frequent monitoring of fibrinogen level in ICU using viscoelastic coagulation tests aids in prompt diagnosis and rapid management with cryoprecipitates or fibrinogen concentrate to improve survival rate.

During the past two decades, there has been an increase in the use of point-of-care ultrasound (POCUS) as a diagnostic tool and procedural adjunct in the ICU. Severe chest trauma involving airway, lungs and cardiac injuries are rapidly identified using ultrasound. In neurocritical care, patient with intracranial hemorrhage can be diagnosed and monitored using POCUS. Whereas, transcranial Doppler (TCD) and optic nerve sheath diameter aid in monitoring raised intracranial pressure.[26] Recently, the use of ultrasound for assessing the cardiac contractility and fluid status during cardiac arrest has also been recommended.

There is a growing evidence suggesting the early use of ECMO in resuscitation of severe trauma and management of secondary complications like cardiac arrest due to acute cardiac injuries and acute respiratory distress syndrome (ARDS). The potential advantages of ECMO in trauma setting include temporary circulatory arrest and neuroprotection after cardiac arrest till definitive management is done. The improvement within the ECMO device (centrifugal pump techniques, complete heparin coated circuits or the use of heparin-free ECMO) has been useful in trauma patients.[27] In a multicenter study by Zonies et al. higher survival rate was observed in traumatic ARDS with the use of ECMO when compared with nontrauma population (65 vs. 26%). The authors concluded that despite high bleeding risk, successful outcome in trauma patients can be attributed to younger age group and better baseline physiological status in the trauma subgroup.[28]

HYBRID OPERATING ROOMS

There is an increased role of interventional radiology in the management of bleeding trauma patient. The key areas include embolization of visceral vascular injuries which has obviated the need for surgical intervention. Endovascular stenting of major vessels such as descending thoracic aorta, subclavian and vertebral artery has replaced open repair of these vessels leading to a reduction in mortality and complications such as stroke and paraplegia. Temporary occlusion of major vessels such as aorta may provide stability pending surgical repair. Further, angiography and embolization is the procedure of choice for vessels which are difficult to access surgically like pelvic vessels.[29]

This has led to the development of hybrid ORs or RAPTORs (Resuscitation with Angiography, Percutaneous Techniques and Operative Repairs) allowing resuscitation, interventional radiology, intensive care and if required open surgery in the same OR using multidisciplinary approach.[5]

Richter et al. shared their orthopedic trauma experience after using a hybrid OR for 1 year. The authors reported that the OR was advantageous for placing implants, performing spine as well as pelvis cases using minimally invasive and conventional approach. Further, appropriate reduction and implant placement could be confirmed in the OR obviating the need for postoperative imaging. They did not find any increase in the perioperative infection rate. Although there is a paucity of literature but hybrid OR is a safe and effective option for trauma management in future.[30]

TRAUMA TRAINING

The trauma team needs to rapidly assess and manage patients to decrease the preventable deaths.[31] Simulation-based medical education (SBME) provides opportunities for training and evaluation of trauma care in prehospital phase, emergency room (ER) and mass casualty scenarios. It is also helpful in other aspects of trauma care like team work, communication and overall performance using trauma team performance observation tool.[32] Recently, a modified nontechnical skills (NOTECHS) scale for trauma (T-NOTECHS) is developed to teach and assess teamwork skills of trauma resuscitation teams. There are reports of improved resuscitation and task performance time using this tool.[31]

A variety of tasks and skills can be acquired and practiced using these modalities. There is a controversy as to which method (manikins or patients or computerized patient simulators) is the best particularly, to improve communication, cooperation and team work. Although, the impact of SBME regarding the improvement of performance is evident in literature but the long-term effects (retention of knowledge and skills) of simulation strategies in trauma needs to be evaluated.[33]

SPECIFIC INJURIES

Chest Trauma

Thoracic trauma is a significant cause of trauma mortality. Fortunately, operative management is required in less than 10% of blunt and 15–30% of penetrating chest injuries. Most chest injuries like tracheobronchial tree injuries, tension pneumothorax, massive hemothorax, open and simple pneumothorax can be managed with airway control, tube thoracostomy and fluid resuscitation. Potentially life-threatening injuries like flail chest and pulmonary contusions can cause respiratory failure for which newer ventilator modes like airway pressure release ventilation (APRV) and even, ECMO are being employed. There has been a dramatic change in the management of traumatic aortic disruption where endovascular repair has largely replaced open repair with good outcomes. Video-assisted thoracic surgery (VATS) is being used in hemodynamically stable patients after both blunt and penetrating trauma including diaphragmatic injury, persistent pneumothorax or retained hemothorax to reduce long-term mortality.[22]

Abdominal Trauma

Solid organ injuries (liver, spleen, and kidney) are the most common abdominal injuries with blunt abdominal trauma. Nonoperative management is the standard of care as long as these patients remain stable. These patients need to be intensely monitored for hemodynamic instability or physiological deterioration to detect missed injury or intraperitoneal bleed. Isolated solid organ injury due to penetrating abdominal trauma was traditionally managed with laparotomy but recently, nonoperative management is preferred in patients without peritonitis. For patients requiring emergency laparotomy, the principles of damage control surgery with minimal manipulation and short duration is recommended.[22]

Head Trauma

The primary goal of treatment for patients with suspected TBI is prevention of secondary brain injury. In patients with TBI, SBP should be aimed at >90 mm Hg to maintain the cerebral perfusion pressure. In TBI patients who are on anticoagulants and antiplatelets, reversal of these agents to achieve INR < 1.6 and platelets >1,00,000 should be targeted to reduce mortality in patients on these medications.

Intracranial pressure (ICP) monitoring is recommended in patients with severe TBI to maintain an ICP < 20 and CPP between 50 and 70 mm Hg. Although, the evidence for use of hyperosmolar therapy is insufficient but still hypertonic saline and mannitol is the primary pharmacologic therapy available to decrease ICP. Decompressive craniectomy is being used to reduce ICP where it is refractory to other measures. The Brain Trauma Foundation (BTF) guidelines recommend the use of seizure prophylaxis to prevent early post-traumatic seizures along with the other deep vein thrombosis (DVT) and stress ulcer prophylaxis.[34]

Pediatric Trauma

Injury is the most common cause of death and disability in childhood. Recent trends in pediatric trauma resuscitation include crystalloid restriction and blood product-based resuscitation as recommended for the adults. Pediatric mass transfusion protocol includes initial 20 mL/kg bolus of isotonic crystalloid followed by weight-based blood product resuscitation with 10–20 mL/kg of PRBCs, FFP and platelets.[35] Most chest trauma can be managed with a combination of supportive care and tube thoracostomy. Severe chest trauma is usually a component of multisystem injury and the management is frequently similar as for the adults. In pediatric abdominal injuries, the presence of intraperitoneal blood on CT or FAST, grade of injury or presence of vascular blush does not mandate a laparotomy, if the patient is fluid responsive. Prompt exploration is indicated only if the patient is hemodynamically unstable or a diagnostic procedure is positive for blood. Angioembolization of solid organ injuries is an option but should be performed only in centers with experience in pediatric interventional procedures and ready access to OR. Management of TBI in children involves early endotracheal intubation, prevention of secondary brain injury and the use of hypertonic saline and mannitol to reduce brain edema.

CONCLUSION

There has been a paradigm shift in the resuscitation of trauma patients. Current practice involves DCR approach with permissive hypotension, balanced resuscitation with a high ratio of blood products, avoidance of crystalloids and early damage control surgery. Management of trauma patients continues to evolve though the basic principles of rapid identification and management remain the same. Operative management of chest and abdominal trauma has been replaced by conservative management and less invasive approach.

This requires close and intense monitoring for the failure of nonoperative management, complications or missed injuries. Further research is required to investigate to role of targeted blood component therapy early in shock resuscitation. The role and effect of ECMO on the outcome in trauma patients also needs to be evaluated so that dedicated trauma ECMO units can be established.

> **KEY POINTS**
> - Goal of trauma care is zero preventable deaths after injury. This can be achieved by standardization of evidence-based care, application of new concepts and innovations of new devices.
> - Prehospital emergency medical services (EMS) are fundamental to trauma care. The ideal system of trauma management is still controversial in terms of prehospital care and needs to be validated.
> - Trauma resuscitation has evolved over time with an understanding of physiology of hemorrhagic shock. Trauma resuscitation is based upon the principles of DCR which aim to maintain and/or rapidly restore hemostasis so the clinical focus has shifted toward coagulopathy.
> - Hybrid ORs with facilities for resuscitation, interventional radiology, intensive care and open surgery are cost-effective and beneficial. In future, there should be setting up of more hybrid ORs, especially in a level 1 trauma center.
> - Trauma training using simulation-based training seems to be a promising educational technique to improve the skills and teamwork required for trauma care.

REFERENCES

1. Koutserimpas C, Samonis G. Machaon: the first trauma surgeon in Western history? J Wound Care. 2018;27(10):659-61.
2. Nathens AB, Brunet FP, Maier RV. Development of trauma systems and effect on outcomes after injury. Lancet. 2004;363(9423):1794-801.
3. Siracuse JJ, Saillant NN, Hauser CJ. Technological advancements in the care of the trauma patient. Eur J Trauma Emerg Surg. 2012;38(3):241-51.
4. Boyd CR, Corse KM, Campbell RC. Emergency interhospital transport of the major trauma patient: air versus ground. J Trauma. 1989;29(6):789-93.
5. Chico-Fernández M, Terceros-Almanza LL, Mudarra-Reche CC. Innovation and new trends in critical trauma disease. Med Intensiva. 2015;39(3):179-88.
6. Khoshmohabat H, Paydar S, Kazemi HM, Dalfardi B. Overview of agents used for emergency hemostasis. Trauma Mon. 2016;21(1):e26023.
7. Smith AH, Laird C, Porter K, Bloch M. Hemostatic dressings in prehospital care. Emerg Med J. 2013;30(10):784-9.
8. McBeth PB, Hamilton T, Kirkpatrick AW. Cost-effective remote iPhone-teathered telementored trauma telesonography. J Trauma. 2010;69(6):1597-9.
9. Dyer D, Cusden J, Turner C, Boyd J, Hall R, Lautner D, et al. The clinical and technical evaluation of a remote telementored telesonography system during the acute resuscitation and transfer of the injured patient. J Trauma. 2008;65(6):1209-16.
10. Strode CA, Rubal BJ, Gerhardt RT, Christopher FL, Bulgrin JR, Kinkler ES Jr, et al. Satellite and mobile wireless transmission of focused assessment with sonography in trauma. Acad Emerg Med. 2003;10(12):1411-4.

11. Latifi R, Hadeed GJ, Rhee P, O'Keeffe T, Friese RS, Wynne JL, et al. Initial experiences and outcomes of telepresence in the management of trauma and emergency surgical patients. Am J Surg. 2009;198(6):905-10.
12. Rogers FB, Ricci M, Caputo M, Shackford S, Sartorelli K, Callas P, et al. The use of telemedicine for real-time video consultation between trauma center and community hospital in a rural setting improves early trauma care: preliminary results. J Trauma. 2001;51(6):1037-41.
13. Bini SA, Schilling PL, Patel SP, Kalore NV, Ast MP, Maratt JD, et al. Digital Orthopaedics: A Glimpse Into the Future in the Midst of a Pandemic. J Arthroplasty. 2020;35(7S):S68-S73.
14. Turolla A, Rossettini G, Viceconti A, Palese A, Geri T. Musculoskeletal physical therapy during the COVID-19 pandemic: is telerehabilitation the answer? Phys Ther. 2020;100(8):1260-4.
15. Dauer E, Goldberg A. What's New in Trauma Resuscitation? Adv Surg. 2019;53:221-33.
16. Spinella PC, Cap AP. Whole blood: back to the future. Curr Opin Hematol. 2016;23(6):536-42.
17. O'Keeffe T, Refaai M, Tchorz K, Forestner JE, Sarode R. A massive transfusion protocol to decrease blood component use and costs. Arch Surg. 2008;143(7):686-90.
18. Vaslef SN, Knudsen NW, Neligan PJ, Sebastian MW. Massive transfusion exceeding 50 units of blood products in trauma patients. J Trauma. 2002;53(2):291-5.
19. Bjerkvig CK, Strandenes G, Eliassen HS, Spinella PC, Fosse TK, Cap AP, et al. "Blood failure" time to view blood as an organ: how oxygen debt contributes to blood failure and its implications for remote damage control resuscitation. Transfusion (Paris). 2016;56(Suppl 2):S182-9.
20. Juffermans NP, Wirtz MR, Balvers K, Baksaas-Aasen K, van Dieren S, Gaarder C, et al. Towards patient-specific management of trauma hemorrhage: the effect of resuscitation therapy on parameters of thromboelastometry. J Thromb Haemost. 2019;17(3):441-8.
21. Tisherman SA, Stein DM. ICU management of trauma patients. Crit Care Med. 2018;46(12):1991-7.
22. Roberts DJ, Ball CG, Feliciano DV, Moore EE, Ivatury RR, Lucas CE, et al. History of the Innovation of Damage Control for Management of Trauma Patients: 1902–2016. Ann Surg. 2017;265(5):1034-44.
23. Harris T, Davenport R, Mak M, Brohi K. The Evolving Science of Trauma Resuscitation. Emerg Med Clin North Am. 2018;36(1):85-106.
24. Holcomb JB, Jenkins D, Rhee P, Johannigman J, Mahoney P, Mehta S, et al. Damage control resuscitation: directly addressing the early coagulopathy of trauma. J Trauma. 2007;62(2):307-10.
25. Moore LJ, Brenner M, Kozar RA, Pasley J, Wade CE, Baraniuk MS, et al. Implementation of resuscitative endovascular balloon occlusion of the aorta as an alternative to resuscitative thoracotomy for noncompressible truncal hemorrhage: J Trauma Acute Care Surg. 2015;79(4):523-30.
26. Johnson GGRJ, Kirkpatrick AW, Gillman LM. Ultrasound in the surgical ICU: uses, abuses, and pitfalls. Curr Opin Crit Care. 2019;25(6):675-87.
27. Della Torre V, Robba C, Pelosi P, Bilotta F. Extra corporeal membrane oxygenation in the critical trauma patient. Curr Opin Anaesthesiol. 2019;32(2):234-41.
28. Zonies D, Merkel M. Advanced extracorporeal therapy in trauma. Curr Opin Crit Care. 2016;22(6):578-83.
29. Harris T, Davenport R, Hurst T, Hunt P, Fotheringham T, Jones J. Improving outcome in severe trauma: what's new in ABC? Imaging, bleeding and brain injury. Postgrad Med J. 2012;88(1044):595-603.

30. Richter PH, Yarboro S, Kraus M, Gebhard F. One year orthopaedic trauma experience using an advanced interdisciplinary hybrid operating room. Injury. 2015;46(Suppl 4):S129-34.
31. Berkenstadt H, Ben-Menachem E, Simon D, Ziv A. Training in trauma management: the role of simulation-based medical education. Anesthesiol Clin. 2013;31(1):167-77.
32. Steinemann S, Berg B, Skinner A, DiTulio A, Anzelon K, Terada K, et al. In situ, multidisciplinary, simulation-based teamwork training improves early trauma care. J Surg Educ. 2011;68(6):472-7.
33. Wisborg T, Brattebø G, Brinchmann-Hansen A, Hansen KS. Mannequin or standardized patient: participants' assessment of two training modalities in trauma team simulation. Scand J Trauma Resusc Emerg Med. 2009;17:59.
34. Vella MA, Crandall ML, Patel MB. Acute management of traumatic brain injury. Surg Clin North Am. 2017;97(5):1015-30.
35. ATLS Subcommittee, American College of Surgeons' Committee on Trauma, International ATLS working group. Advanced trauma life support (ATLS®): the ninth edition. J Trauma Acute Care Surg. 2013;74(5):1363-6.

CHAPTER 3

Anesthesia for Laser Surgery

Soma Ganesh Raja, Senthil Kumar

INTRODUCTION

Light amplification by stimulated emission of radiation (LASER) is used commonly in otorhinolaryngological procedures, thoracic surgeries, ophthalmology, dermatology, dentistry, gynecology, plastic surgery, urology, and neurosurgery, interventional or diagnostic cardiovascular procedures and uncommonly in fetal and neonatal surgeries. Laser offers precise microsurgery, bloodless surgical field, and complete sterility even in difficult locations. Airway surgeries are unique and challenging, as the field is shared by anesthesiologists and surgeons alike and more exigent if laser is used. The ability to focus the laser beam on a minute area concentrates the intensity extensively, allowing precise rapid vaporization of tissue. Laser surgery is relatively dry, providing near instantaneous sealing of lymphatics and small vessels. There is minimal damage to adjacent tissues resulting in less edema, scarring and postoperative pain. The focus of this chapter will be on principles of laser and anesthesia for airway laser surgeries, the principles of which is applicable to most non-airway laser surgeries too.

LASER PHYSICS

Basic understanding of how laser operates helps us to recognize hazards during laser device usage. When a photon interacts with an electron in the outer orbit of an atom, stimulated emission of higher energy photons occurs. When the stimulated emission of photons is enclosed between parallel mirrors, the repeated traversing of these high-energy photons results in formation of laser light. Laser light may be in visible spectrum, invisible infrared or ultraviolet spectrum of electromagnetic radiation. It is monochromatic (of single wavelength or color), coherent (all waves travel together in same phase) and collimated (parallel waves without dispersion).[1]

COMPONENTS OF LASER

The laser machine consists of a laser medium [carbon dioxide (CO_2), argon, etc.] in an optical cavity between two mirrors—one of which is partially

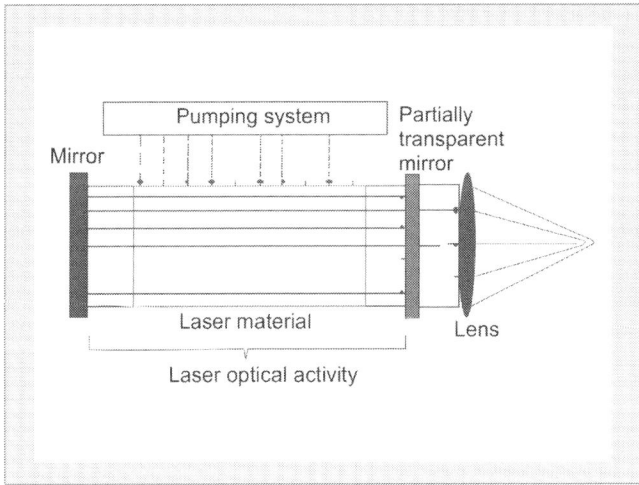

Fig. 1: Components of laser.

reflecting. An external energy source excites the laser medium causing more high intensity photons release. During population inversion (more than 50% of atoms are excited), spontaneous emission of photons occur which strike the mirrors and reflect back causing stimulated emission. The partially reflecting mirror lets a controlled escape through an aperture creating laser beam that is used clinically **(Fig. 1)**.[2,3]

LASER EFFECTIVENESS

The effectiveness of laser is determined by exposure time, spot size, and power. Exposure time is the time that the tissues are exposed to the laser light and is influenced by pulse structure, type and configuration of laser. The pulse structure may be continuous, pulsed or Q switched. In continuous mode, the laser is always on with same instantaneous intensity, where an external shutter controls the exposure time giving a stable operation as in surgical CO_2 or neodymium-doped yttrium aluminum garnet (Nd: YAG) laser. In pulsed mode, laser operates for a fraction of a second with irregular spikes. A high intensity, short-term single or repeated emission of laser radiation causes laser effect ablating tissues quickly. In Q-switched mode, laser output is controlled to produce a single, very short laser pulse, increasing high peak power in regular spikes.

Spot size is the size of laser beam focused through a lens to a very small diameter of 0.1–2 mm. The optical properties (focal length) of the lens determine distance from the lens to target tissue.

Power or power density of laser expressed in watts or watts per square centimeter determines the effects of laser and varies according to spot size and time of exposure.[2-4]

CLINICAL EFFECTS OF LASER

Laser energy is absorbed, reflected, conducted as heat or scattered by tissues causing photothermal (coagulation and vaporization), photochemical (ablation and radiation), photoionizing (disruption) effects. The clinical effects of laser on human tissue depend on laser intensity, frequency of light and degree of absorption. At lower intensities, laser stimulates cells while at higher intensities, cellular activity attenuates, tissue temperature rises causing protein denaturation and photocoagulation. Laser pulsing is utilized to allow heat dissipation between bursts to control thermal energy. "Q switching" is used where laser light aliquots are released in shorter duration bursts of higher energy. The mechanical damage predominates thermal disintegration due to induced vibration in Q-switching.[3,4] There are numerous lasers available for medical use, the properties of which are given in **Table 1**.

LASER CLASSIFICATION

Lasers are classified into four classes according to their power and wavelength as per American National Standards Institute (ANSI). Class 4 lasers alter biological tissue and pose dangers to the eye, skin, and combustible material. All class 3B and class 4 lasers must be operated by trained, authorized personnel, and equipped with a key switch and a safety interlock.[3]

LASER HAZARDS

Atmospheric Contamination

Laser causes smoke plumes and fine particulates, which deposit in alveoli causing reduced mucociliary clearance, inflammation, interstitial pneumonia, bronchiolitis, and emphysema. It may be teratogenic, mutagenic or a vector for viral transmission. Inhaling a gram of tissue has been equated with smoking 3–6 cigarettes. The smoke may carry bacterial spores or viral deoxyribonucleic acid (DNA) as detected in plumes from warts. Efficient smoke evacuators and high efficiency masks are advocated to prevent plume related complications. Special laser masks such as laser plume masks or use of properly fitted filtering facepiece respirator such as an N95 mask (better than laser plume masks) provide better respiratory protection from laser plumes especially when local exhaust ventilation (LEV) is lacking.[4-8]

Gas Embolism

Gas embolism occurs when coaxial gas cooling systems are used in laser probes. There is risk of gas emboli when flexible fiberoptic CO_2 laser is used where helium acts as inert gas for cooling flow to the hollow core or with Nd:YAG laser (caused by the gas coolant for sapphire probe) used during tracheal, laparoscopic or hysteroscopic laser surgeries. Pressurized gas exiting the fiber tip during laser procedure causes gas emboli if the tip is brought in direct

TABLE 1: Characteristics of medical lasers

Laser medium	Type of laser (wavelength in nm)*	Color	Tissue penetration (in mm)	Features	Type of surgery
Gas	CO_2 (10,600)	Invisible	0.2	Rapid vaporization of intracellular water within 1 mm depth, energy in far infrared spectrum, little damage to deep tissues, used as a vaporizer and bloodless cutter can be used with an operating microscope	Laryngeal, tracheobronchial, head and neck procedures, gynecological surgeries
	Argon (488, 514)	Blue-green	0.5–2	Transmitted by water, absorbed by hemoglobin	Retinal, anterior chamber procedures, glaucoma, vascular lesions, laser stapedotomy
	Helium-neon (633)	Red	15	Causes local vascular dilatation, accelerated blood flow, anti-inflammatory effect, and promotes functional recovery	Coaxial laser pointer with CO_2 for red color
Solid	Potassium titanyl phosphate (KTP) (532)	Green	0.5–2	Strongly absorbed by melanin, and hemoglobin	Vascular diseases such as hemangioma, telangiectasia, otolaryngologic lesions and hemorrhages
	Ruby (695)	Red	2.5–3	Absorbed primarily by dark pigments	Retinal surgery, dermatology
	Nd:YAG (1,060)	Invisible	2–6	Uses solid lasing medium, maximal penetration in hemoglobin, melanin and water, greater coagulation versus vaporization	Photocoagulation and deep thermal necrosis for gastrointestinal bleeding, tumor debulking, tracheal procedures
	Diode laser (810, 940)	Invisible	1–3	Photothermal effect on soft tissues, deep penetration through retina	Hyperplastic inferior nasal turbinates, and debulking airway pathology

*All these lasers need fiberoptic transmission except CO_2 laser.

contact with blood vessels. A liquid coolant is strongly preferred else CO_2 can be used as coolant which produces less damage if embolization occurs. Continuous airway CO_2 monitoring is strongly recommended for detection of embolization.[4,9,10]

Organ/Vessel Perforation

Viscus or large blood vessel (>5 mm) can be perforated by a misdirected laser energy. Laser induced pneumothorax has been reported after laryngeal surgery. The depth of damage, perforation and bleeding cannot be assessed immediately with Nd: YAG laser which leads to postoperative complications.[4,9,10]

Inappropriate Heat Transfer

Most medical lasers are reflected by smooth metal surfaces causing inappropriate heat transfer which are discussed here:

Damage to Eyes

Indirect or direct exposure of eyes to laser can cause photokeratitis, photochemical cataract, thermal retinal injuries, corneal burns, and other irreversible serious corneal, and retinal injuries. Corneal injuries are common with laser beam in ultraviolet or infrared spectrum.[3,4] A collimated beam of laser light to a spot 20 microns can be focused by retina which creates risk of visual loss. Eye protection is essential for all personnel within operating room (OR)—including the anesthesiologist, surgeon, scrub nurse, auxiliary nurse, and the patient. Protective eye glasses or metallic eye goggles depending on wavelength and type of laser used to protect eyes during laser surgery. All laser glasses must have clearly labeled optical density value, wavelengths against which protection is offered and maximum irradiance to which eye glasses can be exposed. If many types of laser are used, appropriate eyewear has to be used. Opaque coverings should cover all windows of OR during laser procedures and specific warning signs must be placed outside OR as per ANSI guidelines. Extra goggles must be made available for personnel entering the OR[9,10] (**Table 2**).

Damage to Skin and Drapes

Exposed areas of skin, face and all areas around suspension laryngoscope should be covered completely with wet towels to prevent laser burns. Lips and nose must be included completely while draping as they may be stuck by a reflected laser beam from the proximal rim of the suspension laryngoscope.

All flammable solutions must be avoided inside OR for fear of burns. Though the disposable surgical drapes are water resistant and treated with flame retardant chemicals, they are potentially flammable. It is difficult to extinguish a fire in a disposable surgical drape. So, a CO_2 fire extinguisher must be available. Poor visibility and breathing difficulty occur inside OR

TABLE 2: Eye protection for lasers

Laser (wavelength in nm)	Eye damage	Operating room personnel protection	Patient protection
CO_2 (10,600)	Serious corneal injury	Wrap around clear eye glasses. Optics of microscope provide protection to the surgeon if operating microscope is used	Taping of eyes, using artificial tears, avoiding petroleum-based jelly, saline soaked eye pads, surgical drapes, and another layer of saline-soaked pads
Argon (488,514)	Retinal burns	Amber orange colored eye glasses	
Potassium titanyl phosphate (KTP) (532)	Severe retinal damage	Amber red colored eye glasses. Filter for the bronchoscope to prevent backscatter	
Nd: YAG (1,060)	Irreparable damage to ocular fundus	Green tinted glasses (causes difficult patient assessment), clear lenses coating opaque to near infrared. Risk of backscatter to endoscopist. Filters that absorb 1.06 mcm placed into scopes	

(Nd: YAG: neodymium: yttrium-aluminum-garnet).

once drapes are ignited due to fumes. So, it is important to use moist towels to prevent their flammability.[4,9-11]

Operating room personnel can be exposed to laser in "nominal hazard zone" (up to 1.7 meters around laser) or in "maximal permissible exposure zone" (varies with laser type) and hence must follow all laser safety precautions.[4]

Laser Protocol

Equipment failure and inadequate knowledge of laser equipment can lead to misdirected laser beam, which warrants strict laser safety protocols. A laser safety committee with a liaison officer, anesthesiologist, surgeon, hospital administrators, laser technicians, and biomedical engineers managing a laser register with proper staff education and training is mandatory to avoid laser hazards.

Laser must be in standby mode when not used, used in pulsed mode than in continuous mode, and surgical area must be allowed to cool in between firings. Instrumentation for use with laser must be dull or matt finished to avoid reflection of laser beam. OR windows must be covered by opaque covering to prevent laser penetration. A warning sign on the OR door to alert anyone entering the OR and automatic locking OR doors when OR is in laser mode, is essential to prevent laser hazards.[4,11]

Airway Laser Fire

Airway fire is an important hazard during laser airway surgery with an incidence of 0.5–1.5%. When laser strikes the unprotected endotracheal tube surface, it disintegrates due to laser beam and might catch fire. If fire is unrecognized, a hole in tracheal tube or its cuff occur exposing the oxidant rich anesthetic gases resulting in a life-threatening explosive blowtorch like fire. There will be a total or near total destruction of endotracheal tube with blowtorch fires causing aspiration of molten material, smoke and other particulate matter. 20% of OR fires due to laser cause serious injury to patients.[4,12]

Airway fire occurs as a result of interaction between fuel, oxidizer, and ignition source the fire triad **(Fig. 2)**. The fuel source includes flammable materials inside OR such as endotracheal tubes, gauze, surgical drapes, volatile anesthetics, masks, nasal cannulas, suction catheters, gowns, etc. Oxidant rich atmosphere can occur under drapes or masks where high concentrations of oxygen and nitrous oxide are present. Laser is the high-energy ignition source that can ignite a fire. Other sources such as electrocautery, cables, and heated probes can also ignite fire.[9-14]

Prevention of Airway Fires

Targeting one of the components of fire triad—managing fuel source, minimizing oxidant source, and not using an ignition source prevents laser airway fire.[15-20]

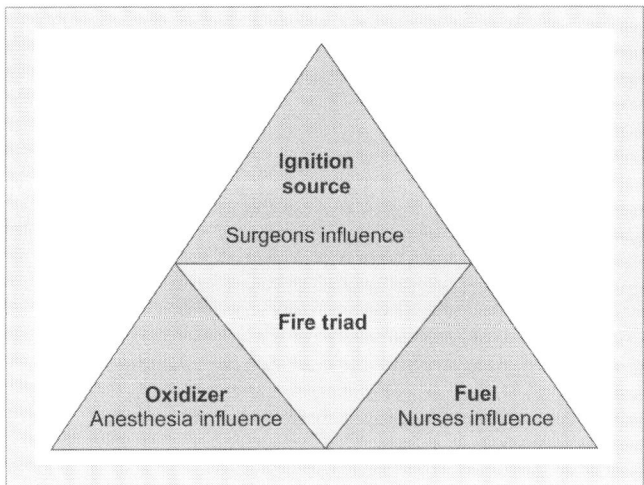

Fig. 2: Fire triad.

Managing fuel source: The common fuel source for an airway fire is endotracheal tube. The safest nonflammable endotracheal tube would be a metallic endotracheal tube-like Norton tube. Though it will not catch fire, its uncuffed nature makes it redundant. A noninflammable shaft and cuff, thin walled tube resistant to different wavelengths of laser, ability to tolerate long exposure times are ideal requisites for a laser safe endotracheal tube. Covering endotracheal tubes with copper, aluminum foil, wet muslin cloth, dental acrylic, merocel laser-guard with 30% overlap to prevent tube exposure have been described but are not approved by Food and Drug Administration (FDA). Moreover, adhesive or benzoin used to stick the foil with tube is also inflammable. Cuff is vulnerable as it cannot be wrapped. These disadvantages lead to development of laser resistant endotracheal tubes.[15-19]

Commercially, available laser resistant tubes are easy to use though expensive. Of all laser resistant tubes, only stainless-steel laser flex tube was found to be safe during CO_2 laser surgery. Cuff is vulnerable for all laser-safe tubes and surgeon must cover the cuff with wet cotton pledgets with their tail threads replaced with thin wires. The cuff should be filled with saline and colored with methylene blue to detect early puncture. Moreover the saline act as a local fire extinguisher and helps avoid fire. The characteristics of laser safe tubes are given in **Table 3**. A metallic tracheostomy tube can be used with jet ventilation if the patient is already tracheostomized.[20,21]

Minimizing oxidant source: Gases used for airway laser surgery such as nitrous oxide, oxygen and inhalational anesthetic gases are combustible. A lower FiO_2 less than 30% with air, nitrogen or helium for dilution is recommended for laser surgery to retard laser fire. Though the minimum flammable concentrations of most inhaled anesthetic agents are well above the alveolar concentrations in clinical practice, sevoflurane is considered as safest when concentration range needed for anesthesia in presence of air,

TABLE 3: Characteristics of laser-safe tubes

Tube name	Characteristics	Laser recommended	Laser contraindicated	Disadvantages
Norton	Matt finished Interlocking spiral-wound stainless steel, thick exterior	CO_2	Nd: YAG	No cuff, needs a separate latex cuff that makes it laser unsafe, causes trauma to larynx while passing
Laser flex	Corrugated stainless steel shaft with proximal and distal cuffs	CO_2, KTP	Nd: YAG	Prolonged laser impingement prevents cuff deflation, increased air flow resistance due to spiral design of tube
Laser trach	Single use red rubber tube with spiral wrapped embossed copper foil	CO_2	Nd: YAG	Needs saline saturation of outer layer before use
Xomed laser shield II	Aluminum foil tape and Teflon wrapped silicon tube	KTP, CO_2	Nd: YAG, Argon	Proximal and distal ends of silicon elastomer shaft and cuff are not laser resistant. Pyrolysis of Teflon can release toxic fumes causing polymer fume fever
Bivona fome cuff	Aluminum spiral with silicon coating, self-inflating polyurethane foam cuff	CO_2	Nd: YAG	Blowtorch airway fires, difficult to deflate the cuff if punctured
Lasertubus	Micro-corrugated silver foil and merocel sponge in a white rubber tube that has cuff within cuff	CO_2, KTP, Nd: YAG, Argon	-	Crimping of the tube can cause hypoxemia

(KTP: potassium–titanyl–phosphate; Nd: YAG: neodymium: yttrium-aluminum-garnet).

oxygen or nitrous oxide is used. Still, when fire occurs, these agents break down to potential toxic compounds.

The anesthesiologist along with team members should take all effective steps to minimize the presence of an oxidizer-enriched environment near the ignition source. Avoiding flammable prepping solutions, use of moistened gauze, and sponges, nonflammable drapes, lowest acceptable power density of laser output, laser in standby mode when not in use, assessment of inspired, exhaled and delivered oxygen concentrations, tubeless anesthetic technique, laser resistant tubes, methylene blue dyed saline filled cuff, minimal FiO_2, closed loop communication between surgeon and anesthetist are suggested to prevent laser fire.[18-20]

Managing ignition source: Knowledge about different types of laser, power settings, and modes of operation, exposure time and spot size will facilitate effective laser use and fire risk reduction.[15-20]

Management of airway fire: All OR personnel must be well trained in management of airway fire with knowledge of location of fire extinguisher inside OR complex. A rehearsed plan of action enhances rapid action. If an airway fire occurs, stop ventilation, disconnect oxygen source and flood the airway with sterile normal saline or water, remove the burnt endotracheal tube after cuff deflation, examine the airway, mask ventilate with Ambu bag and use 100% oxygen once fire is extinguished. Examine and document the extent of airway injuries and presence of remnants of endotracheal tube using a flexible bronchoscope. Reintubate with a fresh endotracheal tube and ventilate. Use steroids to reduce edema and inflammation and monitor the patient for 24 hours for complications. Use of antibiotics and ventilatory support if needed will aid in better recovery.[15-20]

ANESTHETIC CONSIDERATIONS FOR LASER AIRWAY SURGERY

Clear understanding of airway pathology is an important prerequisite for planning anesthetic technique for laser airway surgery. Patients may be young adults with no comorbid conditions or frail elderly with multiple comorbidities. There may be either no anticipated airway problems or significant airway compromise such as stridor due to advanced glottic carcinoma. An ideal anesthetic technique for laser surgery must provide a secure airway without risk of aspiration, adequate ventilation, smooth induction, and maintenance of anesthesia, immobile surgical field free of secretions, adequate depth of anesthesia to suppress hemodynamic response, no risk of laser fire, scavenging of laser plume and safe emergence. A laser proof anesthetic technique by utilizing these conflicting ideal conditions must be provided.[22-29]

Preoperative Care

A proper preoperative care includes assessment by meticulous history with focus on symptoms and signs of airway obstruction such as difficulty in breathing, swallowing, snoring, stridor, wheezing, difficulty in clearing secretions, voice change, position, and breathing pattern during sleep. Stridor indicates a significantly narrowed airway that needs a proper backup plan. Assessment and documentation of airway for difficulty in mask ventilation, intubation, supraglottic device placement, and tracheostomy is mandatory for devising anesthetic plan.

Clear understanding of lesion—its size, location, extent, mobility, associated airway compromise aids smooth anesthetic induction.

While indirect laryngoscopy assesses lesions at the glottic level, chest radiography, three-dimensional reconstruction computed tomography, and magnetic resonance imaging gives accurate anatomical details of subglottic and tracheal lesions. Cross-sectional images provide information on luminal diameter and intrinsic obstruction of airway.

Dynamic assessment of airway during respiration using a flexible nasal endoscopy will give valuable inputs in devising an anesthetic plan along with surgeon.

Assessment of associated comorbidities and involvement of multidisciplinary team help limit errors and aid better performance by preoperative optimization of cardiorespiratory function, nutrition, and other metabolic functions.[22-28]

Premedication

In patients, without compromised airway, premedication with an opioid such as fentanyl, a sedative such as midazolam and an anticholinergic drug like glycopyrrolate to allay anxiety and reduce secretions is safe with appropriate monitoring. Dexmedetomidine is a safe alternative when there is suspected airway compromise as it provides good sedation without respiratory depression. In a compromised airway, no sedative or opioid premedication is advised for fear of airway obstruction.[4,9,22,26]

Intraoperative Care

Intraoperative care should cater to anesthetic goals—profound muscle paralysis for masseter relaxation for introduction of suspension laryngoscope, immobile surgical field, adequate oxygenation, ventilation, analgesia, and cardiovascular stability during surgical stimulation. Profound relaxation till the end of surgery and rapid postoperative recovery is essential. Multiple parameters monitor to analyze heart rate, rhythm, blood pressure, oxygen saturation, end tidal CO_2, temperature and respiration is mandatory. A laser safety checklist can be utilized before switching on laser **(Box 1)**. Using a video monitor during entire laser intervention allows the OR team to observe and anticipate the surgical steps which helps better communication among the team.[4,9,22]

Induction

Standard anesthetic induction using intravenous or inhalational technique is used when there is absence of airway obstruction. In patients with

> **BOX 1:** Laser safety checklist.[29]
>
> *Environmental checks*
> - Doors closed
> - External warning lights on
> - Emergency saline syringe ready?
> - Safety glasses worn by all?
>
> *Patient checks*
> - Wet swabs in place?
> - Flammable objects removed?

compromised airway, nasal endoscopy will aid anesthetic plan. Awake fiberoptic intubation is recommended when there is airway obstruction. A back up plan with armamentarium for execution including video laryngoscopes, cricothyrotomy set, jet ventilator, tracheostomy set in a difficult airway cart along with rigid bronchoscopy and an experienced ear, nose, and throat (ENT) surgeon for emergency tracheostomy should be available before induction. A change in anesthetic plan should be thought about in case an emergency like airway obstruction occurs during induction.

Anesthesia Techniques for Ventilation and Maintenance[30-33]

The various anesthetic techniques of airway management and ventilation depends on degree of airway obstruction, age of the patient and site of surgery—whether it is oral, hypopharyngeal, laryngeal or infraglottic. The various techniques that can be used are:
- Anesthesia with laryngeal mask airway (LMA).
- General anesthesia with endotracheal intubation.
- Tubeless techniques which includes:
  - Intermittent apnea technique.
  - Spontaneous breathing technique.
  - Conventional jet ventilation.
  - High frequency jet ventilation/superimposed high frequency jet ventilation (HFJV/SHFJV).
  - Supraglottic ventilation or transnasal humidified rapid insufflation ventilator exchange (THRIVE).
- Topical/local anesthesia with sedation.

Anesthesia with laryngeal mask airway: Laryngeal mask airway and reinforced LMA can be used for awake and anesthetized patients for fiberoptic bronchoscopy guided laser interventions such as laser pharyngoplasty and for carinal lesions. Since the fiber tip of laser will be away from LMA, laser output will not ignite the LMA or flexible laryngeal mask airway (fLMA) in tracheal or carinal procedures. The only disadvantage is filling of cuff with methylene blue dyed saline than air in a reusable LMA for which complete deflation of cuff will be difficult. It has been described by keeping the cuff above a syringe without plunger that will facilitate gravitational drainage. A disposable single use LMA circumvents this problem.[34]

General anesthesia with endotracheal intubation: This technique is familiar to all anesthesiologists and utilize the laser tubes. Traumatizing laryngeal lesion with the laser tube must be avoided while intubation. Lower FiO_2, cuff inflation with dyed saline and observation of field will aid a successful surgery. It must be remembered that laser tubes have greater external diameter which may limit surgical access and visualization of field necessitating use of smaller tubes.[4,9,10,32,33]

Tubeless Techniques:[34-37]
- *Intermittent apnea technique:* Since smaller airways of children cannot accommodate thick laser tubes, this technique was formulated by Weisberger and Miner. After induction of anesthesia and muscle relaxation, anesthesia is maintained with 100% oxygen. Patient is intubated and extubated intermittently through suspension laryngoscope. Hyperventilation after intubation brings down CO_2 while permissible apnea and hypercapnia occurs during extubated phase, during which surgery is done. 1–5 minutes of apnea can be tolerated during which surgical procedure is done. Apneic period should be shortened when there is reduced functional residual capacity as in small children. Total intravenous anesthesia with propofol and opioids is a better option as it is difficult to maintain anesthetic depth using inhalational agents. It is contraindicated in patients where laryngeal visualization is difficult.[37]
- *Spontaneous breathing technique with insufflation:* This technique is useful in children where it is difficult to pass an endotracheal tube beyond the lesion or the tube obscures the lesion. It allows unrestricted view and surgical access to the larynx. It is accomplished by inhalational agents delivered proximal to larynx—by a nasopharyngeal airway, a tracheal tube beyond the nasopharynx, a small catheter kept above the larynx or via side arm channel of bronchoscope. Intravenous injection of propofol can be used for maintenance. The movement of vocal cords is minimal if anesthetic depth is maintained appropriately. A back up plan of intubation with a laser safe tube must be ready at all times. It is easier in children than in adults as suspension laryngoscope is difficult to use in adults without muscle relaxation. Coughing, lack of ventilatory control, soiling of airway with blood and debris, vocal cord movements due to inadequate anesthetic depth, laryngospasm, OR pollution with anesthetic gases are all complications of this technique and requires continuous closed loop communication with surgeon.
- *Jet ventilation:*[38-41] When prolonged duration of surgery is anticipated and a tubeless field is needed, jet ventilation is appropriate. This technique involves intermittent administration of high-pressure jets of air, oxygen or air-oxygen mixtures that entrain room air and lower the delivered pressures. It allows total view of larynx and trachea and removes the risk of laser fire. A misdirected jet can cause complications such as gastric distension, inadequate ventilation, surgical emphysema, pneumothorax and pneumomediastinum. Moreover the vocal cord movement can interfere with surgeon's focus. The important limitation of jet ventilation

technique is experience of the anesthesiologist. The position of jet nozzle could be supraglottic, infraglottic or transtracheal.

Supraglottic jet ventilation, is delivered via a jet nozzle in lumen of operating microscope and is laser safe as the nozzle is proximal to possible obstruction but is poorly efficient for gas exchange.

Infraglottic jet ventilation is delivered by a laser jet, Hunsaker laser safe subglottic monojet ventilation tube or similar tubes inserted via glottis in mid-trachea before suspension laryngoscope is placed. Though Hunsaker and laser jet catheters are made of noninflammable tetrafluoroethylene, they can degrade and fracture, if their tolerance levels are exceeded during laser use. It gives good surgical field and minimal vocal cord movements. Breath stacking occurs when there is partial airway obstruction necessitating long expiratory pauses. Though gas exchange is better with infraglottic jet ventilation, it is contraindicated when the airway lumen is less than 50% of normal as there is risk of barotrauma.

Transtracheal jet ventilation (TTJV) must be initiated only when there will be unobstructed egress of gases. A partially obstructed airway can cause pneumothorax. Apart from the risk of barotrauma, TTJV catheters are at risk of laser fire as none of the catheters are designed for laser airway surgeries. While low frequency manual jet ventilation can be used for short surgical procedures, automatic jet ventilators with pressure monitoring and capnography can be used for long and difficult procedures. HFJV can be administered through side arm of bronchoscope using an insufflation catheter with side hole for laser airway surgeries. Since small tidal volumes are used in HFJV, the less movement of larynx, trachea, and lungs facilitate precise operation of laser beam.

- *Combined frequency jet ventilation/SHFJV:* Superimposed high frequency jet ventilation is an advanced mode for patients with laryngotracheal stenosis. Two separate jet streams via two injectors of different length is provided by high and low frequency units which open into proximal part of suspension laryngoscope. A third nozzle opening measures the supraglottic pressure near the distal end of the laryngoscope. A high frequency jet stream superimposed on low frequency jet stream is applied simultaneously on the suspension laryngoscope. The distal pressure monitoring port can be used for CO_2 monitoring intermittently **(Fig. 3)**. SHFJV must be utilized when there is severe airway obstruction or pulmonary dysfunction.[42]

- *Supraglottic ventilation or THRIVE:* Transnasal humidified rapid insufflation ventilator exchange maintains oxygenation by a ventilatory mass flow of continuous humidified 100% oxygen at high flow rates up to 120 liters per minute. A patent airway is a prerequisite for THRIVE, and it has been successfully used with CO_2 and potassium titanyl phosphate (KTP) lasers for microlaryngeal surgery.

It does not increase the likelihood of laser airway fire unless a debris or flammable object falls in the "oxygen reservoir" created in the pharynx. THRIVE must be paused, used intermittently or turned off or FiO_2 is reduced to 30% before introduction of laser. Transcutaneous CO_2 monitoring may be used as capnography is not possible. Though there has been a case report

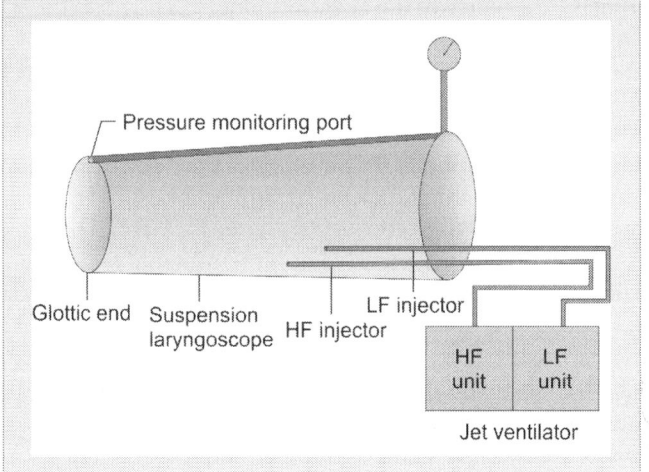

Fig. 3: Illustrative representation of suspension laryngoscopy in superimposed high frequency jet ventilation (SHFJV). (HF: high frequency; LF: low frequency)

of diathermy related fire with THRIVE, fire with laser has not yet been reported. Using THRIVE during laser surgery must be done with caution as there is risk of airway fire, and there is limited data to support its use with laser.[43-45]

Topical/Local Anesthesia with Sedation

Topical anesthesia with sedation may be an appropriate technique for short duration procedure in cooperative adults when laser is used along the side port of flexible fiberoptic scope. It is a useful technique in middle or lower third tracheal lesions. Bleeding is the most severe life-threatening complication with this technique. Sedation can decrease respiratory drive and cause upper airway obstruction. Hypoxemia, hypercarbia, excessive sedation and obstruction of airway in a patient with fixed lesion are all complications that need maneuvers such as jaw thrust, chin lift, positive pressure ventilation to open up airway during procedure followed by securing the airway if needed.

Postoperative Care

A good postoperative care is essential to aid smooth recovery in laser surgery. Patients can be smoothly extubated in an awake state inside OR. Spraying of vocal cords with local anesthetics before extubation will prevent postoperative laryngospasm. The endotracheal tube is inspected postextubation to look for damage by laser if any. A bronchoscopy is needed if there is a missing foil or tape. Postoperative edema, stridor and retractions can occur which needs appropriate treatment. Humidified oxygen and steroids in form of dexamethasone will enhance smooth recovery. Postoperative chest X-ray is mandatory when Venturi is used to rule out pneumothorax.

CONCLUSION

Airway laser surgery is unique as anesthesiologist and surgeon share the same field. Knowledge of basic principles and applications of laser, awareness of general and airway specific laser hazards, management of airway and OR fire will aid a safe anesthetic practice. Proper preoperative assessment of patients, a planned intraoperative anesthetic technique using closed or open system depending on the expertise of the anesthesiologist, immediate recognition of unexpected complications such as airway fire and a good postoperative care will benefit smooth recovery of patients.

ACKNOWLEDGMENTS

The authors are indebted to Dr Aruna Parameswari for her valuable, constructive suggestions, constant support and wise counsel. They are also thankful to Dr Raminder Sehgal for her patient guidance.

KEY POINTS

- Closed loop communication before, during and after any procedure among team members is an indispensable requirement for successful laser surgery.
- The anesthesiologist, surgeon, and the scrub nurse must be familiar with working principles and hazards of laser and management of airway fire.
- The anesthesiologist must be well versed in various anesthetic techniques available for laser airway surgery.
- The triad of fire—fuel, oxidant and ignition source must be known and removal or avoidance of one of the triads prevent risk of fire effectively.
- Clinically, use of low FiO_2 with air rather than nitrous oxide helps avoid airway fire.
- Laser tubes with laser resistant properties impart some degree of protection against laser strike.
- Proper preoperative evaluation of patients, and recognition of compromised airway guides a difficult perioperative course, and aids effective perianesthetic management.
- A closed anesthetic technique with a laser tube is as good as an open anesthetic technique with spontaneous ventilation, intermittent apnea or jet ventilation technique.
- Jet ventilation technique is an appropriate ventilation strategy during adult airway laser surgeries only when the anesthesiologist is experienced and suitable equipment is available.
- Hemodynamic stability, adequate ventilation, and complete immobility are important requirements for successful outcome for laser airway surgery.

REFERENCES

1. Boulnois J. Photophysical processes in recent medical laser developments: a review. Lasers Med Sci. 1986;1(1):47-66.
2. O'Connell Ferster A. Lasers in laryngeal surgery. Operative Techniques in Otolaryngology. Head Neck Surg. 2019;30(4):279-83.

3. Occupational Safety and Health Administration. Hospital eTool: Use of Medical Lasers. [online] Available from https://www.osha.gov/SLTC/etools/hospital/surgical/lasers.html. [Last accessed November, 2020].
4. Dhar P, Malik A. Anesthesia for laser surgery in ENT and the various ventilatory techniques. Trend Anaesth Crit Care. 2011;1(2):60-6.
5. CDC. NIOSH hazard controls HC11—control of smoke from laser/electric surgical procedures. [online] Available from https://www.cdc.gov/niosh/docs/hazardcontrol/pdfs/hc11.pdf?id=10.26616/NIOSHPUB96128. [Last accessed November, 2020].
6. Baggish M, Poiesz BJ, Joret D, Williamson P, Refai A. Presence of human immunodeficiency virus DNA in laser smoke. Lasers Surg Med. 1991;11(3):197-203.
7. Kokosa J, Benedetto MD. Probing plume protection problems in the health care environment. J Laser Appl. 1992;4(3):39-43.
8. Wenig BL, Stenson KM, Wenig BM, Tracey D. Effects of plume produced by the Nd:YAG laser and electrocautery on the respiratory system. Lasers Surg Med. 1993;13(2):242-5.
9. Hemantkumar I. Anesthesia for laser surgery of the airway. Int J Otorhinolaryngol Clin. 2017;9(1):1-5.
10. Sosis M. Anesthesia for laser surgery. J Voice. 1989;3(2):163-74.
11. Sheinbein DS, Loeb RG. Laser surgery and fire hazards in ear, nose, and throat surgeries. Anesthesiol Clin. 2010;28(3):485-96.
12. Bhat AG, Ganapathi P. "Blow-torch phenomenon" during laser assisted excision of a thyroglossal cyst at the base of the tongue. J Anaesthesiol Clin Pharmacol. 2012;28(2):247-8.
13. Perkins SR, Morris JJ, Weidner CD, Barroso SR, Roberts LC, Ramsay M. Surgical laser safety and anesthesiology. BUMC Proceed. 1991;4(4):37-43.
14. Santos P, Ayuso A, Luis M, Martínez G, Sala X. Airway ignition during CO_2 laser laryngeal surgery and high frequency jet ventilation. Eur J Anaesthesiol. 2000;17(3):204-7.
15. Remz M, Luria I, Gravenstein M, Rice SD, Morey TE, Gravenstein N, et al. Prevention of airway fires: do not overlook the expired oxygen concentration. Anesth Analg. 2013;117(5):1172-6.
16. Ahmed F, Kinshuck AJ, Harrison M, O'Brien D, Lancaster J, Roland NJ, et al. Laser safety in head and neck cancer surgery. Eur Arch of Otorhinolaryngol. 2010;267(11):1779-84.
17. Smith LP, Roy S. Operating room fires in otolaryngology: risk factors and prevention. Am J Otolaryngol. 2011;32(2):109-14.
18. Sosis MB. Saline soaked pledgets prevent carbon dioxide laser-induced endotracheal tube cuff ignition. J Clin Anesth. 1995;7(5):395-7.
19. Apfelbaum JL, Caplan RA, Barker SJ, Connis RT, Cowles C, Ehrenwerth J, et al. Practice advisory for the prevention and management of operating room fires: an updated report by the American Society of Anesthesiologists Task Force on Operating Room Fires. Anesthesiology. 2013;118(2):271-90.
20. Dorsch J, Dorsch S. A Practical Approach to Anesthesia Equipment. Philadelphia: Wolters Kluwer/Lippincott Williams & Wilkins Health; 2011.
21. Burns JA, Adlard SD, Kobler JB, Tynan MA, Petrillo RH, Tracy LF. A comparison of laser-protected endotracheal tubes. Otolaryngol Head Neck Surg. 2018;159(5):871-8.

22. Hsu J, Tan M. Anesthesia considerations in laryngeal surgery. Int Anesthesiol Clin. 2017;55(1):11-32.
23. Hofmeyr R, Llewellyn R, Fagan J. Multidisciplinary difficult airway challenges: perioperative management of glottic and supraglottic tumors. Operative Techniques in Otolaryngology. Head Neck Surg. 2020;31(2):120-7.
24. Bradley J, Lee GS, Peyton J. Anesthesia for shared airway surgery in children. Pediatric Anaesth. 2020;30(3):288-95.
25. Best C. Anesthesia for laser surgery of the airway in children. Paediatr Anaesth. 2009;19(Suppl 1):155-65.
26. UpToDate. Anesthesia for laryngeal surgery. Zheng G. Uptodate.com. 2020 [online] Available from https://www.uptodate.com/contents/anesthesia-for-laryngeal-surgery. [Last accessed November, 2020].
27. Thode SA. Laryngo-tracheal laser surgery and general anesthesia. Lasers Surg Med. 1986;6(3):369-72.
28. Mausser G, Friedrich G, Schwarz G. Airway management and anesthesia in neonates, infants and children during endolaryngotracheal surgery. Paediatr Anaesth. 2007;17(10):942-7.
29. Williams SP, Kinshuck AJ, Butler CR, Sandhu GS. Introduction of a laser safety checklist in the ENT operating theatre-our experience across twenty cases. Clin Otolaryngol. 2018;43(5):1357-60.
30. Inglis D, Gilhooly M, Patel A. The simultaneous use of three ventilatory techniques to maintain oxygenation in a patient undergoing tracheal laser resection of tumour. Anaesth Rep. 2019;7(2):70-2.
31. Werkhaven JA. Microlaryngoscopy-airway management with anaesthetic techniques for CO_2 laser. Paediatr Anaesth. 2004;14(1):90-4.
32. Jaquet Y, Monnier P, Van Melle G, Ravussin P, Spahn DR, Chollet-Rivier M. Complications of different ventilation strategies in endoscopic laryngeal surgery: a 10-year review. Anesthesiology. 2006;104(1):52-9.
33. Krespi Y, Kizhner V, Koorn R, Giordano A. Anesthesia and ventilation options for flex robotic assisted laryngopharyngeal surgery. Am J Otolaryngol. 2019;40(6):102105.
34. Deshmukh A, Jadhav S, Wadgoankar V, Takalkar U, Deshmukh H, Apsingkar P, et al. Airway management and bronchoscopic treatment of subglottic and tracheal stenosis using holmium laser with balloon dilatation. Indian J Otolaryngol Head Neck Surg. 2019;71(Suppl 1):453-8.
35. Pearson K, McGuire BE. Anaesthesia for laryngo-tracheal surgery, including tubeless field techniques. BJA Education. 2017;17(7):242-8.
36. Thaung M, Balakrishnan A. A modified technique of tubeless anaesthesia for microlaryngoscopy and bronchoscopy in young children with stridor. Paediatr Anaesth. 1998;8(3):201-4.
37. Weisberger EC, Emhardt JD. Apneic Anesthesia with intermittent ventilation for microsurgery of the upper airway. Laryngoscope. 1996;106(9 Pt 1):1099-102.
38. Hunsaker DH. Anesthesia for microlaryngeal surgery: the case for subglottic jet ventilation. Laryngoscope. 1994;104(8 Pt 2 Suppl 65):1-30.
39. Barakate M, Maver E, Wotherspoon G, Havas T. Anaesthesia for microlaryngeal and laser laryngeal surgery: impact of subglottic jet ventilation. J Laryngol Otol. 2010;124(6):641-5.
40. Gupta S, O'Donnell R. Transtracheal jet ventilation. Anaesth Int Care Med. 2020;21(4):185-9.

41. Bourgain JL, Desruennes E, Fischler M, Ravussin P. Transtracheal high frequency jet ventilation for endoscopic airway surgery: a multicentre study. Br J Anaesth. 2001;87(6):870-5.
42. Rezaie-Majd A, Bigenzahn W, Denk DM, Burian M, Kornfehl J, Grasl MCh, et al. Superimposed high-frequency jet ventilation (SHFJV) for endoscopic laryngotracheal surgery in more than 1500 patients. Br J Anaesth. 2006;96(5):650-9.
43. Flach S, Elhoweris A, Majumdar S, Crawley S, Manickavasagam J. Transoral laser microsurgery using high-flow nasal cannula oxygenation: our experience of 21 cases. Clin Otolaryngol. 2019;44(5):871-4.
44. Huang L, Dharmawardana N, Badenoch A, Ooi E. A review of the use of transnasal humidified rapid insufflation ventilatory exchange for patients undergoing surgery in the shared airway setting. J Anesth. 2020;34(1):134-43.
45. Ward P. THRIVE and airway fires. Anaesthesia. 2017;72(8):1035.

CHAPTER 4

Anesthesia Circuits: Bain and Closed

Swati Chhabra, Sadik Mohammed

INTRODUCTION

Anesthesia circuits are the "means of connect" between the anesthesia machine and the patient. They serve the purpose of ventilation [providing oxygen and removing carbon dioxide (CO_2)] and delivering anesthetic agents. The breathing circuits have a history of more than 170 years. A plethora of devices has been introduced ranging from Morton's ether inhaler to the modern day closed circle systems. The properties of an ideal anesthesia circuit are listed in **Box 1**.

Various classification systems have been introduced by many researchers such as Dripps, Eckenhoff and Vandam, Moyers, Collins, Adriani, etc. The most commonly used classification system classified the anesthesia circuits as open, semi-open, semi-closed and closed.[1] Open systems were used for open-drop anesthesia with ether or chloroform, where gauzes over masks (such as Schimmelbusch mask, and Yankauer mask) were dripped with anesthetic agent. Semi-open systems are the Mapleson circuits. In 1954, Mapleson introduced breathing systems A to E, to which F was later added and a few modifications to these were introduced as well. These systems rely on the continuous fresh gas flow (FGF) to eliminate CO_2.[2,3] Semi-closed and closed systems utilize unidirectional valves and CO_2 absorbers in a circle system. When the FGF is more than the patient's requirement, it is a semi-closed circuit while the FGF is equal to the patient's requirement in a closed circuit.

Such classifications are frequently confusing and a simpler classification would be according to the method of CO_2 elimination, such as:

BOX 1: Properties of an ideal anesthesia circuit.

An ideal anesthesia circuit should:
- Be simple to use and portable
- Work efficiently for spontaneous, assisted and controlled ventilation
- Reliable and safe in all age groups
- Be able to effectively remove carbon dioxide with no or minimal rebreathing
- Allow for scavenging of exhaled gases
- Offer low resistance to gas flow
- Conserve heat and moisture

- Circuits with CO_2 washout (open and semi-open systems).
- Circuits with CO_2 absorption (semi-closed and closed systems).

The efficiency of an anesthesia circuit is determined by the lowest FGF that prevents rebreathing of CO_2. An efficient system avoids high fresh gas requirement and reduces wastage of anesthetic agents and other gases. The two anesthesia circuits that have stood the test of time and are widely used are the Bain circuit and circle system (both semi-closed and closed), which are elaborately discussed in this chapter.

BAIN CIRCUIT

Bain circuit was introduced by Bain and Spoerel in 1972. It is a modified Mapleson D circuit and has a coaxial arrangement **(Figs. 1A and B)**.

Configuration

The various components of the Bain circuit are coaxial tubing, reservoir bag, and an adjustable pressure limiting (APL) valve **(Fig. 2)**. Usually, the length of coaxial tubing is 180 cm; however, the length could be 270 or 540 cm for use in dental, ophthalmology, and magnetic resonance imaging (MRI) suite. The lengthier versions have higher compliance such that lesser tidal volume is delivered than the set value on the ventilator. In addition, positive end expiratory pressure (PEEP) and resistance during spontaneous ventilation are increased.[4,5] The fresh gas enters the system through the inner tube that is of 6 mm diameter. The outer tube is corrugated and is 22 mm in diameter. The tube is wide enough for a minimal resistance to airflow and the corrugations prevent kinking upon bending and collapse at subatmospheric pressures. The inner tube is for inspiratory gases while the outer tube is for both inspiratory and expiratory gases.

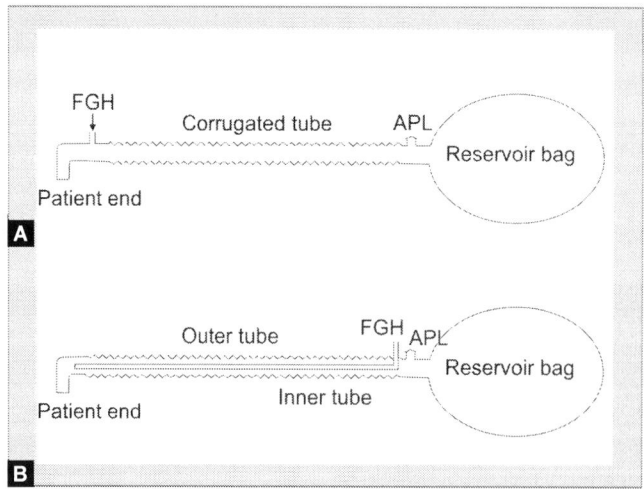

Figs. 1A and B: (A) Mapleson D circuit; (B) Its coaxial modification, the Bain circuit. (FGF: fresh gas flow; APL: adjustable pressure limiting)

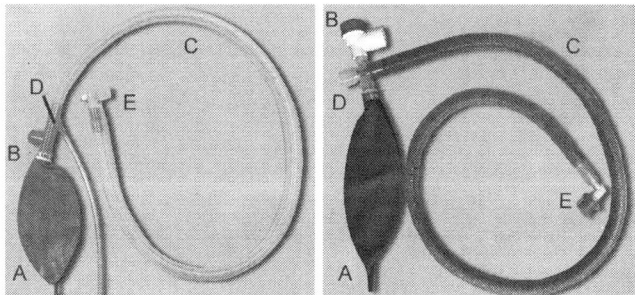

Fig. 2: Components of the Bain circuit depicted in two different looking Bain circuit having same configuration. A: Reservoir bag; B: Adjustable pressure limiting (APL) valve; C: Corrugated outer tube with a coaxial inner tube; D: Fresh gas inlet; E: Patient's end.

The reservoir bag is at the machine end of the circuit and its material could be antistatic rubber, plastic or latex-free rubber. The usual capacity for use in adults is 2 L. In addition to assisting or controlling the ventilation, the purpose of the reservoir bag is to accommodate fresh gas during expiration for the subsequent inspiration. If this bag is removed from the circuit's design and patient has to breathe directly from the fresh gas source, the FGF should at least match the peak inspiratory flow rate of the patient (30 L/min). The bag can also be used to assess the breathing pattern of the patient, although judging the tidal volume could be erroneous.

The APL valve is positioned away from the patient's end. As the name suggests, it is an adjustable valve and is one-way and spring loaded. During spontaneous respiration, there is positive pressure inside the system at expiration and with the valve open, a pressure of 1 cmH$_2$O is required to actuate the valve. During controlled ventilation, appropriate adjustment of the valve is recommended to control the leak through the valve thus, controlling the airway pressure.

Flow Mechanics

The ventilation is divided into phases, viz., first inspiration, expiration, and expiratory pause, subsequent inspiration to understand the mechanics during spontaneous and controlled ventilation. During spontaneous ventilation, the FGF should be 1.5–3 times the minute ventilation to prevent rebreathing while during controlled ventilation FGF 1–2 times the minute ventilation is required. Hence, Bain circuit is more efficient for controlled ventilation.

Spontaneous Ventilation (Figs. 3A to D)

The APL valve should be fully open and the exhaled gases are vented during expiration.

First inspiration: The circuit is filled with just the fresh gas and thus the patient's inspiratory gas is all fresh gas (**Fig. 3A**).

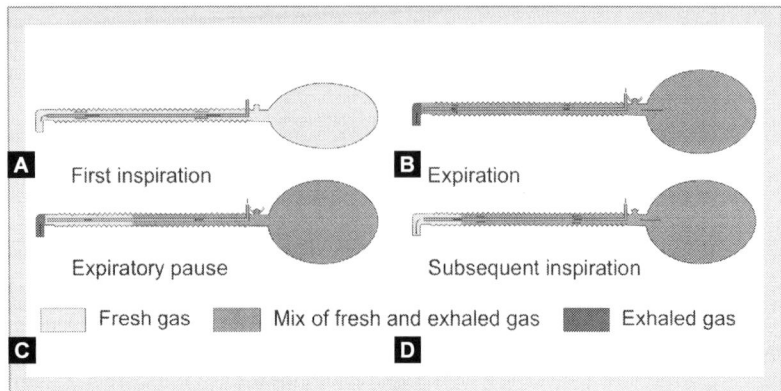

Figs. 3A to D: Diagrammatic representation of flow mechanics of Bain circuit during spontaneous ventilation.

Expiration: The exhaled gases and the fresh gas mix up in the outer tubing and fill up the reservoir bag. When the bag fills up, APL valve opens. Mix of fresh and exhaled gas is then vented out **(Fig. 3B)**.

Expiratory pause: The fresh gas continues to flow from the inner tubing to the outer tubing and displaces the mix of exhaled and fresh gas. Since the reservoir bag is already full, the mixture of gases is vented through the APL valve. The patient side of the outer tube is thus filled with fresh gas for the subsequent inspiration **(Fig. 3C)**. In spontaneous ventilation with the patient under the effect of anesthetic agents, expiratory pause might be short and might lead to rebreathing of exhaled gases. To prevent this, very high FGF are required to flush out the exhaled gases.

Subsequent inspiration: The patient inhales fresh gas from both inner and outer tubing followed by mixture of gases from outer tubing and reservoir bag depending on the tidal volume **(Fig. 3D)**.

Controlled Ventilation (Figs. 4A to D)

The APL valve should be partially closed and venting of the gases occurs during expiration.

First inspiration: The circuit is filled up with fresh gas. When the reservoir bag is squeezed, fresh gas is passed from the outer tubing as well as from inner tube to the patient while some of the fresh gas is also vented out through the APL valve that is partially closed **(Fig. 4A)**.

Expiration: A mix of fresh and exhaled gas enters the outer tubing and refills the reservoir bag **(Fig. 4B)**.

Expiratory pause: The fresh gas continues to flow from the inner tubing to the outer tubing and displaces the mix of fresh and exhaled gas. Since the reservoir bag is already full, the mix of gases is vented through the APL valve. Longer the expiratory pause more is the amount of fresh gas in the outer tubing for the subsequent inspiration **(Fig. 4C)**.

Anesthesia Circuits: Bain and Closed

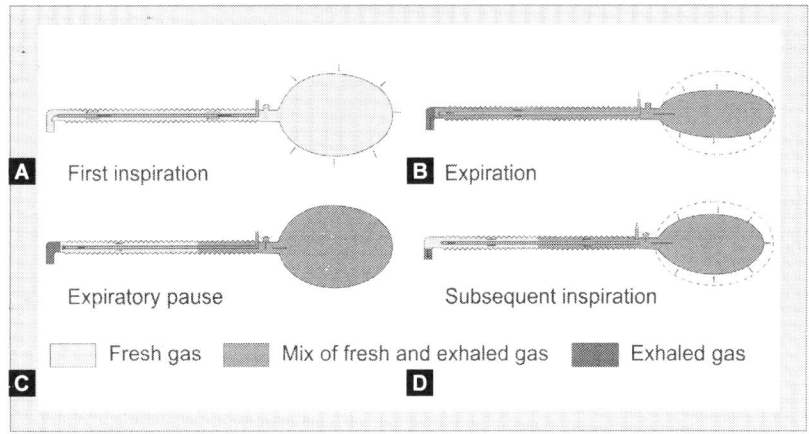

Figs. 4A to D: Diagrammatic representation of flow mechanics of Bain circuit during controlled ventilation.

Subsequent inspiration: When the reservoir bag is squeezed, fresh gas from the inner and outer tubing and then the mix of the fresh and exhaled gas is passed to the patient while some mixed gas in the reservoir bag is vented out from the partially closed APL valve **(Fig. 4D)**.

Preuse Checks

Safe delivery of anesthesia mandates checking the equipment prior to use and Bain circuit is no exception.[6] At first, it should be visually inspected for the structural integrity of the inner tube which if kinked/disconnected/obstructed could lead to fatal hypoxia and hypercapnia.[7-10] The functional integrity can be checked with the following tests:

- *Occlusion test.*
    - It was first described by Foex and Crampton-Smith in 1977. For the test, the inner tube is occluded with either a dedicated device or a plunger from a 2 mL syringe and start a FGF of 6 L/min with the APL valve fully closed. If the Bain circuit is functioning correctly, a dip in bobbin on the rotameter will be observed. If the anesthesia machine/workstation does not support this, there is another way to perform the occlusion test. The inner tube is occluded, the APL valve is closed and FGF is set to 6 L/min. Once the reservoir bag is full and the machine reads pressure of 30 cmH$_2$O, decrease the FGF to the minimum possible. If the abovementioned pressure is sustained for 5 seconds, the Bain circuit is working fine. However, the circuit is faulty if either the pressure of 30 cmH$_2$O is not attained or not sustained for 5 seconds.
- *Pethick test.*
    - It was described by Pethick in 1975. The patient end of the circuit is occluded, the APL valve is closed and the oxygen flush is activated. When the reservoir bag is inflated, the patient end is opened while continuing the flush. If the inner tube is intact, high flow of gases

will lower the pressure at the patient end and thus, the reservoir bag will collapse. However, if the inner tube is faulty or disconnected, the collapse will not be observed or rather the bag might inflate.

Of the two, occlusion test is much more sensitive than Pethick test.[11] Capnography can also be utilized in testing the integrity of inner tube.[12]

Advantages and Disadvantages of Bain Circuit

Advantages

- It is lightweight and convenient to use in operating room as well as during transport of patients.
- At the FGFs used in clinical practice, it offers very low resistance to breathing.
- Due to coaxial structure, exhaled gases in the outer tubing provide warmth to the gases in the inner tubing by counter current heat exchange mechanism.
- Since the APL valve is located far from the patient end, scavenging of the exhaled gases is possible by connecting the scavenging tubing to the 30 mm male connector at the machine end **(Fig. 5)**.
- Some ventilators (Penlon Nuffield 200) can be attached in place of the reservoir bag for mechanical ventilation with APL valve fully closed **(Fig. 5)**.[13]

Disadvantages

- It can be uneconomical because of the high FGF requirement especially with spontaneous ventilation.
- Unrecognized disconnections, kinking or obstruction of the inner tube may result in catastrophe.

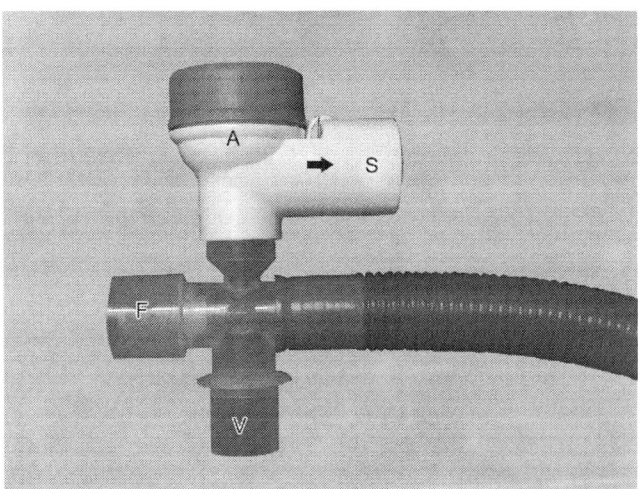

Fig. 5: Machine end of Bain circuit. A: APL valve; F: fresh gas inlet; S: attachment for scavenging; V: attachment for ventilator as replacement for reservoir bag (APL: adjustable pressure limiting).

- Optimal FGF is difficult to determine and may need to change with spontaneous, assisted or controlled ventilation in the same patient. Monitoring of end tidal CO_2 is helpful in this and should be used.

CIRCLE SYSTEM

A circle system has separate inspiratory and expiratory channels and rather than relying on the FGF for flushing out CO_2, it has a CO_2 absorber in the expiratory limb. The unidirectional valves assist in achieving a circular and unidirectional flow. The more commonly used circle system is a semi-closed one that utilizes more FGF than the requirement of the patient and some of the gas is vented out from the system. A closed system on the other hand utilizes FGF in the amount required for consumption. A closed circle system is quite close to the concept of an ideal breathing circuit. It efficiently conserves the anesthetic gases, heat and moisture, thus reducing the cost and environmental pollution.

The essential components of a classic circle system **(Fig. 6)** are:
- CO_2 absorber.
- Corrugated tubing.
- Y-piece connector for the patient's end.
- Two unidirectional valves (one inspiratory and one expiratory).
- Fresh gas inlet.
- Reservoir bag.
- Adjustable pressure limiting valve.

CO_2 Absorbers

The semi-closed and closed operation is not possible without a CO_2 absorber. The absorbent is held in canisters having transparent sidewalls so that

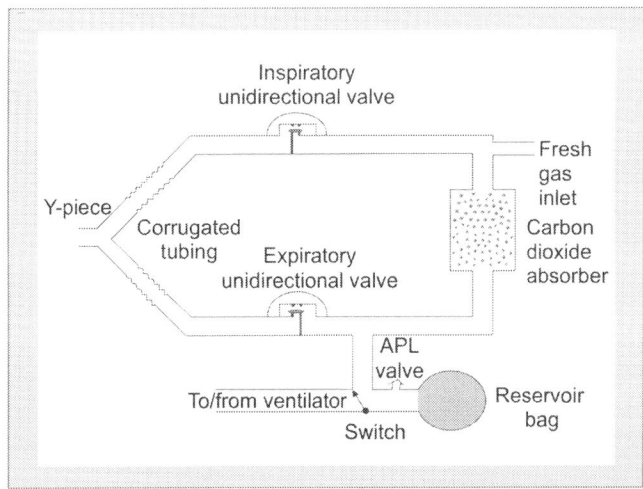

Fig. 6: Diagrammatic representation of a classic circle system.
(APL: adjustable pressure limiting)

absorbent color can be monitored **(Fig. 7A)**. Initially, absorption in the canister occurs at the inlet and along the canister sides. As this absorbent becomes exhausted, CO_2 will be absorbed farther downstream in the canister. Baffles or annular rings are mounted in the canister to direct the gas flow toward the central part of the canister and to increase the travel path for gases that otherwise tend to preferentially pass along the sides of the canister.[14]

The main constituent of commercially available absorbents is calcium hydroxide. To this, other metallic bases are added to accelerate the chemical reaction that leads to removal of CO_2 from the exhaled gases. Soda lime contains 1.5–5% of sodium hydroxide in addition to calcium hydroxide while barium lime consists of about 85% calcium hydroxide, 11% barium hydroxide and 4% potassium hydroxide. The chemical reaction **(Fig. 8)** requires 14–16% water content in the absorbent and desiccation results in production of carbon monoxide. Characteristically, the reaction is exothermic and involves a change in the pH. Modern day absorbents no longer contain potassium hydroxide and contain reduced concentrations of sodium hydroxide. Potassium hydroxide is the primary cause of reactions that cause high internal temperatures and reactions that produce carbon monoxide, formaldehyde, and compound A. While sodium hydroxide does react with agents when the absorbent is desiccated, its lower concentration does not produce dangerous amount of toxic substances or high temperatures enough to cause damage to the canister. There is a notable amount of literature analyzing the effect of various constituents of absorber and its desiccation on concurrent use of inhalational anesthetic agents.[15-18]

Alkali-free absorbents consist mainly of calcium hydroxide, with small amounts of other agents added to accelerate CO_2 absorption and bind water. With these absorbents, there is no evidence of carbon monoxide formation with any anesthetic agent, even if the absorbent becomes desiccated. There is little or no compound A or formaldehyde formation with sevoflurane even with low FGFs and desiccated absorbent. The CO_2 absorption capacity of these

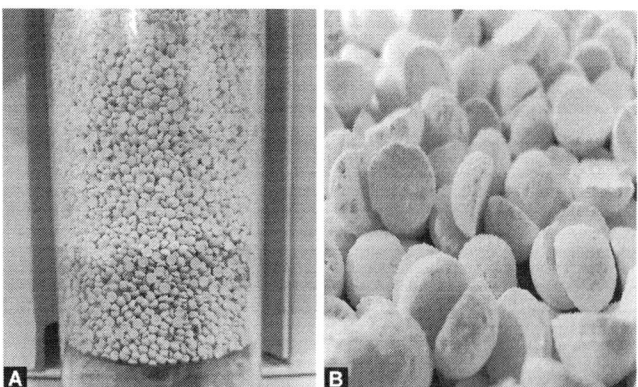

Figs. 7A and B: (A) A transparent canister to aid in visualization of color change of absorbent; (B) Irregular pellets to increase surface area for CO_2 absorption.

absorbents is less than that of absorbents containing strong alkali but does not deteriorate when moisture is lost.

Shape and Size

Absorbents are supplied as pellets or granules with irregular surface shape to enhance absorptive area **(Fig. 7B)**. Pellets and small granules provide larger surface area and decrease gas channeling along low-resistance pathways. However, they may cause more resistance and caking. The optimum size of the granules of the absorbent is 4–8 mesh. Larger size will lead to inefficient CO_2 absorption due to decreased contact area.

Indicator

An indicator is an acid or base whose color depends on pH. It is added to the absorbent to indicate when the absorbent's ability to absorb CO_2 is exhausted. Therefore, it is necessary to know which indicator is being used and what color change is expected when the absorption capacity is exhausted or the absorbent is desiccated. Some of the commonly used indicators and their colors when fresh and exhausted are listed in **Table 1**.

$$CO_2 + H_2O = H_2CO_3$$

$$H_2CO_3 + 2NaOH - Na_2CO_3 + H_2O + Heat$$
(Fast reaction)

$$Na_2CO_3 + Ca(OH)_2 = CaCO_3 + 2NaOH$$
(Slow reaction)

Fig. 8: Chemical reaction in a CO_2 absorbent.

TABLE 1: Color characteristics of indicators in CO_2 absorbents

Indicator	Color when fresh	Color when exhausted or desiccated
Phenolphthalein	White	Pink
Ethyl violet	White	Purple
Ethyl orange	Orange	Yellow
Mimosa Z	Red	White

Corrugated Tubing

The corrugations help in making the tubing flexible without kinking. The diameter of the tubing is 22 mm that minimizes resistance to gas flow (<1 cm H_2O/L/min of flow). The corrugations result in turbulent flows in the circuit and any changes in the anesthetic gas composition in the anesthesia machine is reflected in the inspired concentration according to FGF rate (faster at higher flows and vice versa).[19] The tubing in the early days were made up of rubber, however, currently available ones are made up of autoclavable silicone or disposable plastic **(Figs. 9A and B)**. The volume of the circuit is about 500 mL/m of length. The compliance of the circuit is variable and ranges from 0 to 6 mL/m/mm Hg of pressure applied. The peak inspiratory pressures during lung inflation compress some gas volume in the tubing that is measured by the spirometer although not delivered to the patient, thus contributing to the apparatus dead space. For pediatric age groups, smaller diameter tubings are used though the resistance is not increased significantly **(Figs. 10A and B)**. Less gas is compressed in such circuits leading to more accurately measured tidal volume and minute ventilation.

Increasing the length of the tubing does not increase the resistance but increases the apparatus dead space as per the compliance of the system. In addition to the simple tubing, coaxial (concentric or side by side) and concertina type tubing are also used **(Figs. 11 and 12)**. The circuit leak test is performed by the anesthesia machine by pressurizing the system at 30 cm H_2O and determining FGF required to maintain the pressure.

Y-Piece

A Y-piece connects the inspiratory and expiratory tubing to the patient interface. It might or might not be detachable. It is a three-way connector; two for the tubing and one at the patient's end. The site of attachment is a

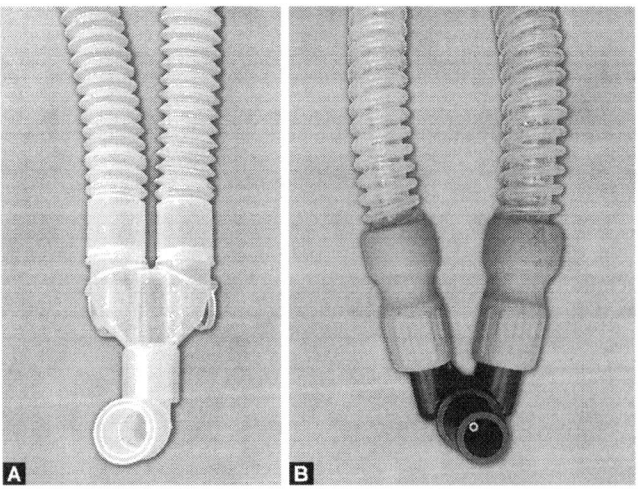

Figs. 9A and B: Corrugated tubing with Y-piece. (A) Plastic; (B) Silicone.

Anesthesia Circuits: Bain and Closed

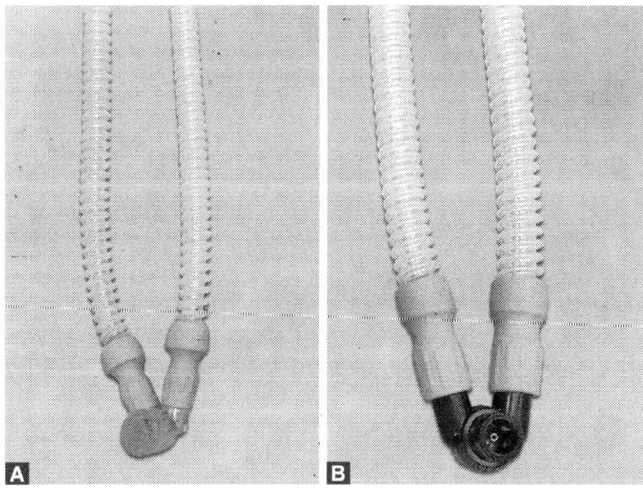

Figs. 10A and B: (A) Pediatric corrugated tubing with Y-piece; (B) Adult corrugated tubing with Y-piece.

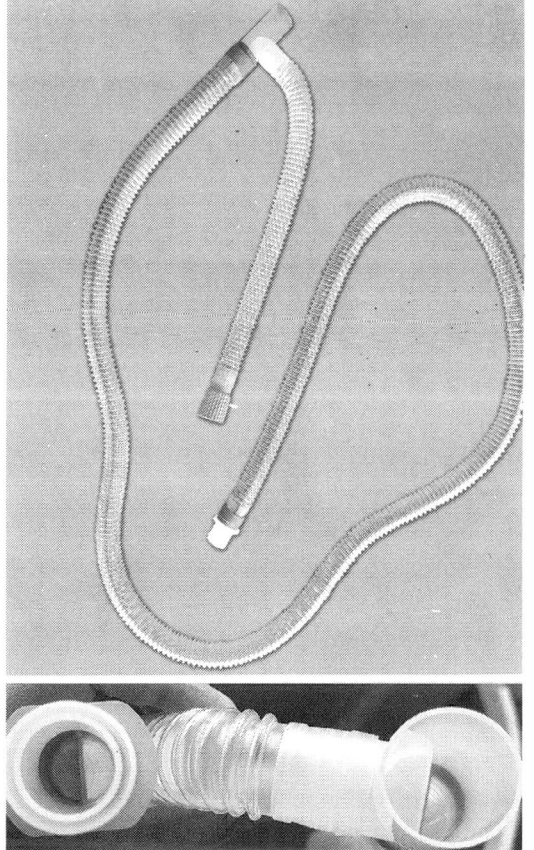

Fig. 11: Coaxial corrugated tubing (side-to-side type). Note that, a single tubing is divided into two by a septum for inspiratory and expiratory gases. There are two ports for the machine end.

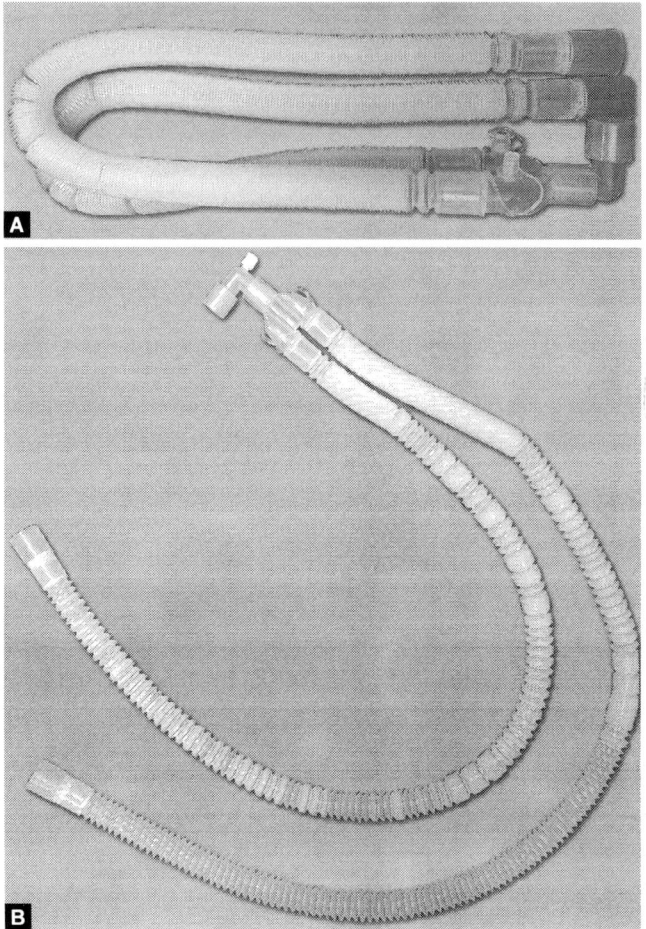

Figs. 12A and B: Concertina type corrugated tubing. Its length can be contracted (A) or expanded (B) as per requirement.

common site for a leaking circuit. The dead space of the circuit extends from the Y-piece to the patient.

Unidirectional Valves

A circle system consists of two unidirectional valves; one inspiratory (opens with inspiration and closes with expiration) and one expiratory (opens with expiration and closes with inspiration). Visible markings or words indicating inspiratory or expiratory connections are mandatory as per safety standards **(Fig. 13)**. Most commonly used valves have disk on knife-shaped edges that are encased in a clear dome-shaped structure for easy visualization of the disk. The disk is made up of hydrophobic plastic so that it does not stick owing to moisture content of the gases. The valves have low resistance and high competence which implies that they open with minimal pressure ($<0.3 \, cmH_2O$) and close rapidly and completely to prevent any backflow.

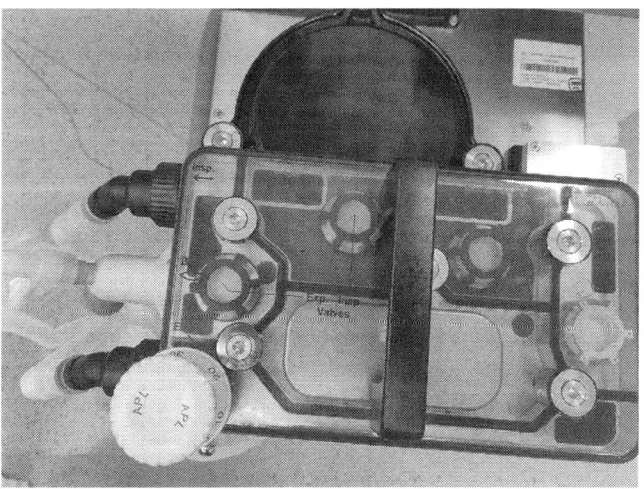

Fig. 13: Top view of a circle system assembly showing markings for inspiratory and expiratory unidirectional valves.

Fresh Gas Inlet

It is connected to the common gas outlet of the anesthesia machine by a flexible tube. On most of the modern anesthesia workstation, there is a direct connection between machine's gas outlet and anesthesia circuit and the fresh gas inlet is not visible to the operator. For achieving better efficiency, the best site for fresh gas inlet is between CO_2 absorber and inspiratory unidirectional valve. The problems with the alternative positions are discussed later.

Reservoir Bag

Reservoir bag, also known as breathing bag or counter lung, contains oxygen and anesthetic gases for inspiration. This is important since the maximum FGF on anesthesia machines might not provide enough for a patient's peak inspiratory gas flow requirements during spontaneous breathing. The ideal bag volume should be more than the patient's inspiratory capacity so that bag is not emptied with maximal inspiratory effort. It is available in volumes of 500 mL to 3 L **(Fig. 14)**. With gradual distension of the bag, the pressure peaks at around 50–70 cmH_2O with a fall in pressure observed with further distension of the bag. It can also be used for assessing the spontaneous ventilation. While the presence of spontaneous breaths can be ascertained with experience, the visual tidal volume estimation is frequently not accurate and depends on the FGF rate. Lower the rate, better the excursion of the bag since patient is inhaling from the bag. Conversely, with higher FGF rate, excursion is less since patient is breathing from the fresh gas entering the system.

Adjustable Pressure Limiting Valve

These are also known as outflow, spill or pop off valves. The basic design of APL valve could be spring loaded disk type (Datex Ohmeda) or needle type

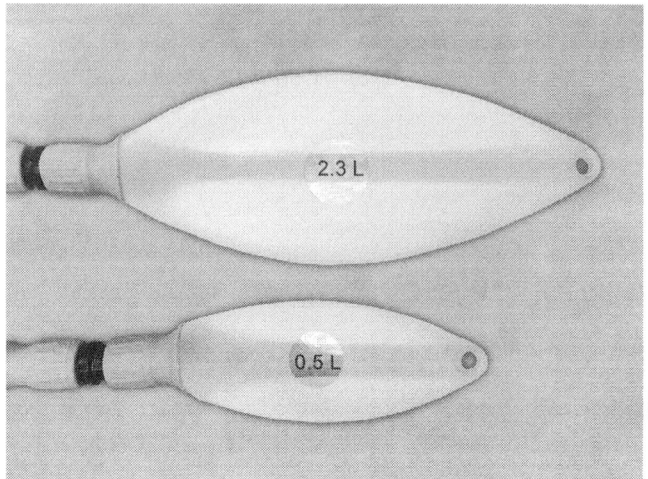

Fig. 14: Pediatric and adult sizes of reservoir bag.

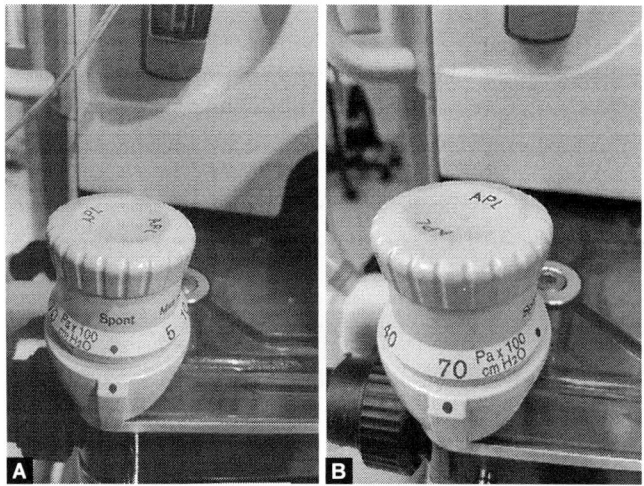

Figs. 15A and B: Fully open (A) and fully closed (B) adjustable pressure limiting (APL) valve.

(Draeger). For spontaneous respiration, valve should open and actuate at a pressure of 1 cm H_2O or even lesser. The valve is to be rotated clockwise to close it and more pressure is required to open it, which thus provides a PEEP. Just one or two turns should be able to turn the valve from open to closed position **(Figs. 15A and B)**. The exhaled gases enter the scavenging system at the APL valve location.

Advancement in technologies, need for enhanced efficiency in terms of reduced anesthetic gas usage and safety requirements have transformed a classic circle design to more complex ones **(Fig. 16)**. Apart from the basic components, some additional components are frequently part of a circle

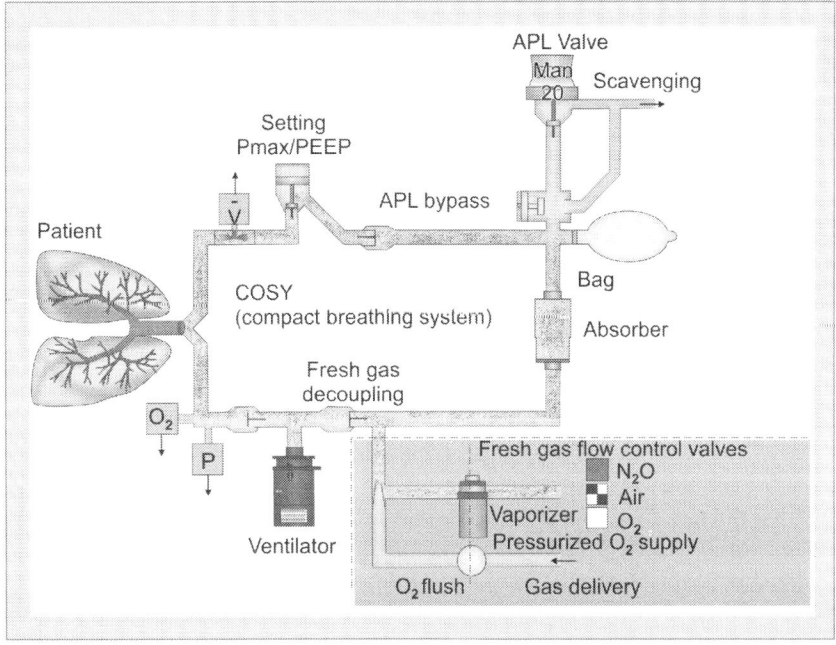

Fig. 16: Diagrammatic representation of a complex circle system.
Courtesy: Draeger India Pvt Ltd.

system in order to monitor the gas delivery, assist or control ventilation and to enhance the safety[20]:

- *Pressure gauge:* It measures the pressure in the circuit and could be analog or digital.
- *Pressure sensor for the circuit:* It is usually integrated into the absorber assembly.
- *Oxygen sensor:* It should be placed in the inspiratory limb of the circuit.
- *Capnometer:* It could be main stream or side stream and should be as close to the patient as possible.
- *Agent monitor:* It is side stream and should be close to the patient for reliable readings of both inspiratory and expiratory agent concentrations.
- *Ventilator:* In earlier systems, ventilators replaced the reservoir bag by attachment to bag mount, however, they are integrated into the system in current systems.
- *Bag/ventilator selector switch:* It is a convenient and rapid method to switch from spontaneous or manual ventilation to mechanical ventilation. The position of the switch is marked to indicate the mode. When the switch is in ventilator mode, both the APL valve and reservoir bag are bypassed from the circuit.
- *Positive and expiratory pressure valve:* It can be an integral part of the circle system or added as and when required. It should be in the expiratory limb of the circuit.

- *Humidification devices and filters*: Heated humidifiers are positioned on the inspiratory limb while the heat and moisture exchangers can be positioned between the Y-piece and patient interface. Filters are used to protect equipment from the patient or vice versa.

Flow Mechanics

Once the gas flows through the classic breathing system are understood, it is easy to determine the gas flows through other advanced systems. During inspiratory phase of spontaneous ventilation, the inspiratory unidirectional valve is open and the mixture of fresh and exhaled gas from the reservoir bag pass through the absorber and joins the fresh gas and flows toward the patient **(Fig. 17)**. During expiratory phase, the expiratory unidirectional valve is open and the exhaled gases pass into the reservoir bag until it is full. The excess gas is vented through the APL valve. Since the inspiratory unidirectional valve is closed, fresh gas entering the system flows retrograde toward the absorber, pushing the gas in the absorber toward the APL valve **(Fig. 18)**. If the FGFs are higher, some fresh gas might be vented through the APL valve.

During inspiratory phase of the manual or assisted ventilation, excess gases are vented through the partially opened APL valve. The inhaled mixture is a combination of fresh gas and previously exhaled gas from which the CO_2 has been removed **(Fig. 19)**. During expiratory phase, exhaled gases flow into the reservoir bag. FGFs retrograde through the absorber. The longer the exhalation time and the higher the FGF, the more likely it is that fresh gas will pass retrograde into the absorber **(Fig. 20)**.

Arrangement of Components

The various components are arranged in a particular configuration to achieve the following goals although not all are achievable with any particular arrangement:

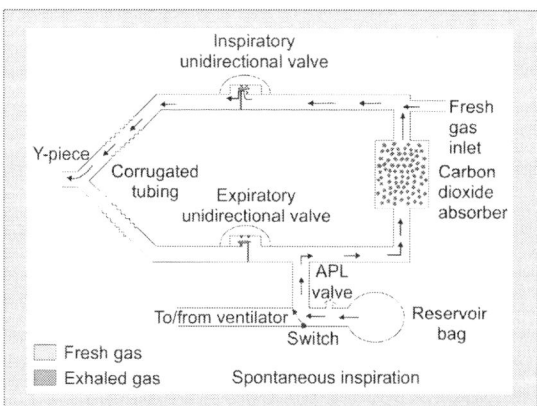

Fig. 17: Diagrammatic representation of flow mechanics of a circle system during inspiratory phase of spontaneous ventilation *(For color version see Plate 1)*.

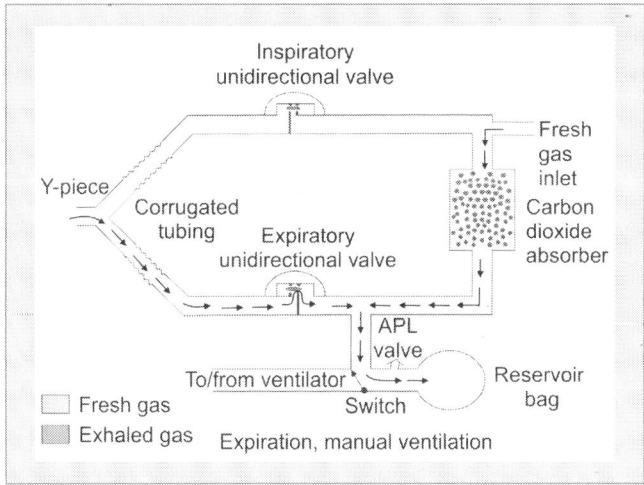

Fig. 18: Diagrammatic representation of flow mechanics of a circle system during expiratory phase of spontaneous ventilation *(For color version see Plate 2)*.

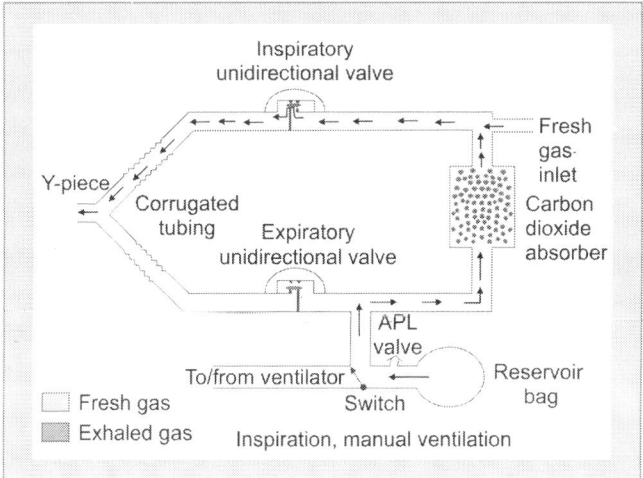

Fig. 19: Diagrammatic representation of flow mechanics of a circle system during inspiratory phase of manual ventilation *(For color version see Plate 2)*.

- Decrease the requirement and wastage of anesthetic gases and volatile agents.
- Decrease desiccation of CO_2 absorber.
- Increase humidification of inspired gases.
- Accurate readings from spirometer.
- Avoid increase in resistance during both spontaneous and controlled respiration.
- Fresh gas flow rate decoupling during mechanical ventilation.
- Low resistance with minimal dead space.
- Ease of design.

Anesthesia Circuits: Bain and Closed

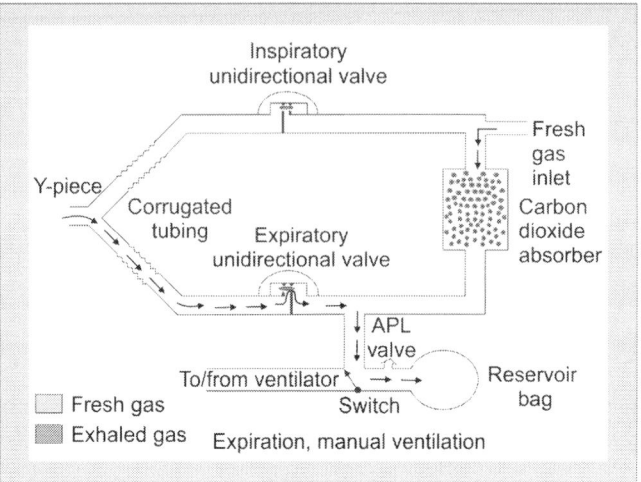

Fig. 20: Diagrammatic representation of flow mechanics of a circle system during expiratory phase of manual ventilation *(For color version see Plate 2).*

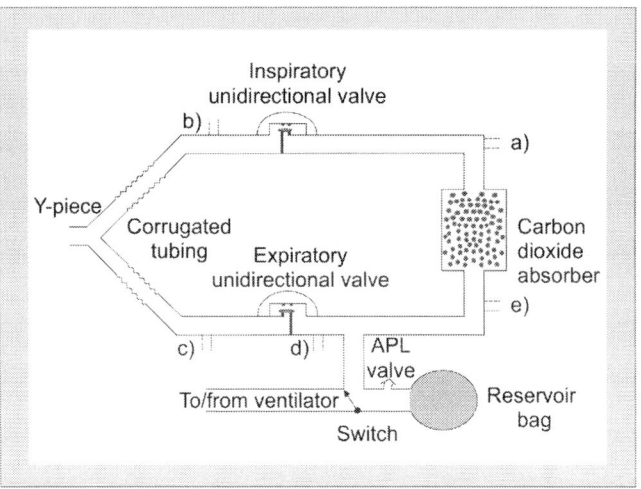

Fig. 21: Alternate arrangements of fresh gas inlet in a circle system. See text for details.

Numerous alternative arrangements of the various components are possible with each arrangement having its own advantages and disadvantages.[14] The manufacturing companies design the circuit based on the above-mentioned goals.

An example of alternative arrangement and its consequences about fresh gas inlet is described below with diagrammatic representation in **Figure 21**.

"a": Positioned between inspiratory unidirectional valve and CO_2 absorber
- Most commonly used.
- During expiration and expiratory pause, fresh gas passing through the CO_2 absorber may cause its desiccation or is vented out through the APL valve depending upon the flow rate.

"b": Positioned between inspiratory unidirectional valve and Y-piece
- No retrograde flow through the CO_2 absorber.
- Changes in fresh gas constituents reflect faster in inspired concentrations.
- During expiration, the fresh gases mix with exhaled gases without being delivered to the patient.
- Might lead to erroneous readings like end-tidal volumes and agent concentrations due to fresh gas mixing.

"c": Positioned between Y-piece and expiratory unidirectional valve
- Exhaled gases might be forced toward the patient leading CO_2 rebreathing.
- Increased venting of fresh gas through the APL valve.
- Better humidification of inspired gas but more desiccation of CO_2 absorber.

"d": Positioned between expiratory unidirectional valve and APL valve-bag assembly
- Increased venting of fresh gas through the APL valve.
- Better humidification of inspired gas but more desiccation of CO_2 absorber.
- Possibility of absorber dust being blown into inspiratory limb with the use of "oxygen flush".

"e": Positioned between CO_2 absorber and APL valve-bag assembly
- Increased venting of fresh gas through the APL valve.
- Better humidification of inspired gas but more desiccation of CO_2 absorber.
- Possibility of absorber dust being blown into inspiratory limb with the use of "oxygen flush".
- On similar pattern, if concept of flow through a classic circle system is understood, the pros and cons of alternate arrangements of other components such as APL valve, reservoir bag, etc., can be inferred.

Low-flow Anesthesia and Totally Closed System

The technique of low flow anesthesia involves FGF requirement less than the alveolar ventilation and there is rebreathing of at least 50% of the exhaled gases by the patient after absorption of CO_2 by the absorber.[21] However, in general terms, utilization of a FGF less than 2 L/min may qualify as low-flow anesthesia. The flows are further classified as metabolic flow (about 250 mL/min), minimal flow (250–500 mL/min), low flow (500–1000 mL/min) and medium flow (1–2 L/min). These are attained with the help of semi-closed circle system.

Recently totally closed systems (e.g., Draeger Zeus® Infinity® Empowered anesthesia device) have been introduced as high-end automatic systems.[22] With these systems, the anesthesiologist simply sets targets for each phase of the anesthesia process and lets the device calculate a reasonable and effective dose. This provides the most cost-effective anesthesia possible by keeping gas consumption to an absolute minimum. After initial few minutes of high FGFs, a totally closed system works to achieve a desired inspired oxygen concentration and end-tidal concentration/minimum alveolar concentration of volatile anesthetic agent. To balance with the uptake of the gases and anesthetic agents by the patient, the system allows FGFs only when required and volatile anesthetic agents are injected into the system as per the target values set by the operator. There is complete rebreathing of the exhaled gases leading to retention of heat, moisture and better economy. However, the operator has to have a thorough knowledge of the uptake and distribution of the agents along with continuous monitoring of oxygen in inspired gases and capnography.

Advantages and Disadvantages of Circle System

Advantages

- Helps conserve anesthetic gases, heat and moisture.
- Allows for low flow anesthesia and permits a stable agent concentration in inspired gases.
- Has less dead space.
- Decreases atmospheric pollution by recycling anesthetic gases. While the absorbent removes the CO_2, waste/excess gases is scavenged.

Disadvantages

- It is bulky, has complex design and multiple connections, prone to disconnections, misconnections, leaks and obstructions.
- Due to large volume of a circle system, any changes made in the dial settings of the vaporizer takes time to equilibrate and deliver, especially at low flows.[19]
- After being at low flow for some time, there is a potential for hypoxia due to dilution of fresh gases by exhaled gases. Oxygen sensor is mandatory to prevent this complication.
- Reaction of CO_2 absorbents with volatile anesthetic agents could be deleterious.

CONCLUSION

Bain circuit and circle system are commonly used circuits in anesthesia practice. While the Bain circuit relies on the FGF for the elimination of CO_2, the circle system achieves this by incorporating a CO_2 absorber. Each of the two has its own sets of advantages and disadvantages. These have peculiar flow mechanics during spontaneous and controlled ventilation and its thorough knowledge is mandatory for safe clinical application. Another important aspect is to utilize these circuits in a technique that is cost efficient with less wastage of anesthetic agents, decreased environmental pollution while addressing to the patient safety recommendations.

ACKNOWLEDGMENT

We acknowledge the contribution of Dr Nehal Singh (Postgraduate student, Department of Anesthesiology and Critical Care, AIIMS, Jodhpur) in drawing the diagrams for the chapter.

KEY POINTS

- Bain circuit is a modified Mapleson D circuit and has a coaxial arrangement.
- Exhaled gases in the outer tubing provide warmth to the gases in the inner tubing by counter current heat exchange mechanism.
- During spontaneous ventilation, the fresh gas flow should be 1.5–3 times the minute ventilation to prevent rebreathing while during controlled ventilation, fresh gas flow 1–2 times the minute ventilation is required. Hence, Bain circuit is more efficient for controlled ventilation.
- Preuse checks for Bain circuit is mandatory and can be done using occlusion test and Pethick test.
- A circle system has separate inspiratory and expiratory channels and rather than relying on the fresh gas flow for flushing out CO_2, it has a CO_2 absorber in the expiratory limb.
- The essential components of a circle system are Y-piece connector at the patient's end, two unidirectional valves (one inspiratory and one expiratory), fresh gas inlet, adjustable pressure limiting (APL) valve, reservoir bag, CO_2 absorber and corrugated tubing to connect the various components.
- A semi-closed circle system utilizes more fresh gas flow than the patient's requirements while a closed circle system utilizes fresh gas flow equal to patient's requirement.

REFERENCES

1. Dorsch JA, Dorsch SE. Mapleson breathing system. In: Understanding Anaesthesia Equipment, 5th edition. New Delhi: William and Wilkins; 2008. pp. 276-96.
2. Mapleson WW. Editorial I: Fifty years after–reflections on 'The elimination of rebreathing in various semi-closed anaesthetic systems'. Br J Anaesth. 2004;93(3):319-21.
3. Kaul TK, Mittal G. Mapleson's Breathing Systems. Indian J Anaesth. 2013;57(5): 507-15.
4. Sellers WF, Dykes S. Don't pre-oxygenate with a 3-metre Bain circuit. Anaesthesia. 2003;58(9):916.
5. Sweeting CJ, Thomas PW, Sanders DJ. The long bain breathing system: an investigation into the implications of remote ventilation. Anaesthesia. 2002; 57(12):1183-6.
6. Hartle A, Anderson E, Bythell V, Gemmell L, Jones H, McIvor D, et al. Checking anaesthetic equipment 2012: Association of anaesthetists of Great Britain and Ireland. Anaesthesia. 2012;67(6):660-8.
7. Singh I, Gupta M, Singh TK. Hypercapnia resulting from a faulty co-axial (Bain) circuit. Indian J Anaesth. 2011;55(4):402-4.
8. Jaideep C. Another circuit block: this time the actual Bain circuit. Indian J Anaesth. 2014;58(6):778-9.
9. Gooch C, Peutrell J. A faulty Bain circuit. Anaesthesia. 2004;59(6):618.
10. Ghai B, Makkar JK, Bhatia A. Hypercarbia and arrhythmias resulting from faulty Bain circuit: a report of two cases. Anesth Analg. 2006;102(6):1903-4.
11. Szypula KA, Ip JK, Bogod D, Yentis SM. Detection of inner tube defects in co-axial circle and Bain breathing systems: a comparison of occlusion and Pethick tests. Anaesthesia. 2008;63(10):1092-5.
12. Kataria S, Subramanyam R. Capnography to check the safety of Bain circuit. J Clin Monit Comput. 2010;24(1):71-2.

13. Al-Shaikh B, Stacey SG. Breathing systems. In: Essentials of Equipment in Anaesthesia, Critical Care, and Peri-operative Medicine, 5th edition. Edinburgh: Elsevier; 2019. pp. 53-65.
14. Dorsch JA, Dorsch SE. The circle system. In: Understanding Anaesthesia Equipment, 5th edition. New Delhi: William and Wilkins; 2008. pp. 297-375.
15. Kharasch ED, Powers KM, Artru AA. Comparison of Amsorb, sodalime, and Baralyme degradation of volatile anesthetics and formation of carbon monoxide and compound A in swine in vivo. Anesthesiology. 2002;96(1):173-82.
16. Knolle E, Linert W, Gilly H. The color change in CO_2 absorbents on drying: an in vitro study using moisture analysis. Anesth Analg. 2003;97(1):151-5.
17. Baum JA, Woehlck HJ. Interaction of inhalation anaesthetics with CO_2 absorbents. Best Pract Res Clin Anaesthesiol. 2003;17(1):63-76.
18. Castro BA, Freedman LA, Craig WL, Lynch C 3rd. Explosion within an anesthesia machine: Baralyme, high fresh gas flows and sevoflurane concentration. Anesthesiology. 2004;101(2):537-9.
19. Sobolev I, Sellers WF. Rate of change in gas concentrations in a charged circle system with absorber. Anaesthesia. 2001;56(4):380-1.
20. Davey AJ. Breathing systems and their components. In: Davey AJ, Diba A (Eds). Ward's Anaesthetic Equipment, 6th edition. Philadelphia: Elseiver; 2012. pp. 107-38.
21. Nunn G. Low-flow anaesthesia. Contin Educ Anaesth Crit Care Pain. 2008;8(1):1-4.
22. Parthasarathy S. The closed circuit and the low flow systems. Indian J Anaesth. 2013;57(5):516-24.

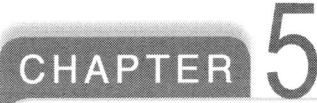

What's New in the Management of Vasodilatory Shock?

Shyam Madabhushi

INTRODUCTION

Vasodilatory shock or distributive shock is an entity characterized by low systemic vascular resistance (SVR), thereby lowering the arterial pressure. In a purist's sense, vasodilatory shock is not accompanied by cardiac dysfunction. However, the dominant etiology of vasodilatory shock being sepsis, cardiac dysfunction may accompany vasodilatory shock and contribute to end-organ dysfunction.

Management strategies for vasodilatory shock adopt one, or a combination, of the following:
- Vasopressors.
- Intravenous fluid administration.
- Adding adjuncts such as steroids.
- Extracorporeal cytokine removal strategies.
- Mechanical circulatory support.

The discussion in this article will center upon advances in each of these strategies.

VASOPRESSORS

Classical vasopressors for management of vasodilatory shock include catecholamines and the noncatecholamine vasopressin. Given the dominance of sepsis, noradrenaline is usually the first choice of vasopressor (also endorsed by international guidelines).[1,2] Vasopressin and adrenaline are used as additional vasopressors. Adrenaline continues to retain its position as the agent of choice for anaphylactic shock, while vasopressin is used in addition to norepinephrine in refractory shock.

Catecholamines unfortunately have their set of side effects, e.g., tachycardia, increased myocardial oxygen demand, lactic acidosis, reduced renal perfusion, etc. Tachyphylaxis due to internalization of receptors is an additional issue. Catecholamine-sparing strategies are therefore needed. We shall now examine some of these strategies.

Timing of Vasopressin

Vasopressin is frequently used as the second vasopressor of choice in addition to norepinephrine in vasodilatory shock and has been recommended by the Surviving Sepsis Guidelines.[1] It is relevant here that high doses of norepinephrine are independently associated with mortality, as demonstrated by Schmittinger et al.[3] Although, by no means a new agent in the management of septic shock, the timing and use of vasopressin is under review. The Vasopressin and Septic Shock Trial (VASST)[4] provides evidence that vasopressin when added early during an escalating dose of norepinephrine (NE < 15 µg/min) improves 28- and 90-day survival when compared to late addition to norepinephrine (NE >15 µg/min). This implies that adding vasopressin early in cases where the norepinephrine is being titrated upward may offer a survival benefit.

Avoidance of hemodynamic instability and minimizing the duration of hypotension is also important in preventing organ dysfunction. There is evidence to indicate that even relatively small periods of hypotension during surgery are associated with organ dysfunction in the postoperative period.[5] Hypotension during downward titration of vasopressors is common. Studies have explored the effect of preferentially titrating off vasopressin versus norepinephrine first in the intensive care unit (ICU). Wu and colleagues in their recently published meta-analysis[6] explored the incidence of hypotension between both strategies. The incidence of hypotension was significantly lower when norepinephrine was discontinued first than when vasopressin was discontinued first (OR 0.3, CI 0.1–0.86, p = 0.02). However, there was no difference in ICU mortality or ICU length of stay (LOS).

In summary, the evidence favors earlier addition of vasopressin to norepinephrine and titrating it off later than norepinephrine in vasodilatory shock.

Angiotensin II

Angiotensin II (AT-II) is a noncatecholamine, naturally occurring vasopressor synthesized in the liver as angiotensinogen. Angiotensinogen is sequentially acted upon by renin and angiotensin-converting enzyme (ACE) to generate AT-II, which then binds to type 1 receptors (AT_1R). The AT_1R is associated with multiple downstream signaling pathways resulting in vasoconstriction and sympathetic nervous system activation with its attendant effects on multiple systems, including secretion of aldosterone and vasopressin. AT-II was first synthesized in the 1950s.

The AT-II for the treatment of High-Output Shock III (ATHOS-3)[7] trial was a multicentric, randomized, placebo-controlled trial designed in collaboration with the La Jolla pharmaceutical company. Eligibility criteria included adults with vasodilatory shock that did not respond to at least 25 mL/kg of volume resuscitation over 24 hours and the administration of high-dose vasopressors, defined as norepinephrine or equivalent of >0.2 µg/kg/min. Patients were assigned to receive either AT-II (to a maximum of 200 ng/kg/min) or saline placebo in a 1:1 ratio. The primary end-point was mean atrial pressure (MAP) at hour 3 of infusion, with response defined as MAP > 75 mm Hg or an increase in MAP of at least 10 mm Hg from baseline without an increase in the dose of background vasopressors. Multiple secondary end-points were also assessed. A total of 163 patients received AT-II. 69.9% of patients in the AT-II arm attained the primary outcome compared to 23.4% in the placebo arm, which was statistically significant. At 48 hours, improvement in the cardiovascular sequential organ failure assessment (SOFA) scores in the AT-II arm, although, there was no overall difference in mortality. The data presented indicate that AT-II holds promise as a vasopressor for refractory shock.

INTRAVENOUS FLUID ADMINISTRATION AND TIMING OF VASOPRESSORS

The survival sepsis guidelines advocate administration of a large bolus of crystalloids (30 mL/kg BW) in patients with an elevated lactate or hypotension. It is germane here to mention that the guidelines are absolute about the quantity without adjusting for cardiac or renal disease. This one-size-fits-all strategy has been criticized.[8] In addition, dangers of fluid overload have been well-publicized. Alternative protocols for fluid administration assisted by lung ultrasound were developed in response to these complications [FALLS (Fluid Administration Limited by Lung Sonography) protocol].[9]

In response to this, it is being explored whether vasopressors must be started early, even preceding the completion of a fluid bolus. The CENSER trial[10] conducted in Thailand by Permpikul and colleagues-enrolled patients to early norepinephrine or standard treatment groups within 1 hour of diagnosing hypotension (MAP < 65 mm Hg) in patients with sepsis. The median time to initiation of norepinephrine in the early group was 1 hour 10 minutes compared to 2 hours 47 minutes in the standard treatment group. Shock control at 6 hours (primary outcome) was achieved in 76.1% patients in the Early group, compared to 48.4% ($p < 0.001$) in the control group. Although, there was no statistically significant difference in mortality, ICU or hospital LOS, the early norepinephrine group achieved target urine output, improvements in tissue perfusion and lactate clearance more often than in the usual therapy group. The incidence of pulmonary edema and new-onset arrhythmias were higher in the usual care group. This study demonstrated that an early vasopressor strategy might be more appropriate than the fluid-first strategy recommended by the surviving sepsis guidelines.

In a propensity-matched trial by Ospina-Tascon et al.,[11] patients were managed with an early vasopressor (<1 h) compared to a delayed vasopressor strategy. Patients in both the groups were 1:1 propensity matched for age, comorbidities, heart rate (HR), lactate, etc. Patients in the early vasopressor strategy received considerably less fluid when compared to the delayed vasopressor strategy. The overall mortality of the early vasopressor group was lower when compared to the delayed vasopressor group.

Both these studies demonstrate the potential of adopting an early vasopressor strategy, thereby limiting the potentially harmful effects of excess intravenous fluids.

ADJUNCTIVE THERAPIES: STEROIDS AND VITAMINS

Fludrocortisone

Fludrocortisone as an adjunct to hydrocortisone has emerged from the Activated Protein C and Corticosteroids for Human Septic Shock (APROCCHSS) trial.[12] The trial was a 2 × 2 factorial design randomized control trial designed to investigate the role of steroids and activated protein C. After the withdrawal of activated protein C, the trial progressed with two groups, with one group receiving hydrocortisone and fludrocortisone (50 µg tablet/day, delivered via a nasogastric tube, for 7 days), while the other group received the placebos for these two groups. Eligible patients had sepsis and hypotension needing vasopressor therapy.

The primary outcome was mortality. The experimental group had 43% mortality at D90 compared to 49% in the placebo group. Some caveats with the study design were the fact that the trial enrolled patients over a considerable period of time (2008–2015), required change in protocol (due to withdrawal of activated protein C), and that mortality is high when compared to other trials investigating the role of steroids (such as the ADRENAL trial).[13] However, this aspect of adding fludrocortisone probably merits further investigation.

Thiamine and Vitamin C

Thiamine and vitamin C both are essential vitamins not synthesized by the body but are required as cofactors for a variety of biological processes. Specifically, vitamin C is a potent antioxidant. The role of thiamine and vitamin C is specific to vasodilatory shock caused by sepsis, where reactive oxygen species (ROS) induce further inflammation by generating damage-associated molecular patterns (DAMPs). By acting as a free-radical scavenger, vitamin C administration seeks to address the pathogenesis of the cytokine storm in sepsis that leads to vasodilatory shock.[14] Studies have demonstrated ascorbic acid deficiency in sepsis.[15]

Thiamine is a precursor of thiamine pyrophosphate (TPP), which is an essential coenzyme involved in energy metabolism. It also has a role in suppressing the activation of NF-κB. Evidence suggests that the prevalence of thiamine deficiency in sepsis is between 20 and 70%.[16,17] Given this data, it is logical that thiamine and vitamin C supplementation would lead to benefit.

In a study published by Marik and colleagues,[18] a combination of thiamine (200 mg IV q12 hourly for 4 days, ascorbic acid 1.5 g IV q6 hourly for 4 days, hydrocortisone 50 mg IV q6 hourly for 7 days) demonstrated, among others, a reduction in duration of vasopressor infusions, need for renal replacement therapy (RRT) and mortality (8.5% in experimental group vs. 40.4% in standard care). However, methodological issues with the trial—retrospective in nature, propensity-matched design, etc. have prompted a large North American randomized controlled trial (RCT)—the VICTAS (Vitamin C, Thiamine and Steroids in Sepsis) trial.[19,20] The data and results of this trial will hopefully address the role of thiamine and vitamin C in sepsis.

Cytokine Removal Strategies

Cytokine adsorption and removal techniques have been used for almost two decades now. Candidates include the polymyxin B hemoperfusion system by the Toray Medical Corp., and the CytoSorb cartridge. The premise of all cytokine adsorption/removal techniques is attenuation of the inflammatory milieu, thereby reducing vasodilatation and improving shock.[21] Case reports for both these systems are aplenty. However, there is a paucity of well-designed clinical trials to address their utility. The EUPHRATES trial[22] was an important step in this direction. Adult patients with septic shock and an endotoxin assay activity of 0.60 or higher were enrolled in this multicentric North American trial. Patients in the intervention group received two sessions (of 90–120 minutes) of polymyxin B hemoperfusion plus standard therapy within 24 hours of enrollment, while the placebo group received sham hemoperfusion plus standard therapy. The primary outcome of interest was 28 days mortality among patients randomized with a multiple organ dysfunction score (MODS) > 9. The outcome, however, was of no difference in the primary outcome.

The newest member of this category of therapy is the oXiris membrane, manufactured by Baxter, which has an additional polyimine ethylene layer with greater endotoxin adsorption capacity. The efficacy of this filter system was studied in a crossover study involving patients with proven or suspected Gram-Negative sepsis and Kidney Disease: Improving Global Outcomes (KDIGO)—stage 3 acute kidney injury (AKI), with an endotoxin level of 0.03 EU/mL or greater.[23] Two treatment groups were created: initial continuous renal replacement therapy (CRRT) session (24 hours) with the oXiris filter followed by CRRT with a standard filter for the next 24 hours, or the reverse order in the second group. A significant reduction in the endotoxin levels, TNF-α concentrations, blood lactate levels and requirements of norepinephrine. The literature demonstrates that this is still an active modality, with newer materials being created to address the cytokine storm associated with sepsis.

MECHANICAL CIRCULATORY SUPPORT FOR DISTRIBUTIVE SHOCK

Extracorporeal membrane oxygenation (ECMO) for distributive shock is gaining traction. Postulated mechanisms conferring benefit include augmented oxygen delivery (mitigating tissue hypoxia) and improving tissue perfusion. In sepsis, myocardial dysfunction is an additional mechanism for shock. ECMO is eminently suited to provide circulatory support to this category of patients.

Randomized trials for ECMO for distributive shock are not available. A retrospective review by Falk and colleagues from a dedicated high-volume ECMO referral center in Sweden reported on ECMO outcomes in septic shock over a 5-year time period.[24] Inclusion criteria were adults with septic shock requiring a high level of vasopressors and inotropes [compounded into a score called the vasoactive inotropic score-(VIS)]. A total of 37 patients were included for analysis, of which 10 were commenced on venovenous (VV) ECMO and 27 on venoarterial (VA) ECMO. Hospital survival was higher in the VA ECMO group, both for LVF (94.4% vs. 50%) and non-LVF patients (66.7% vs. 62.5%). The data demonstrated that ECMO can be a viable option for patients with septic shock (with and without LVF).

CONCLUSION

Vasodilatory shock is a clinical entity of enormous significance. Newer strategies are aimed at either utilizing existing therapies for vasodilatory shock in novel ways or use of therapies that are totally new. Studies have focused on different strategies of using vasopressin and noradrenaline or altering the timing of crystalloids. Among newer therapies, the role of thiamine, vitamin C, fludrocortisone and AT-II are under investigation. Extracorporeal therapies include the use of cytokine removal cartridges and the use of ECMO.

KEY POINTS

- Therapies for distributive shock are evolving.
- A growing body of literature supports starting vasopressors early for septic shock reversal.
- Vasopressin may be added earlier to norepinephrine than later, and probably must be titrated off later than norepinephrine on resolution of shock.
- Angiotensin II is the newest vasopressor found to be effective in reversal of refractory shock.
- ECMO is being investigated for the management of vasodilatory shock. Data suggests a greater role for VA than VV ECMO.
- Extracorporeal cytokine removal strategies are theoretically attractive and are supported by case reports. Newer membranes such as oXiris® are being developed.
- The abundance of literature points to the grim reality that mortality and morbidity from distributive shock, especially sepsis, is still considerable and presents a formidable public health challenge.

REFERENCES

1. Rhodes A, Evans LE, Alhazzani W, Levy MM, Antonelli M, Ferrer R, et al. Surviving Sepsis Campaign: International Guidelines for Management of Sepsis and Septic Shock: 2016. Intensive Care Med. 2017;43(3):304-77.
2. Levy MM, Evans LE, Rhodes A. The Surviving Sepsis Campaign Bundle: 2018 update. Intensive Care Med. 2018;44(6):925-8.
3. Schmittinger CA, Torgersen C, Luckner G, Schröder DC, Lorenz I, Dünser MW. Adverse cardiac events during catecholamine vasopressor therapy: a prospective observational study. Intensive Care Med. 2012;38(6):950-8.
4. Russell JA, Walley KR, Singer J, Gordon AC, Hébert PC, Cooper DJ, et al. Vasopressin versus norepinephrine infusion in patients with septic shock. N Engl J Med. 2008;358(9):877-87.
5. Walsh M, Devereaux PJ, Garg AX, Kurz A, Turan A, Rodseth RN, et al. Relationship between intraoperative mean arterial pressure and clinical outcomes after noncardiac surgery: toward an empirical definition of hypotension. Anesthesiology. 2013;119(3):507-15.
6. Wu Z, Zhang S, Xu J, Xie J, Huang L, Huang Y, et al. Norepinephrine vs. vasopressin: which vasopressor should be discontinued first in septic shock? A meta-analysis. Shock. 2020;53(1):50-7.

7. Khanna A, English SW, Wang XS, Ham K, Tumlin J, Szerlip H, et al. Angiotensin II for the treatment of vasodilatory shock. N Engl J Med. 2017;377(5):419-30.
8. Marik PE, Byrne L, van Haren F. Fluid resuscitation in sepsis: the great 30 mL per kg hoax. J Thorac Dis. 2020;12(Suppl 1):S37-47.
9. Lichtenstein D. FALLS-protocol: lung ultrasound in hemodynamic assessment of shock. Heart Lung Vessel. 2013;5(3):142-7.
10. Permpikul C, Tongyoo S, Viarasilpa T, Trainarongsakul T, Chakorn T, Udompanturak Set. Early Use of Norepinephrine in Septic Shock Resuscitation (CENSER). A Randomized Trial. Am J Respir Crit Care Med. 2019;199(9):1097-105.
11. Ospina-Tascón GA, Hernandez G, Alvarez I, Calderón-Tapia LE, Manzano-Nunez R, Sánchez-Ortiz AI, et al. Effects of very early start of norepinephrine in patients with septic shock: a propensity score-based analysis. Crit Care. 2020;24(1):52.
12. Annane D, Renault A, Brun-Buisson C, Megarbane B, Quenot JP, Siami S, et al. Hydrocortisone plus fludrocortisone for adults with septic shock. N Engl J Med. 2018;378(9):809-18.
13. Venkatesh B, Finfer S, Cohen J, Rajbhandari D, Arabi Y, Bellomo R, et al. Adjunctive glucocorticoid therapy in patients with septic shock. N Engl J Med. 2018;378(9):797-808.
14. Marik PE. Hydrocortisone, ascorbic acid and thiamine (HAT therapy) for the treatment of sepsis. Focus on ascorbic acid. Nutrients. 2018;10(11):1762.
15. Carr AC, Rosengrave PC, Bayer S, Chambers S, Mehrtens J, Shaw GM. Hypovitaminosis C and vitamin C deficiency in critically ill patients despite recommended enteral and parenteral intakes. Crit Care. 2017;21(1):300.
16. Cruickshank AM, Telfer AB, Shenkin A. Thiamine deficiency in the critically ill. Intensive Care Med. 1988;14(4):384-7.
17. Donnino MW, Carney E, Cocchi MN, Barbash I, Chase M, Joyce N, et al. Thiamine deficiency in critically ill patients with sepsis. J Crit Care. 2010;25(4):576-81.
18. Marik PE, Khangoora V, Rivera R, Hooper MH, Catravas J. Hydrocortisone, vitamin C, and thiamine for the treatment of severe sepsis and septic shock: a retrospective before-after study. Chest. 2017;151(6):1229-38.
19. Hager DN, Hooper MH, Bernard GR, Busse LW, Ely EW, Fowler AA, et al. The Vitamin C, Thiamine and Steroids in Sepsis (VICTAS) protocol: a prospective, multi-center, double-blind, adaptive sample size, randomized, placebo-controlled, clinical trial. Trials. 2019;20(1):197.
20. Lindsell CJ, McGlothlin A, Nwosu S, Rice TW, Hall A, Bernard GR, et al. Update to the Vitamin C, Thiamine and Steroids in Sepsis (VICTAS) protocol: statistical analysis plan for a prospective, multicenter, double-blind, adaptive sample size, randomized, placebo-controlled, clinical trial. Trials. 2019;20(1):670.
21. Honore PM, Hoste E, Molnár Z, Jacobs R, Joannes-Boyau O, Malbrain MLNG, et al. Cytokine removal in human septic shock: where are we and where are we going?. Ann Intensive Care. 2019;9(1):56.
22. Dellinger RP, Bagshaw SM, Antonelli M, Foster DM, Klein DJ, Marshall JC, et al. Effect of Targeted Polymyxin B Hemoperfusion on 28-day Mortality in Patients with Septic Shock and Elevated Endotoxin Level: The EUPHRATES Randomized Clinical Trial. JAMA. 2018;320(14):1455-63.
23. Broman ME, Hansson F, Vincent JL, Bodelsson M. Endotoxin and cytokine reducing properties of the oXiris membrane in patients with septic shock: a randomized crossover double-blind study. PLoS One. 2019;14(8):e0220444.
24. Falk L, Hultman J, Broman LM. Extracorporeal membrane oxygenation for septic shock. Crit Care Med. 2019;47(8):1097-105.

CHAPTER 6

Controversies and Gray Zones in Regional Anesthesia

Raj Tobin

INTRODUCTION

Regional anesthesia (RA) has always been an integral part of anesthesia. There has been a notable resurgence since, the introduction of sonography guidance. The technique has moved several notches up in terms of safety and success rate. No longer are we dependent on anatomical landmarks or struggling blindly for the most appropriate response to nerve stimulation but sonography still requires considerable evidence to get anointed as the savior of all complications in RA. Despite this resurgence of RA in the day to day practice of anesthesia, there remain some gray areas and controversies. But as William Hazlitt, one of the greatest critics of English language has said "when a thing ceases to be a subject of controversy, it ceases to be a subject of interest".

Majority of these controversies are about neuraxial anesthesia as therein lie the dreaded complication of spinal hematoma and neurological deficits. But it is equally worrying if a patient develops new onset paresthesia or deficit after a peripheral nerve block. This is where an anesthetist has to perform a very rigorous "risk benefit analysis" as the practice of medicine is based on the foundation of "First Do No Harm".

Some of the controversies like RA and anticoagulants (old or new) and antiplatelets, RA in immunosuppressed and infected patients, prevention and management of infectious complications of neuraxial and patients with preexisting neurological disease have been covered under very robust practice advisories by the American Society of Regional Anesthesia (ASRA) and the European Society of Regional Anesthesia (ESRA) and Pain Medicine.

In this chapter, we shall be touching upon areas which are still contested despite practice advisories as also RA in diabetics as we have a huge burden of this disease in our country. So, in that spirit, let us look at some areas in the practice of RA which continue to challenge us and make us pause and think twice when we choose regional over general anesthesia.

NEURAXIAL ANESTHESIA IN THROMBOCYTOPATHY AND THROMBOCYTOPENIA

Anesthesiologist's world over tread very cautiously when neuraxial anesthesia is contemplated in a patient with low platelet counts. Invariably, it is dropped in favor of general anesthesia or there is insistence on platelet transfusions followed by test for platelet count or platelet function before neuraxial is given. The American College of Obstetrics and Gynecology recommends platelet count of 75–80 × 10^9/L as the acceptable level for neuraxial technique in parturient[1] and there is a very detailed guideline by ASRA[2] about the time gap between the antiplatelet medication and neuraxial techniques. However, there is a risk of spinal hematoma even in patients with normal baseline hemostatic parameters, and a Swedish study has penned the risk as 8:260,000 (risk 0.00003; 95% CI 0.00001–0.00006).[3] What contributes to these cases is that one checks the platelet count but not the quality of platelets. Thromboelastography is not done routinely before every neuraxial, and there is an invisible dagger hanging over us every time we provide neuraxial anesthesia to a patient. Data from oncology offers us another perspective and is very heartening. In oncology many patients of leukemia and lymphoma are under the care of oncologists for several years requiring multiple transfusions of blood products. This increases the risk of alloimmunization so there is a wariness and reluctance for transfusion of blood products in oncology. The threshold for platelet count before a neuraxial procedure is considerably lower for oncologists. A threshold of 50 × 10^9/L for adults has been suggested by the American Association of Blood Banks.[4] After considering the safety record of neuraxial procedures in oncology patients with low platelets and acknowledging the issues associated with exposure to blood products in leukemia and lymphoma, Pediatric Oncology Group of Ontario, recommends a threshold of 20 × 10 /L for children.[5] But the fear of dreaded spinal hematoma will continue to deter the practice of neuraxial anesthesia till considerable data emerges about neuraxial anesthesia in patients with low platelets. This will not be coming for a long time as worldwide there is a very strong inhibition towards this.

NEURAXIAL ANESTHESIA IN PATIENTS UNDER GENERAL ANESTHESIA/DEEP SEDATION

Today a majority of neuraxial and peripheral nerve blocks are performed in awake patients. The presumption is that an "awake patient" will respond to an intraneural placement and also, verbalize the typical symptoms of local anesthetic systemic toxicity (LAST). Medical literature suggests that merely one-third of needle-to-nerve contacts are actually noticed by the individuals.[6] Secondly, if LAST occurs when patient is under general anesthesia then only mild symptoms of LAST like metallic taste, excitation or circumoral numbness will be missed, but on the other hand, patient will be better prepared for cardiopulmonary resuscitation with a secured airway and with low oxygen consumption by tissues.[7] Despite these opinions, ASRA 2015 practice advisory[8] has held on to its 2008 advisory that neuraxial procedures and interventional pain procedures done under deep sedation or under general anesthesia takes away the safety of patient reporting warning signs. The advisory suggests appropriate risk benefit analysis in patients with certain specific conditions like developmental delay or multiple bone trauma who may not permit an awake neuraxial. In pediatric population, the benefit of a cooperative, immobile infant or child outweighs the risk of performing neuraxial RA under general anesthesia or deep sedation. This has been reiterated by the joint ASRA/ESRA practice advisory on controversial topics in pediatric population too.[9]

EPIDURAL BLOOD PATCH

Epidural blood patch is the recommended treatment for postdural puncture headache if other methods of management fail. Various authors have advocated the use as a single or repeat procedure with acceptable success rates[10-14] and it has been in practice for more than 50 years. But neurological complications and subdural hematoma have been reported after this procedure in parturient.[15,16] In an article published in 2019, in RA and pain medicine, the author has rightly expressed that an epidural blood patch is an iatrogenic epidural hematoma and so the potential is always there for it to become symptomatic. The author further suggests that along with pressure effect of blood volume which has been injected, the reduced compliance of the epidural space or a combination of both can contribute to neurological symptoms. The article is focused mostly on use of epidural blood patch for management of spontaneous intracranial hypotension.[17] Considering the increase in the number of elderly parturient, some of the recommendations of the author can be extrapolated to parturient and other postoperative patients. These involve eliciting history of back pain, spinal interventions, review of images, informed consent documenting the risks such as backpain, radiculopathy, arachnoiditis, marking the site of leak, and a very vigilant postprocedure care.

EPIDURAL TEST DOSE

The main aim of using an epidural test dose is to detect inadvertently placed intravascular, intrathecal or subdural epidural needle or catheter, so that a major mishap (high spinal block if in subarachnoid space, LAST if intravascular) may be avoided.

Moore and Batra proposed 45 mg of lidocaine with 15 μg of epinephrine as the ideal epidural test dose.[18] There have been strong advocates in anesthesia fraternity both for and against its use. However, its utility has been debated maximally in labor epidurals and pediatric patients.

In patients in labor, serious adverse events like severe hypotension, total spinal anesthesia with respiratory paralysis and fetal bradycardia have been reported with the use of a test dose of local anesthetic. Physiological changes of pregnancy like an increase in stroke volume as well as heart rate and varying heart rates and tachycardia during labor due to uterine contraction and/or anxiety render a test dose with 15 μg of epinephrine very difficult to decipher. Additionally, if a functioning epidural analgesia has to be converted to epidural

TABLE 1: Recommendations regarding epidural test dose in pediatric patients[9]	
Recommendations	Level of evidence
Test dose should be discretionary. *Regarding epinephrine*: Partially administered dose of epinephrine or general anesthesia can blunt the response and give a false negative result which will be falsely reassuring *Regarding LA*: LA should be injected slowly in small aliquots (0.1–0.2 mL/kg) and with intermittent aspiration. ECG should be monitored continuously while injecting	Case reports (B4)
After the injection of a test dose of LA with epinephrine, any change in T wave or in heart rate within 30–90 seconds of the injection of test dose should be interpreted as an accidental IV injection unless proved otherwise	Noncomparative observational studies with descriptive statistics (B3)
Data is lacking in pediatric regional anesthesia regarding the use of sonography, fluoroscopy to visualize accidental intravascular needle placement	Expert opinion

(LA: local anesthesia; ECG: electrocardiogram; IV: intravenous)

anesthesia then there is always a niggling fear of migration of catheter into the dural space. In a survey conducted across 209 maternity units in the United Kingdom, 34% administered a proper test dose while others injected the therapeutic dose slowly while monitoring the patient continuously.[19] There are no established guidelines today for patients in labor. In a review published in 2019, authors have suggested that in present day practice of low dose, low concentration epidurals, just the analgesic dose or a fraction of it may be considered as an appropriate test dose.[20]

As regards to test dose before epidurals in pediatric, the joint ASRA-ESRA recommendations have been summarized in **Table 1**.

REGIONAL ANESTHESIA AND ACUTE COMPARTMENT SYNDROME

Acute compartment syndrome (ACS) is a feared but uncommon orthopedic emergency. The traditionally believed symptom of pain, paresis and paresthesia in a patient is not reliable for diagnosis.

Intracompartment pressure monitoring is considered the "gold standard" for the diagnosis of ACS and the normal intracompartment pressure is below 10–12 mm Hg.[21] Pain is invariably present when the pressure exceeds 20 mm and a pressure of over 30 mm is an indication for decompressive fasciotomy.[22-24] Identified risk factors for ACS are listed in **Table 2**.

The treatment of ACS is urgent fasciotomy and the best results without neurologic consequences are achieved when fasciotomy is performed as

TABLE 2: Risk factors for acute compartment syndrome (ACS)[22,25,26]

Patient factors	- Male gender - Age <35 years - Anticoagulation therapy - Hemophilia - Hypothyroidism - Exercise-related - Snake bites
Surgical factors	- Intramedullary nailing - Open fracture - High energy and penetrating trauma - Vascular injuries - Tourniquet use - Complications of intravenous, intraosseous infusions - Revascularization - Casts and circular dressings - Pulsatile irrigation

soon as possible after diagnosis. The guidelines issued by BOAST 2014 (British Orthopaedic Association Standard for Trauma 2014) documents ACS as a surgical emergency and recommends that the surgery should occur within an hour of diagnosis.[27] In patients with etiology of revascularization following acute limb ischemia, delayed fasciotomy increased the likelihood of major amputation within 30 days.[28]

The apprehension that RA may mask the pain caused by ACS has been a reason of discord between orthopedic surgeons and anesthesiologists regarding the practice of RA. However, this masking can occur with any other mode of pain management too. "An indictment is not a conviction" as quoted by Howard Coble and several systemic reviews done toward this have not found any convincing evidence that RA delays the diagnosis of ACS.[26,29]

The focus on children has always been more regarding ACS as they are a vulnerable group unable to express the pain and distress or distinguish between the surgical and ischemic pain. Another vulnerable group being patients with altered sensorium. While the jury is still out there, a review article on ESRA and ASRA practice advisory for pediatric patients mentions in its key points that no current evidence supports the thinking that RA increases the incidence of ACS in children. Several recommendations mentioned in the key points include a detailed informed consent, use of lower concentration of local anesthetics in both single shot and continuous peripheral catheters, restriction of volume and concentration in sciatic nerve catheters, cautious use of adjuvants, follow up by "Acute Pain Services" in high-risk group and institution of compartment pressure monitoring whenever there is a suspicion of ACS.[30]

ADJUVANTS IN NERVE BLOCKS

The intent in adding an adjuvant to a regional block is to prolong the sensory and/or motor block by acting synergistically with local anesthetics thereby reducing the dose and hence the toxicity of the local anesthetics particularly in infusions. A wide range of adjuvants have been tried in the last three decade including fentanyl, midazolam, neostigmine, clonidine, dexamethasone, dexmedetomidine, buprenorphine, ketamine, tramadol, magnesium, etc. Even neuromuscular blocking drugs have been used in peribulbar blocks and intravenous RA but with a major concern of toxicity and prolonged motor blockade, they are not used at present time. Most of these drugs do not have Food and Drug Administration (FDA) approval to be used as an adjuvant in neuraxial block except clonidine and preservative free morphine.

Food and Drug Administration Act does not limit the use of these drugs by physicians for off label use if the physician considers it appropriate and rational. Serendipitous observations and therapeutic innovations confirmed by well planned and executed investigations help in discovering new uses of existing drugs.[31] But literature shows that off label use does not guarantee safety as seen with high dose long-term opioids resulting in intrathecal granulomas[32] and grave neurological, respiratory and hemodynamic effects of intrathecal tramadol.[33,34] Special mention of use of an off-label drug is not required in the informed consent if there is strong scientific literature and mention in textbooks, however drugs such as adenosine, calcitonin, and cannabinoid receptor agonists will require robust support with appropriate documentation and consents mentioning investigational new drug applications.[35]

In India, opioids are used widely in combination with local anesthetics for neuraxial blocks and the most commonly used opioids are morphine and fentanyl. However, unlike preservative free morphine, fentanyl has not been approved by FDA for intrathecal use. Side-effect of nausea, sedation and pruritus with opioids continue to be worrisome whether used in neuraxial block or peripheral nerve block.

The analgesic effect of neuraxial midazolam is caused by the spinal suppression of sensory functions and its antinociceptive effect mediated by GABAergic and opioid receptor mechanisms. In a study conducted on 1100 patients, authors concluded that neuraxial midazolam is not associated with any bladder bowel symptoms or adverse neurological symptoms[36] but midazolam is currently not recommended for peripheral nerve block.[37]

Clonidine has approval of FDA for use in epidural space and this approval has been assumed to be acceptable for use of dexmedetomidine as both are α2 adrenergic receptor agonist. The most commonly used adjuvants in peripheral nerve block today are dexmedetomidine, clonidine and dexamethasone.

In a review published in 2016, authors concluded that preclinical and clinical studies have demonstrated the efficacy of dexmedetomidine without neurotoxicity and that 100 µg may be the ideal dose for peripheral nerve block. In key points they further mentioned that it acts not centrally or by causing vasoconstriction but at the nerve level by causing hyperpolarization. Caution is warranted in patients with bradycardia.[38]

A multicenter randomized trial comparing 2, 5 and 8 mg of perineural dexamethasone for ultrasound guided infraclavicular block found all three dosages to be equivalent in terms of sensorimotor and analgesic durations.[39] In another randomized prospective study, 120 patients undergoing upper limb surgery with ultrasound-guided infraclavicular block (using 35 mL of lidocaine 1% and bupivacaine 0.25% with epinephrine 5 μg/mL) were given either perineural dexamethasone (5 mg) or dexmedetomidine (100 μg) and the patients in dexamethasone group had longer duration of analgesia and sensorimotor block and a decreased level of sedation.[40] There have been attempts to combine two adjuvants for a better outcome. In a randomized prospective study done with 80 patients undergoing thoracoscopic pneumonectomy, dexmedetomidine (1 μg/kg) and dexamethasone (10 mg) were added to 0.5% ropivacaine for intercostal nerve block. The patients were found to have prolonged analgesia, reduced postoperative fentanyl requirement with no notable adverse effects.[41]

Combined ASRA/ESRA recommendations were published in 2018 for pediatric population regarding the use of adjuvants.[42] Along with the level of evidence based on which these recommendations were made, the recommendations have been summarized in **Table 3**.

TABLE 3: American Society of Regional Anesthesia/European Society of Regional Anesthesia and Pain Therapy (ASRA/ESRA) recommendations for use of adjuvants in regional anesthesia

Adjuvant	Type of regional anesthesia	Level of evidence
Clonidine (1–2 μg/kg) and morphine (10–30 μg/kg). Minimal possible dose as toxicity data are limited	Intrathecally	Several randomized controlled trials but not sufficient to conduct meta-analysis (A2)
Ketamine	Neuraxial-but not recommended for intrathecal use because of the potential to cause neuronal apoptosis Epidural dose used must be minimally necessary	Based on noncomparative studies with descriptive statistics (B3)
Dexamethasone	Not recommended for neuraxial	Based on observational studies with associative statistics (B2)
Dexmedetomidine	Can be used in neuraxial and peripheral nerve blocks but minimally necessary dose should be used	Neuraxial recommendation is based on several randomized controlled trials but not sufficient to conduct meta-analysis (A2) and recommendations on peripheral nerve blocks is based on sufficient number of randomized controlled trials to conduct a meta-analysis (A1)
Fentanyl, Sufentanil (Synthetic opioids)	No benefit in caudal epidurals	Based on several randomized controlled trials but not sufficient to conduct meta-analysis (A2)

REGIONAL ANESTHESIA AND PERIPHERAL NERVE INJURY

Perioperative nerve injuries have multifactorial cause and may result due to improper positioning, surgical insult, tourniquet, underlying patient factor, preexisting nerve injury or can be a combination of these. Many a times the preexisting nerve injuries/deficits due to diabetes, chemotherapy, etc., are missed if special focus is not given to elicit the history preoperatively. When detected after the surgery, invariably the suspicion falls first on the regional technique. This happens despite evidence in medical literature against this tendency to hold regional block as the culprit. In a study conducted in Veterans Affairs inpatient surgical population with the hypothesis that peripheral nerve blocks do not increase peripheral nerve injury, the incidence of new peripheral nerve injury (PNI) was found to be 1.2% (114/9,558 cases). Out of 3,380 patients who were given nerve blocks, 30 experienced new peripheral nerve injury (0.9%) compared with 84 of 6,178 patients who were not given any block (1.4%; p = 0.053). A very interesting fact in this study is that only 8 cases out of 30 were considered to be potentially related to the block. The authors concluded that peripheral nerve block is not an independent risk factor for PNI but added that younger and healthier patients and those undergoing minimally invasive abdominal or urological procedures are at a higher risk.[43]

In a prospective audit of more than 7000 peripheral nerve and plexus blocks for neurologic and other complications, the results showed that incidence of serious complications after peripheral nerve blockade is uncommon. The audit further added that the neurologic symptoms/signs in the postoperative period were in all probability unrelated to nerve blockade.[44] In the same year in a retrospective analysis of 380,680 cases during a 10 year period performed in the University of Michigan, peripheral nerve block was not found to be an independent risk factor for PNI.[45] Three studies published in RA and pain medicine concluded that the choice of RA does not increase the risk of PNI in total knee replacement,[46] total hip replacement[47] and total shoulder replacement.[48]

Considering the potential of a nerve injury to impact the quality of life and precipitate litigations, the Second ASRA Practice Advisory on Neurologic Complications associated with RA and Pain Medicine, has put forth extensive evidence-based practice advisory regarding patient factor, choice of anesthetic, intraoperative blood pressure, surgical factors, diagnosis and management of perioperative neuraxial/PNI.[49]

REGIONAL ANESTHESIA AND REBOUND PAIN

The entire foundation of RA is based on its ability to give succor to patients after a painful surgery, but "Rebound Pain" continues to challenge the perioperative pain management teams especially in ambulatory day care patients.[50] Suggested definition of "Rebound Pain " is the difference in pain score reported by a patient when the block is effective versus when the block has resolved.[51] A simple explanation one tends to believe is that once the effect of the peripheral block wears off, patients begin to experience the nociceptive

> **BOX 1:** Suggested recommendations for preventing rebound pain.[51-53,55]
> - Focus on patient education to prevent or mitigate the incidence of rebound pain. Surgeons must take a lead in the preoperative period in counseling the patient. In order to reduce anxiety and catastrophizing thoughts, patients should be advised to compare the intensity of RP to their preoperative pain and not to the completely pain free status when the block was working
> - Patients should be encouraged to take oral multimodal analgesics on a regular schedule and not wait for the offset of PNB
> - Peripheral nerve blocks must be performed safely
>
> (RP: rebound pain; PNB: peripheral nerve block)

stimuli of the surgical trauma. It has been variously described as burning, and sometimes as dull aching pain,[51] pain can be at rest or may be evoked pain, lasts for about 2 hours and does not respond to intravenous opioids.[52,53] The pathophysiology is still not understood completely. Most commonly seen in younger age (<60 years), female gender and patients with heightened pain susceptibility depending on individual psychophysical factors. Various studies have been done on the impact of single shot versus continuous peripheral nerve blocks,[54] effect of adjuvants and some such but none is conclusive. Two well-known inflammatory conditions, diabetes and obesity, did not increase the incidence of rebound pain.[52] Some suggestions to prevent rebound pain are listed in **Box 1**.

REGIONAL ANESTHESIA IN DIABETICS

In diabetes country profiles 2016, WHO has stated the burden of diabetes mellitus as 7.8% of the total population in India which is huge proportion of our population. Hence, many of them with this comorbidity will present for surgery and may require RA. Diabetics suffer from various types of neuropathy but the most common is the distal symmetrical sensorimotor polyneuropathy.

Susceptibility to injury is more in diabetic nerves because of chronic ischemic hypoxia. Along with this there is decreased perineural blood flow so the nerves get exposed to a larger concentration of local anesthetics which can result in injury.[56] In a study conducted during sonography guided popliteal sciatic nerve block 15 out of 55 diabetic patients required more than 0.5 mA to elicit a motor response and 4 out of 15 had intraneural placement. The rest of the 11 patients required currents ≥2 mA despite needle-nerve contact but in the nondiabetic group of 52 patients, there were three such patients (1 intraneural, 2 with ≥2 mA).[57] Hence, keeping the current low can result in intraneural injection and keeping the current high can cause failed block if only a nerve stimulator is used. In this study, the advantage offered by sonography was that the needle tip could be visualized.

It has been postulated that since the neuropathic nerves are more sensitive to local anesthetics, the duration of block will be prolonged. In an animal study, attenuation of neuropathy as seen with long-term glucose control, normalized the duration of block but an acute control of hyperglycemia had no impact on the duration of block.[58] No practice advisory has so far stated that RA should

> **BOX 2:** Suggestions for safe practice of regional anesthesia in patients with diabetes/diabetic neuropathy.[59-61]
> - Proper preoperative evaluation eliciting history suggestive of autonomic or peripheral neuropathy. Mapping of sensory motor deficits in the preoperative charts and appropriate informed consent explaining the risks and benefits
> - Due to increased risk of infection in perineural catheters, strict asepsis must be followed
> - Diabetic neuropathy increases the duration of block hence appropriate adjustments in dose is advisable
> - Amongst the adjuvants, epinephrine must be avoided
> - Ultrasound guidance is recommended to monitor the distance between tip of the needle and the nerve

not be used in diabetics. Some of the suggestions pertaining to practice of RA in diabetics have been summarized in **Box 2**.

CONCLUSION

Regional anesthesia is a major component of the practice of anesthesia. It offers the promise of a comfortable pain-free postoperative period, low cost and comparatively less strain on facilities with resource crunch. Quite often, during a risk benefit analysis RA comes out a winner and in many ways, it has stood the test of time. In the eternal quest for safer practices, there will always be controversies and gray areas and as newer evidence emerge, the path will become smoother and safer.

> **KEY POINTS**
> - Regional anesthesia has always been an integral part of the practice of anesthesia.
> - Advent of sonography, safer local anesthetics, adjuvants, technically advanced catheters and local anesthetic infusion systems have made regional techniques safer and their use more widespread than ever before.
> - Incidentally, the rise in its use in everyday practice since last two decades has coincided with stringent patient safety parameters, medicolegal responsibilities and an increase in the use of anticoagulants and antiplatelets for stroke, atrial fibrillation (AF), stents, and prophylaxis or treatment of deep vein thrombosis.
> - Though a boon for pain management and ambulatory anesthesia practice, a stringent risk benefit analysis is must before every procedure.
> - The crux of a safe regional anesthesia practice is a very thorough evaluation of patient, documentation of relevant findings and obtaining informed consent stating the risks and benefits before any procedure.

REFERENCES

1. American College of Obstetricians and Gynecologists' Committee on Practice Bulletins—Obstetrics. Practice Bulletin No. 166: thrombocytopenia in Pregnancy. Obstet Gynecol. 2016;128(3):e43-53.
2. Horlocker TT, Vandermeuelen E, Kopp SL, Gogarten W, Leffert LR, Benzon HT. Regional Anesthesia in the Patient Receiving Antithrombotic or Thrombolytic

Therapy: American Society of Regional Anesthesia and Pain Medicine Evidence-Based Guidelines (Fourth Edition). [published correction appears in Reg Anesth Pain Med. 2018;43(5):566. Vandermeuelen, Erik (corrected to Vandermeulen, Erik)]. Reg Anesth Pain Med. 2018;43(3):263-309.
3. Moen V, Dahlgren N, Irestedt L. Severe neurological complications after central neuraxial blockades in Sweden 1990-1999. Anesthesiology. 2004;101(4):950-9.
4. Kaufman RM, Djulbegovic B, Gernsheimer T, Kleinman S, Tinmouth AT, Capocelli KE, et al. Platelet transfusion: a clinical practice guideline from the AABB. Ann Intern Med. 2015;162(3):205-13.
5. Guideline for platelet transfusion thresholds for pediatric hematology/oncology patients: complete reference guide. Edmonton, AB: The C17 Guidelines Committee; 2010.
6. Perlas A, Niazi A, McCartney C, Chan V, Xu D, Abbas S. The sensitivity of motor response to nerve stimulation and paresthesia for nerve localization as evaluated by ultrasound. Reg Anesth Pain Med. 2006;31(5):445-50.
7. Marhofer P. Regional blocks carried out during general anesthesia or deep sedation: myths and facts. Curr Opin Anaesthesiol. 2017;30(5):621-6.
8. Neal JM, Barrington MJ, Brull R, Hadzic A, Hebl JR, Horlocker TT, et al. The Second ASRA Practice Advisory on Neurologic Complications Associated With Regional Anesthesia and Pain Medicine: Executive Summary 2015. Reg Anesth Pain Med. 2015;40(5):401-30.
9. Ivani G, Suresh S, Ecoffey C, Bosenberg A, Lonnqvist PA, Krane E, et al. The European Society of Regional Anaesthesia and Pain Therapy and the American Society of Regional Anesthesia and Pain Medicine Joint Committee Practice Advisory on Controversial Topics in Pediatric Regional Anesthesia. Reg Anesth Pain Med. 2015;40(5):526-32.
10. Crawford JS. Experience with epidural blood patch. Anesthesia. 1980;61:304-2.
11. Bucklin BA, Hawkins JL, Anderson JR, Ullrich FA. Obstetric anesthesia workforce survey: twenty-year update. Anesthesiology. 2005;103(3):645-53.
12. Paech MJ, Doherty DA, Christmas T, Wong CA, Epidural Blood Patch Trial Group. The volume of blood for epidural blood patch in obstetrics: a randomized, blinded clinical trial. Anesth Analg. 2011;113(1):126-33.
13. Martin JA, Hamilton BE, Osterman MJ, Curtin SC, Matthews TJ. Births: final data for 2013. Natl Vital Stat Rep. 2015;64(1):1-65.
14. van Kooten F, Oedit R, Bakker SL, Dippel DW. Epidural blood patch in post dural puncture headache: a randomised, observer-blind, controlled clinical trial. J Neurol Neurosurg Psychiatry. 2008;79(5):553-8.
15. Iga K, Murakoshi T, Kato A, Kato K, Terada S, Konno H, et al. Repeat epidural blood patch at the level of unintentional dural puncture and its neurologic complications: a case report. JA Clin Rep. 2019;5(1):14.
16. Verduzco LA, Atlas SW, Riley ET. Subdural hematoma after an epidural blood patch. Int J Obstet Anesth. 2012;21(2):189-92.
17. Narouze S. Epidural blood patch is an iatrogenic epidural hematoma: asymptomatic or symptomatic? This is the question. Reg Anesth Pain Med. 2019;rapm-2019-100851.
18. Moore DC, Batra MS. The components of an effective test dose prior to epidural block. Anesthesiology. 1981;55(6):693-6.
19. Regan KJ, O'Sullivan G. The extension of epidural blockade for emergency Caesarean section: a survey of current UK practice. Anaesthesia. 2008;63(2):136-42.
20. Massoth C, Wenk M. Epidural test dose in obstetric patients: should we still use it? Curr Opin Anaesthesiol. 2019;32(3):263-7.

21. Tuckey J. Bilateral compartment syndrome complicating prolonged lithotomy position. Br J Anaesth. 1996;77(4):546-9.
22. McQueen MM, Gaston P, Court-Brown CM. Acute compartment syndrome. Who is at risk? J Bone Joint Surg Br. 2000;82(2):200-3.
23. Blick SS, Brumback RJ, Poka A, Burgess AR, Ebraheim NA. Compartment syndrome in open tibial fractures. J. Bone Joint Surg Am. 1986;68(9):1348-53.
24. McQueen MM, Christie J, Court-Brown CM. Acute compartment syndrome in tibial diaphyseal fractures. J Bone Joint Surg Br. 1996;78(1):95-8.
25. Bae DS, Kadiyala RK, Waters PM. Acute compartment syndrome in children: contemporary diagnosis, treatment, and outcome. J Pediatr Orthop. 2001;21(5):680-8.
26. Mar GJ, Barrington MJ, McGuirk BR. Acute compartment syndrome of the lower limb and the effect of postoperative analgesia on diagnosis. Br J Anaesth. 2009;102(1):3-11.
27. British Orthopaedic Association. BOAST: Diagnosis and Management of Compartment Syndrome of the Limbs. [online] Available from https://www.boa.ac.uk/resources/boa-standards-for-trauma-and-orthopaedics/boast-10-pdf.html. [Last accessed October, 2020].
28. Rothenberg KA, George EL, Trickey AW, Chandra V, Stern JR. Delayed fasciotomy is associated with higher risk of major amputation in patients with acute limb ischemia. Ann Vasc Surg. 2019;59:195-201.
29. Llewellyn N, Moriarty A. The national pediatric epidural audit. Paediatr Anaesth. 2007;17(6):520-33.
30. Lönnqvist PA, Ecoffey C, Bosenberg A, Suresh S, Ivani G. The European society of regional anesthesia and pain therapy and the American society of regional anesthesia and pain medicine joint committee practice advisory on controversial topics in pediatric regional anesthesia I and II: what do they tell us?. Curr Opin Anaesthesiol. 2017;30(5):613-20.
31. Department of Health and Human Services. Food and Drug Administration Drug Bulletin. 1982;12:4-5
32. De Andrés J, Tatay Vivò J, Palmisani S, Villanueva Pérez VL, Mínguez A. Intrathecal granuloma formation in a patient receiving long-term spinal infusion of tramadol. Pain Med. 2010;11(7):1059-62.
33. Barrett NA, Sundaraj SR. Inadvertent intrathecal injection of tramadol. Br J Anaesth. 2003;91(6):918-20.
34. Ouro-Bang'na Maman AF, Ahouangbévi S, Chobli M. [Respiratory depression after intrathecal injection of tramadol with hyperbaric bupivacaine]. Can J Anaesth. 2006;53(11):1161-2.
35. Singh S, Bansal P, Dureja J. Off-label use of drugs in regional anesthesia: A need for setting up policies. J Anaesthesiol Clin Pharmacol. 2017;33(4):448-9.
36. Tucker AP, Lai C, Nadeson R, Goodchild CS. Intrathecal midazolam I: a cohort study investigating safety. Anesth Analg. 2004;98:1512-20.
37. Kirksey MA, Haskins SC, Cheng J, Liu SS. Local Anesthetic Peripheral Nerve Block Adjuvants for Prolongation of Analgesia: A Systematic Qualitative Review. PLoS One. 2015;10(9):e0137312.
38. Marhofer P, Brummett CM. Safety and efficiency of dexmedetomidine as adjuvant to local anesthetics. Curr Opin Anaesthesiol. 2016;29(5):632-7.
39. Bravo D, Aliste J, Layera S, Fernández D, Leurcharusmee P, Samerchua A, et al. A multicenter, randomized comparison between 2, 5, and 8 mg of perineural dexamethasone for ultrasound-guided infraclavicular block. Reg Anesth Pain Med. 2019;44(1):46-51.

40. Aliste J, Layera S, Bravo D, Fernández D, Jara Á, García A, et al. Randomized comparison between perineural dexamethasone and dexmedetomidine for ultrasound-guided infraclavicular block. Reg Anesth Pain Med. 2019;rapm-2019-100680.
41. Zhang P, Liu S, Zhu J, Rao Z, Liu C. Dexamethasone and dexmedetomidine as adjuvants to local anesthetic mixture in intercostal nerve block for thoracoscopic pneumonectomy: a prospective randomized study. Reg Anesth Pain Med. 2019;rapm-2018-100221.
42. Suresh S, Ecoffey C, Bosenberg A, Lonnqvist PA, de Oliveira GS Jr, de Leon Casasola O, et al. The European Society of Regional Anesthesia and Pain Therapy/American Society of Regional Anesthesia and Pain Medicine Recommendations on Local Anesthetics and Adjuvants Dosage in Pediatric Regional Anesthesia. Reg Anesth Pain Med. 2018;43(2):211-6.
43. Yajnik M, Kou A, Mudumbai SC, Walters TL, Howard SK, Edward Kim T, et al. Peripheral nerve blocks are not associated with increased risk of perioperative peripheral nerve injury in a Veterans Affairs inpatient surgical population. Reg Anesth Pain Med. 2019;44(1):81-5.
44. Barrington MJ, Watts SA, Gledhill SR, Thomas RD, Said SA, Snyder GL, et al. Preliminary results of the Australasian Regional Anaesthesia Collaboration: a prospective audit of more than 7000 peripheral nerve and plexus blocks for neurologic and other complications. Reg Anesth Pain Med. 2009;34(6):534-41.
45. Welch MB, Brummett CM, Welch TD, Tremper KK, Shanks AM, Guglani P, et al. Perioperative peripheral nerve injuries: a retrospective study of 380,680 cases during a 10-year period at a single institution. Anesthesiology. 2009;111(3):490-7.
46. Jacob AK, Mantilla CB, Sviggum HP, Schroeder DR, Pagnano MW, Hebl JR. Perioperative nerve injury after total knee arthroplasty: regional anesthesia risk during a 20-year cohort study. Anesthesiology. 2011;114(2):311-7.
47. Jacob AK, Mantilla CB, Sviggum HP, Schroeder DR, Pagnano MW, Hebl JR. Perioperative nerve injury after total hip arthroplasty: regional anesthesia risk during a 20-year cohort study. Anesthesiology. 2011;115(6):1172-8.
48. Sviggum HP, Jacob AK, Mantilla CB, Schroeder DR, Sperling JW, Hebl JR. Perioperative nerve injury after total shoulder arthroplasty: assessment of risk after regional anesthesia. Reg Anesth Pain Med. 2012;37(5):490-4.
49. Neal JM, Barrington MJ, Brull R, Hadzic A, Hebl JR, Horlocker TT, et al. The Second ASRA Practice Advisory on Neurologic Complications Associated With Regional Anesthesia and Pain Medicine: Executive Summary 2015. Reg Anesth Pain Med. 2015;40(5):401-30.
50. Williams BA, Bottegal MT, Kentor ML, Irrgang JJ, Williams JP. Rebound pain scores as a function of femoral nerve block duration after anterior cruciate ligament reconstruction: retrospective analysis of a prospective, randomized clinical trial. Reg Anesth Pain Med. 2007;32(3):186-92.
51. Henningsen MJ, Sort R, Moller AM, Herling SF. Peripheral nerve block in ankle fracture surgery: a qualitative study of patients' experiences. Anaesthesia 2018; 73(1):49-58.
52. Williams BA, Ibinson JW, Mangione MP, Modrak RT, Tonarelli EJ, Rakesh H, et al. Research priorities regarding multimodal peripheral nerve blocks for postoperative analgesia and anesthesia based on hospital quality data extracted from over 1,300 cases (2011-2014). Pain Med. 2015;16(1):7-12.
53. Lavand'homme P. Rebound pain after regional anesthesia in the ambulatory patient. Curr Opin Anaesthesiol. 2018;31(6):679-84.

54. Youm YS, Cho SD, Cho HY, Hwang CH, Jung SH, Kim KH. Preemptive Femoral Nerve Block Could Reduce The Rebound Pain After Periarticular Injection in Total Knee Arthroplasty. J Arthroplasty. 2016;31(8):1722-6.
55. Nobre LV, Cunha GP, Sousa PCCB, Takeda A, Cunha Ferraro LH. [Peripheral nerve block and rebound pain: literature review]. Rev Bras Anestesiol. 2019;69(6):587-93.
56. Kalichman MW, Calcutt NA. Local anesthetic-induced conduction block and nerve fiber injury in streptozotocin-diabetic rats. Anesthesiology. 1992;77(5):941-7.
57. Heschl S, Hallmann B, Zilke T, Gemes G, Schoerghuber M, Auer-Grumbach M, et al. Diabetic neuropathy increases stimulation threshold during popliteal sciatic nerve block. Br J Anaesth. 2016;116(4):538-45.
58. Kroin JS, Buvanendran A, Tuman KJ, Kerns JM. Effect of acute versus continuous glycemic control on duration of local anesthetic sciatic nerve block in diabetic rats. Reg Anesth Pain Med. 2012;37(6):595-600.
59. Ten Hoope W, Looije M, Lirk P. Regional anesthesia in diabetic peripheral neuropathy. Curr Opin Anaesthesiol. 2017;30(5):627-31.
60. Kopp SL, Jacob AK, Hebl JR. Regional Anesthesia in Patients With Preexisting Neurologic Disease. Reg Anesth Pain Med. 2015;40(5):467-78.
61. Neal JM, Barrington MJ, Brull R, Hadzic A, Hebl JR, Horlocker TT, et al. The Second ASRA Practice Advisory on Neurologic Complications Associated With Regional Anesthesia and Pain Medicine: Executive Summary 2015. Reg Anesth Pain Med. 2015;40(5):401-30.

CHAPTER 7

Intraoperative Blood Conservation Strategies

Jyotsna Goswami, Rudranil Nandi

INTRODUCTION

Anemia increases postoperative morbidity and mortality substantially. Around 20–40% of all surgical patients develop anemia during their perioperative journey.[1] As per World Health Organization (WHO), anemia is defined by hemoglobin (Hb) concentration less than 13 g/dL in male, less than 12 g/dL in female and less than 11 g/dL in pregnant women. Blood transfusion has been used liberally in perioperative period even few years ago. But recent evidences suggested that restricted use of packed red blood cells (PRBCs) transfusion is as effective and sometimes superior to liberal use of PRBCs.[2] In 2010, WHO introduced the concept of patient blood management (PBM) to avoid unnecessary transfusion and thus to improve patient outcome. PBM essentially consists of following pillars—(1) diagnosis and treatment of anemia, (2) prevention of coagulopathy, (3) applying modalities of blood conservation, (4) delaying transfusion till body homeostasis is preserved, and (5) multimodal team approach including shared decision.[1] WHO has urged all its 194 member states to implement PBM in their medical institutes and hospitals. It also ensures uniform decision-making related to blood transfusion management in perioperative period across the departments within an institute.[3] After implementation of PBM algorithm, it was found that prevalence of anemia at the time of surgery dropped from 26 to 10%, perioperative blood loss was reduced by 20% and transfusion rate for total hip arthroplasty came down from 23 to 8% and for total knee arthroplasty it came down from 8 to 0%.[4]

For decades, the cut off value of Hb level and hematocrit for perioperative blood transfusion was 10.0 g/dL and 30% respectively. However later on, many authors did not support the idea of a single transfusion trigger and advised against it. They suggested the use of a range of Hb values between 6.0 and 10.0 g/dL taking consideration of associated comorbidities. Although two types of PBM strategies are described such as restrictive and liberal, the definition of each one is not very clear. Transfusion threshold in restrictive strategy is Hb of 8 g/dL and hematocrit value of 25%. There is evidence that restrictive PBM strategies were associated with lesser PRBC transfusion compared to liberal

PBM strategies without any difference in mortality, morbidity and length of hospital stay. Hence, different guidelines strongly recommend restrictive strategy to reduce transfusion requirements, which is facilitated by various blood conservation modalities that can be adopted during preoperative and intraoperative period. Cell salvage and autologous donations are two most important blood conservation strategies described in literature. Cell salvage was first used in 1818 in an obstetric patient after postpartum hemorrhage.[5] Since then many researchers and clinicians used this technique. Eventually in 1970 modern cell saver was produced and became commercially available.

PREOPERATIVE ASSESSMENT AND OPTIMIZATION TO REDUCE INTRAOPERATIVE BLOOD LOSS

An assessment for possibility and risk of transfusion should be carried out for all patients. Cardiac surgery, spine surgery, liver surgery, major oncosurgery and orthopedic surgeries are frequently associated with massive bleeding. These patients should undergo early screening for anemia and evaluation of other systemic comorbidities. Preoperative routine hematological testing should include Hb, hematocrit, coagulation profile, prothrombin time (PT), activated partial thromboplastin time (aPTT) and international normalized ratio (INR). Multispecialty (anesthesiologist, surgeon, hematologist, and radiologist) involvement in the preoperative period, for the decision making regarding appropriate surgical approach is necessary for management of this high-risk group of patients. Radiological interventions, minimally invasive procedures and staging procedures help to reduce surgical bleeding. Involvement of bigger surgical team is preferred to reduce the surgical duration. If possible, preoperative evaluation should be performed weeks before the procedure to allow adequate time for optimization before the procedure. Optimization include following measures:

Therapeutic Interventions for Anemia

Preoperative anemia is associated with increased risk of postoperative infection leading to increased morbidity, mortality and prolonged hospital stay. Effective preoperative management of anemia improves surgical outcome.[6] Preoperative erythropoietin injection and iron supplementation reduce perioperative blood transfusions. Patients with iron deficiency anemia are benefited with preoperative iron supplementation, if time permits. Iron is the most common and widespread nutritional deficiency worldwide and occurs in association with chronic conditions. It plays a key role in erythropoiesis. True iron deficiency can occur due to increased need, limited intake and blood loss. Patients can also have a functional iron deficiency in chronic disease and aging despite adequate total body stores. In case of true low iron levels, early correction with iron replacement is the optimal treatment. This can be oral iron formulations such as ferrous sulfate, ferrous fumarate or ferrous gluconate and the body can absorb up to 6 mg/day. Parenteral iron therapy can be used in case of following conditions: (1) functional iron deficiency, (2) oral iron is not tolerated, (3) oral treatment is ineffective, or (4) when time is limited for adequate replacement. Hb is usually increased by 2 weeks of parenteral iron therapy and becomes maximum at 6 weeks. Single-dose parenteral iron according to iron requirements and body weight is sufficient most of the time.[7]

Other causes of anemia can be treated with replacement of the relevant component, for example, vitamin B_{12} or folic acid. Although, healthy subjects are able to tolerate Hb values below 6 g/dL, older patients and those with significant comorbidities cannot tolerate such a low Hb level. Preoperatively red blood cells (RBCs) should be transfused to maintain an Hb level between 6.0 and 10 g/dL.[8] Patients' age, comorbid burden, hemodynamic and oxygenation status, preoperative Hb levels and the complexity of surgical intervention should be taken into consideration before transfusing preoperatively.

Management of Ongoing Anticoagulants and Antiplatelet Agents

Risk of thrombosis should be balanced with the risk of bleeding in perioperative period. Patients with prosthetic heart valve or with history of venous thromboembolic (VTE) event within the last 3 months are usually on oral anticoagulant therapy. In those patients, bridging anticoagulation should be started with heparin or low molecular weight heparin (LMWH). The effect of warfarin can be reversed with prothrombin complex concentrate (PCC) 50 IU/kg. Intravenous vitamin K (10 mg) is also helpful. If PCC is not available, fresh frozen plasma (FFP) can be used. Dabigatran, rivaroxaban and apixaban are three new novel oral anticoagulants. In case of major elective surgery, when neuraxial blockade planned or in patients with renal dysfunction, dabigatran should be stopped 5 days before surgery whereas, apixaban and rivaroxaban should be stopped 3 days before. Otherwise, dabigatran can be stopped 3 days before and apixaban-rivaroxaban 24–48 hours before surgery **(Table 1)**.

Irreversible antiplatelet drug like aspirin can be continued till the day before surgery. But it should be discontinued 5 days before any major surgery in a patient with very low risk of cardiovascular events or high-risk procedures like intracranial surgery. Prasugrel and ticlopidine should be stopped 7 days before any surgical intervention **(Table 1)**.[9,10] In patients, who have coronary stents, antiplatelet drug management may differ depending on the type of stent, time interval from the coronary event and type of surgery. After a bare metal stent placement elective surgery is postponed for 30 days whereas after a drug-eluting stent (DES) placement elective surgery is postponed for 6 months. But a time sensitive surgery may be performed after 3 months of DES placement if needed.[11] The abovementioned time durations were decided depending upon the requirement of minimum duration of uninterrupted dual antiplatelet therapy. If a patient is on dual antiplatelet therapy, elective surgery is contraindicated.

Autologous Blood Donation

Preoperative autologous blood donation (PAD) significantly reduces the requirement of allogenic blood transfusion. Donation of autologous blood

TABLE 1: Time gap to stop a drug before surgery

Anticoagulant and antiplatelet drugs	Cessation prior to surgery
Antiplatelets	
• Aspirin (COX 1 inhibitor)	• Continue except in identified surgery
• Clopidogrel (P2Y12 blocker)	• 5–7 days
• Ticlopidine (P2Y12 blocker)	• 10 days
• Prasugrel (P2Y12 blocker)	• 7–10 days
• Ticagrelor (P2Y12 blocker)	• 5 days
• Cilostazol (phosphodiesterase inhibitor)	• 2 days
• Tirofiban (GP IIb IIIa inhibitor)	• 4–8 hours
• Eptifibatide (GP IIb IIIa inhibitor)	• 4–8 hours
• Abciximab (GP IIb IIIa inhibitor)	• 24–48 hours
Anticoagulants	
Injectable	
• Heparin (thrombin + factor Xa inhibitor)	• 6 hours
• LMWH (thrombin + factor Xa inhibitor)	• 12–24 hours
• Fondaparinux (factor Xa inhibitor)	• 36–42 hours
• Argatroban (thrombin inhibitor)	• 4 hours
• Hirudins (thrombin inhibitor)	• 8–10 hours
Oral	
• Warfarin (Vitamin K antagonist)	• 5 days
• Rivaroxaban (factor Xa inhibitor)	• 3 days
• Apixaban (factor Xa inhibitor)	• 3 days
• Endoxaban (factor Xa inhibitor)	• 3 days
• Dabigatran (thrombin inhibitor)	• 5 days

(LMWH: low-molecular-weight heparin)

assures the availability of blood and blood components if required. If time permits, all suitable patients should be counseled and offered the option of PAD. Patients' blood donation starts 1 month before scheduled date of surgery. One unit or 450 mL of blood in each week maximum up to 4 units can be collected. Last collection should be 72 hours prior to surgery, so that lost red cells can be regenerated before the surgery. The blood is collected and stored conventionally. This blood should be kept separate in the blood bank with proper documentation and readily available during surgery if required.[12] Oral or IV iron and erythropoietin therapy are continued during the time interval between the last donation and the surgery, to facilitate erythropoiesis. Depletion of 2,3-diphosphoglycerate (2,3 DPG) and reduced ability of erythrocytes to deliver oxygen to tissue are common feature of autologous blood as with stored allogenic blood.

Advantages

Unlike allogenic blood, autologous blood transfusion is associated with minimal risk of viral transmission and hemolytic, febrile or allergic reaction mediated by immunologic reaction. It does not cause transfusion-related immune-modulation (TRIM), which is associated with cancer recurrence.[13]

Disadvantages

Preoperative autologous blood donation needs lots of planning for logistics, so it is difficult before emergency or semiemergency surgery. Autologous blood needs to be stored with proper identification, which may be vulnerable due to human error. As more than 50% of autologous blood remain unused and wasted, running a PAD programs is less cost-effective than transfusion of allogenic blood.[13] Some patients may not tolerate the preoperative donation. Iron therapy and erythropoietin that are used after PAD also add more cost to the treatment.[14]

Precautions and Contraindications

Repeated blood donations may cause cardiovascular adverse events, especially in patients with anemia, cardiac disease, uncontrolled hypertension, etc., PAD is not used in these patients. In practice, when preoperative donations are done weekly, it becomes very difficult to maintain hemoglobin level with iron and erythropoietin therapy. As a result, although patients have reserved blood, they had lower hemoglobin level before surgery, making them more vulnerable to transfusion. So, PAD should be reserved for only those who have rare blood group.

INTRAOPERATIVE STRATEGIES

Reducing blood loss intraoperatively involves a multidisciplinary approach and ongoing communication with the surgical team. These include combined consideration of patient positioning, thermoregulation, regional anesthesia, blood pressure management, operative techniques, hemodilution, cell salvage, and the use of antifibrinolytics.

Patient Positioning

Patient should be positioned in such manner so that venous drainage axes are compressed, as this can lead to increased blood loss. Maintaining the surgical field above the heart where possible, for example, in head and neck surgery, can also reduce bleeding at operative sites. Twisting the neck should be avoided during head and neck surgery as it interferes with jugular venous drainage.[15]

Thermoregulation

Hypothermia (core temperature <36.8°C) may cause altered function of coagulation factors and reduced platelet function and thus resulting increased risk of intraoperative bleeding. Decrease in temperature by 1°C is associated with 16% increased risk of hemorrhage and 22% increased incidence of transfusion.[16] Temperature is an important monitor intraoperatively and proactive measures such as hot air blanket, fluid warmer, increasing OR temperature should be used to prevent hypothermia.

Regional Anesthesia

Loss of sympathetic tone as a result of neuraxial and regional anesthesia help to reduce the arterial and peripheral venous blood pressure in the surgical field, resulting in less intraoperative blood loss compared to general anesthesia.[17]

Operative Techniques

A proactive management of surgical bleeding is an important blood conservation strategy. Preventive measures such as tourniquets can be considered, especially with lower-limb surgery. Vessel ligation should be proactive rather than reactive. Other methods to stop bleeding early include pressure, ligation, diathermy, and topical vasoconstrictors (e.g., use of adrenaline-soaked swabs and the use of fibrin glues), staged approaches to surgery, laparoscopy and extended surgical team (reduced duration of surgery).

Cell Salvage

The surgeries, where major blood loss is expected, re-transfusion of salvaged autologous blood can be planned. Cell salvage has three steps: (1) collection, (2) washing, and (3) re-infusion. Blood that is lost during surgery is collected from the surgical field with a separate double-lumen suction device. Blood is sucked through one lumen and predetermined volume of heparinized saline is taken through the other lumen. They are mixed and this heparinized saline mixed blood is then collected in a reservoir after passing through a filter. Blood components are then separated by centrifugation. The RBCs are then passed through semipermeable membrane to remove free Hb, white blood cell (WBC), plasma and heparin. This salvaged RBCs are then mixed with normal saline, so that the hematocrit becomes 50–80%. It should be transfused within 6 hours.[18] Red cell survival, pH, 2,3-DPG, and potassium levels in salvaged red cells are almost similar to banked homologous blood. Cell salvage is now gradually becoming popular.[19] Patients with rare blood group, patients who does not want allogenic transfusion and when blood loss more than 1,000 mL or 20% of total blood volume are expected cell salvage should be considered if available.[19] Most commonly it is used in neurosurgery, cardiovascular surgery, joint replacement surgery, liver transplant surgery, etc. The disadvantages are equipment cost and the need for trained operators. Previously cell salvage was considered unsafe in oncosurgery, bowel surgery and obstetric surgery in fear of contamination with cancer cells, bowel content and amniotic fluid respectively. But after introduction of leukocyte depletion filters (LDFs) which can remove contaminants, cell salvage can be safely used in above mentioned surgeries.

Risks

Hemolysis not immune-mediated, nonhemolytic febrile reactions, air embolism, error of transfusion, coagulation abnormalities can occur with cell salvage. Contamination with drugs, cleansing solutions, infectious agents, activated leukocytes, cytokines, and other microaggregates are some side-effects. Improved technology and training of the operators and increasing experience reduce the possibility of these complications. Salvaged blood is devoid of coagulation factors and platelets, thus resulting in coagulopathy. Salvage process may cause shear stress injury to RBCs, resulting in hemolysis. By minimizing suction pressure, RBC hemolysis can be reduced. Use of variable-pressure suction devices can reduce this stress injury to RBCs and minimize RBC hemolysis. Shear stress injury also shortens the lifespan of the RBC by causing sublethal damage. Mixing normal saline with the blood while suction helps to reduce stress injury on RBC by 60%. Evidence suggests that the incidence of complications is much less in case of autotransfusion than allogeneic blood transfusion.[20]

Benefits

Salvaged blood has more erythrocyte viability as high as 88% in comparison to allogenic blood. Besides, 2,3-DPG and adenosine triphosphate (ATP) levels are also higher in salvaged blood. As they are freshly collected, the biconcave shape of salvaged RBCs remain unaltered and thus can pass through capillaries easily as opposed to allogenic blood, which is stored for quite some time and RBCs lose their elasticity. So, autologous blood has better oxygen carrying capacity and oxygen delivery than allogenic blood. Autologous transfusion is reported to be associated with increased survival after esophagectomy in comparison with allogenic blood transfusion.[21] This favorable result is probably due to lack of immune modulation after autologous transfusion. Besides, salvaged RBCs cause immune stimulation which has protective role to postoperative infection. Cell salvage reduces number of allogeneic blood transfusion by 39%.[22] Use of salvaged blood is associated with reduced incidence of perioperative myocardial infarction and postoperative infections.

Antifibrinolytics

Perioperative use of antifibrinolytics helps to reduce blood loss and allogenic transfusion. Tranexamic acid is commonly used antifibrinolytic. It prevents the breakdown of fibrin and promotes the maintenance of blood clots. Many trials have demonstrated its effectiveness; the WOMAN trial published in April 2017, was an international or multicentric randomized controlled trial looking at postpartum hemorrhage in more than 20,000 women. They compared tranexamic acid with placebo (1.5% vs. 1.9%) and found a significant reduction in death due to bleeding in patients, who received tranexamic acid especially when given within 3 hours of delivery.[23] The CRASH-2 (Clinical Randomization of an Antifibrinolytic in Significant Hemorrhage 2) trial in 2011 assessed tranexamic acid in trauma patients and found that early administration within 1 hour significantly reduced the risk of death due to bleeding (7.7% in the placebo group vs. 5.3% in the tranexamic acid group).[24] Recommended dose for adult patients is 1 g bolus and infusion of 500 mg/h if needed.

Controlled Hypotensive Techniques

Lowering the mean arterial pressure (MAP) in a controlled way reduces end-organ blood flow and thus helps to decrease blood loss. Meticulous hemodynamic monitoring is required during this technique. It is most commonly used in high bleeding risk surgeries like hip, spinal and open prostate surgeries. The risks of inducing hypotension must be tailored for an individual patient and balanced to ensure appropriate vital organ perfusion. A reduction of MAP by 30% of baseline is thought to be clinically acceptable for American Society of Anesthesiologists (ASA) I patients. The methods that can be used to lower MAP are increasing the concentration of inhalational anesthetics, extra dose of IV anesthetics or opioid, additional antihypertensives such as labetalol, esmolol, sodium nitroprusside, glyceryl trinitrate, clonidine, etc. Controlled hypotensive techniques are contraindicated in ischemic heart disease, uncontrolled hypertension, cerebrovascular disease and anemia.[25]

Acute Normovolemic Hemodilution

Acute normovolemic hemodilution (ANH) is used when high to moderate blood loss is anticipated in case of major surgeries like cardiac, orthopedic, thoracic or liver surgery. Hemodilution is of two types: (1) normovolemic, and (2) hypervolemic.

As the name indicates, in normovolemic hemodilution, normal blood volume is maintained by initial removal of patient's blood followed by replacement of the volume with crystalloid. Hematocrit values are preferred to be 20–30%. Low hematocrit reduces plasma viscosity and thus improves tissue perfusion and blood flow. Reduced hematocrit also ensures reduced loss of RBCs and plasma constituent during surgical bleeding. So, ANH creates an intraoperative anemia, which is well tolerated. Eventually this fresh whole blood is transfused back after surgical control of bleeding. Thus, all blood components are replaced when they are needed the most.[26]

In hypervolemic hemodilution, blood is not withdrawn first. Instead fluid administration leads to hemodilution and drop in hematocrit value. So, surgical bleeding causes loss of lesser number of RBCs. But in patients with reduced cardiac function, care must be taken to prevent decompensatory cardiac state.

Unlike PAD, ANH can be used in nonelective surgery. ANH also avoids blood storage related issues and clerical errors. ANH is found to reduce the rate of transfusion by <10% and has modest hemostatic benefit.[27] ANH reduces amount of allogenic blood transfused after major surgeries like cardiac, neurological, orthopedic, and spine surgeries. After induction of anesthesia, blood is collected from central venous cannula (CVC). Usually the volume to be collected, is decided preoperatively based on maximum allowable blood loss (MABL). The lumen of CVC has a rubber blocker, which can be pierced by a large bore needle and attached to blood collecting bag obtained from blood bank. While collecting, the bag is usually placed at the lower level than the patient and intermittent rocking movement is performed to prevent clot formation. This collected blood can be kept at the OR temperature for 8 hours.

Alternatively, a large-bore cannula is inserted in large vein and 15–20 mL/kg of blood is collected before the surgery starts. The collected blood is kept inside operating room after proper labeling in room temperature, which is transfused back after the hemostasis is achieved. Aggressive hemodilution is required to hematocrits of approximately 20% to achieve maximum efficacy in terms of Hb spared that can be calculated as follows:

$$\text{Amount of Hb spared} = (Hb_I - Hb_{ANH}) \times V_{BL}$$

where Hb_I = Initial [Hb] (g dL^{-1}), Hb_{ANH} = [Hb] following ANH and V_{BL} = volume of blood lost during surgery (dL).

For example, if one patient had Hb of 10 g/dL after ANH from 14 g/dL initial Hb and suffered 1,000 mL blood loss, then amount of Hb spared is = (14–10) × 10 = 40 g.

Advantages

It is inexpensive compared to PAD as there is no need to store the autologous blood. Besides as the blood is kept inside OR, blood is easily available if required and associated with no risk of blood mismatch. As ANH transfuse whole blood, patient also gets platelets and clotting factors.

Disadvantages and Complications

As ANH is associated with sudden decrease of hematocrit, it may lead to hemodynamic instability that may cause myocardial ischemia in susceptible patients. Anesthetic personnel need to be very cautious during the procedure. Complications may arise because of the physiological effects of the acute hemodilution. Literature regarding effectiveness of the technique is very limited.

Transfusion of Blood Components

Red blood cells are transfused whenever Hb level drops below the predetermined cutoff level. If patients do not have other comorbidities, restrictive transfusion threshold (Hb 7–8 g/dL) of RBCs is safer than liberal transfusion threshold (Hb > 9 g/dL).

Fresh frozen plasma (FFP) is leukodepleted plasma that contains all the factors of the soluble coagulation system. It is rapidly frozen to maintain the integrity of coagulation factors. The recommended dose is 15 mL/kg. Cryoprecipitate is also a leukodepleted plasma derived from FFP containing von Willebrand factor, factor VIII, fibrinogen, factor XIII and fibronectin in concentrated amount. Volume of one unit of cryoprecipitate is 20–40 mL that contains 400–450 mg of fibrinogen. One pool of five units contains 2 g of fibrinogen. Usually, two pools of cryoprecipitate are transfused when required. During major hemorrhage, fibrinogen should be maintained >1.5 g/L.

Platelets can be administered in two ways—(1) platelet rich plasma (PRP) and (2) single donor platelets (SDP). Buffy coat platelets of four different whole blood donations are mixed with plasma of one donation and some platelet additive solution to produce one-unit PRP. Whereas, SDP is produced from apheresis donation of single donor. Each SDP pack containing 250–350 mL increases the platelet count by approximately 30,000/µL.

During massive bleeding, FFP and platelets are transfused in a ratio of 1:1:1 with RBC. After initial rapid transfusion of four units each of RBCs and FFPs, platelet concentrate are transfused. Later thromboelastography (TEG)-guided replacement of individual blood products should be considered.[28]

INTRAOPERATIVE MONITORING

Patient should be monitored for organ perfusion and blood loss, anemia, coagulopathy and adverse effects of transfusion.

Monitoring of Perfusion of Vital Organs and Blood Loss

Standard ASA recommended monitoring like heart rate, blood pressure, oxygen saturation, capnography and urine output should be performed to ensure perfusion of vital organs. Inspection of the surgical field is important to assess any excessive bleeding. Blood loss can be assessed by measurement from suction bottle, surgical sponges and surgical drains. Estimation of Hb concentration by arterial blood gas (ABG) analysis and point of care (POC) testing by HemoCue (HemoCue, a Danaher company. © 2019 HemoCue India, a division of DHR Holding India Pvt Ltd., New Delhi) is useful. ABG helps to detect acidosis, anemia and hypocalcemia. It also shows lactate level which is a surrogate marker of tissue perfusion and volume status. Invasive hemodynamic monitoring like arterial blood pressure, central venous pressure and pulmonary artery catheter-based parameters should be used when indicated.

Monitoring of Coagulation

Intraoperative monitoring of coagulation parameters helps in diagnosis and management of any coagulation abnormality contributing to excessive bleeding. It includes assessment of oozing of blood from mucosal and serosal surfaces, catheter insertion sites and wounds. Coagulation tests such as PT, INR, aPTT, platelet count and fibrinogen levels may be asked depending on suspected coagulopathy. When intraoperative heparin is used, activated clotting time (ACT) is monitored. TEG and rotational thromboelastometry (ROTEM) are two commonly used POC testing for coagulation status, which measures the dynamics of clot development, stabilization/strength and dissolution. The rate of transfusion and the total cost of treatment can be reduced by introduction of the PBM algorithm.[29]

Monitoring Adverse Effects of Transfusion

There may be different types of transfusion reactions with different manifestations. ABO incompatibility may present with hyperthermia, hemoglobinuria or microvascular bleeding. Hypoxemia, respiratory distress

TABLE 2: Adverse effects of blood transfusion	
Immune-mediated	*Nonimmune-mediated*
• Allergic • Anaphylactic reaction • Transfusion-associated lung injury (TRALI) • Transfusion-related immune modulation (TRIM) • Hemolytic reaction acute or delayed • Febrile nonhemolytic • Graft versus host disease • Post-transfusion purpura	• Infectious (e.g., hepatitis, bacterial infection, parasites) • Coagulopathy (after massive transfusion) • Circulatory overload • Metabolic derangements (e.g., hyperkalemia, hypocalcemia) • Errors handling/storage of blood • Delayed wound healing • Hypothermia • Thrombophlebitis • Citrate toxicity • Iron overload

and increased peak airway pressure are characteristic features of transfusion-related acute lung injury (TRALI) or transfusion-associated circulatory overload (TACO). There may be hyperthermia and hypotension due to bacterial contamination, urticaria due to allergic reactions and hypocalcemia due to citrate toxicity **(Table 2)**. Patient should be monitored for all these above-mentioned manifestations. If signs of a transfusion reaction are present, immediately stop the transfusion, give supportive therapy, order appropriate diagnostic testing and notify the blood bank. Management includes the administration of antihistamine, steroids. If transfusion reaction is life-threatening, there should not be any delay in administering adrenaline. Faulty in-patient identity check may lead to ABO incompatibility resulting into transfusion reactions, which is the most serious adverse outcome of blood transfusion.

BIOLOGICAL AND CLINICAL CONSEQUENCES OF PERIOPERATIVE ALLOGENIC BLOOD TRANSFUSION

Allogenic blood transfusion has been the conventional treatment for perioperative anemia and is associated with various adverse events such as hemolytic, allergic and febrile reactions, TRALI, TACO, TRIM, etc. The estimated risks of infection per blood unit range from 1/1–400,000 for hepatitis B (HBV), 1/1.6–3.1 million for hepatitis C virus (HCV), 1/1.4–4.7 million for human immunodeficiency virus (HIV) and 1/0.5–3.0 million for human T-cell lymphotropic virus. Life-threatening reactions are estimated to occur in 1 in 150,000 patients transfused. Besides, blood transfusion is independently associated with increased length of hospital stay and increased mortality. One of the immediate biological consequences of the administration of packed RBCs, FFP and/or platelets is immune suppression due to TRIM. In the patients who are transfused, TRIM can have a negative impact on short- and long-term surgical outcomes. Transfusion-related immune suppression can cause cancer recurrence,[30] postoperative infection[31] and acute lung injury.[32]

The timing of transfusion may also have different effects on the inflammatory and immune response. Thus, when blood products are administered during or immediately after surgery ("second hit"-first hit being surgical trauma), the so-called systemic inflammatory response syndrome can be further exaggerated by transfusions delaying mechanisms of resolutions of inflammation, which can also participate in the pathogenesis of transfusion-related adverse outcomes. Allogenic blood transfusions may cause perioperative myocardial ischemia, low-output cardiac failure, increased morbidity and mortality.

CONCLUSION

Blood conservation strategies should begin well in advance from the day of surgery and should include a multimodal, multispecialty approach throughout the patient's perioperative journey. Cell salvage is a very good option in cases where major intraoperative blood loss is anticipated, especially in patients, who refuse allogeneic blood products. Introduction of LDFs facilitates use of cell salvage in obstetrics, oncosurgery and gastrointestinal (GI) surgery. Autologous blood transfusion in the form of PAD and ANH can be useful especially in patients with rare blood groups and surgeries with high risk of bleeding. Autologous transfusion is an important component of a comprehensive blood transfusion strategy.

KEY POINTS

- Allogenic transfusion is associated with many immune-mediated adverse effects which eventually affect patient outcome.
- Preoperative and intraoperative blood conservation strategies reduce requirement of allogenic transfusion in perioperative period.
- Preoperative strategies include treatment of preoperative anemia, preoperative blood donations and optimization of other systemic factors.
- Intraoperative measures include cell salvage, acute normovolemic hemodilution (ANH), coagulation monitoring and timely intervention to correct coagulation abnormalities.
- In cell salvage, the RBCs that are lost during surgery are collected, washed in saline and then transfused back to the patient.
- Acute normovolemic hemodilution withdraws blood from patient just before the initiation of the surgical procedure reducing the hematocrit of the blood that is lost during surgery. Withdrawn blood is again transfused to the patient after the surgical procedure.

REFERENCES

1. Spahn DR, Theusinger OM, Hofmann A. Patient blood management is a win-win: a wake-up call. Br J Anaesth. 2012;108(6):889-92.
2. Hébert PC, Wells G, Blajchman MA, Marshall J, Martin C, Pagliarello G, et al. A multicenter, randomized, controlled clinical trial of transfusion requirements in critical care. Transfusion Requirements in Critical Care Investigators, Canadian Critical Care Trials Group. N Engl J Med. 1999;340(6):409-17.
3. Sullivan HC, Roback JD. The pillars of patient blood management: key to successful implementation (Article, p. 2840). Transfusion. 2019;59(9):2763-7.

4. Kotzé A, Carter LA, Scally AJ. Effect of a patient blood management programme on preoperative anemia, transfusion rate, and outcome after primary hip or knee arthroplasty: a quality improvement cycle. Br J Anaesth. 2012;108(6):943-52.
5. Blundell J. Experiments on the transfusion of blood by the syringe. Med-Chir Trans. 1818;9(Pt 1):56-92.
6. Ng O, Keeler BD, Mishra A, Simpson JA, Neal K, Al-Hassi HO, et al. Iron therapy for preoperative anaemia. Cochrane Database Syst Rev. 2019;12:CD011588.
7. Spahn DR, Zacharowski K. Non-treatment of preoperative anaemia is substandard clinical practice. Br J Anaesth. 2015;115(1):1-3.
8. Kozek-Langenecker SA, Afshari A, Albaladejo P, Santullano CA, De Robertis E, Filipescu DC, et al. Management of severe perioperative bleeding: guidelines from the European Society of Anaesthesiology. Eur J Anaesthesiol. 2013;30(6):270-382.
9. Koenig-Oberhuber V, Filipovic M. New antiplatelet drugs and new oral anticoagulants. Br J Anaesth. 2016;117(Suppl 2):ii74-84.
10. American Society of Regional Anesthesia and Pain Medicine. Anticoagulation Guidelines: Regional Anesthesia in the Patient Receiving Antithrombotic or Thrombolytic Therapy. American Society of Regional Anesthesia and Pain Medicine Evidence-Based Guidelines (Fourth Edition). Regional Anesthesia and Pain Medicine 2018;43:263-309. Available from https://www.asra.com/advisory-guidelines/ article/9/regional-anesthesia-in-the-patient-receiving-antithrombotic-orthrombolytic-ther. [Last accessed November, 2020].
11. Levine GN, Bates ER, Bittl JA, Brindis RG, Fihn SD, Fleisher LA, et al. 2016 ACC/AHA Guideline Focused Update on Duration of Dual Antiplatelet Therapy in Patients With Coronary Artery Disease: A Report of the American College of Cardiology/American Heart Association Task Force on Clinical Practice Guidelines: An Update of the 2011 ACCF/AHA/SCAI Guideline for Percutaneous Coronary Intervention, 2011 ACCF/AHA Guideline for Coronary Artery Bypass Graft Surgery, 2012 ACC/AHA/ACP/AATS/PCNA/SCAI/STS Guideline for the Diagnosis and Management of Patients With Stable Ischemic Heart Disease, 2013 ACCF/AHA Guideline for the Management of ST-Elevation Myocardial Infarction, 2014 AHA/ACC Guideline for the Management of Patients With Non-ST-Elevation Acute Coronary Syndromes, and 2014 ACC/AHA Guideline on Perioperative Cardiovascular Evaluation and Management of Patients Undergoing Noncardiac Surgery. Circulation. 2016;134(10):e123-55.
12. Singbartl G. Pre-operative autologous blood donation: clinical parameters and efficacy. Blood Transfus. 2011;9(1):10-8.
13. Walunj A, Babb A, Sharpe R. Autologous blood transfusion. Contin Educ Anaesth Crit Care Pain. 2006;6(5):192-6.
14. Transfusion Guidelines. Autologous blood transfusion (collection and reinfusion of the patient's own red blood cells). [online] Available from https://www.transfusionguidelines.org/transfusion-handbook/6-alternatives-and-adjuncts-to-blood-transfusion/6-1-autologous-blood-transfusion-collection-and-reinfusion-of-the-patient-s-own-red-blood-cells. [Last accessed October, 2020].
15. Manjuladevi M, Vasudeva Upadhyaya K. Perioperative blood management. Indian J Anaesth. 2014;58(5):573-80.
16. Rajagopalan S, Mascha E, Na J, Sessler DI. The effects of mild perioperative hypothermia on blood loss and transfusion requirement. Anesthesiology. 2008;108(1):71-7.
17. Richman JM, Rowlingson AJ, Maine DN, Courpas GE, Weller JF, Wu CL. Does neuraxial anesthesia reduce intraoperative blood loss?. A meta-analysis. J Clin Anesth. 2006;18(6):427-35.

18. Allam J, Cox M, Yentis SM. Cell salvage in obstetrics. Int J Obstet Anesth. 2008;17(1):37-45.
19. Klein AA, Bailey CR, Charlton AJ, Evans E, Guckian-Fisher M, McCrossan R, et al. Association of Anaesthetists guidelines: cell salvage for peri-operative blood conservation 2018. Anesthesia. 2018;73(9):1141-50.
20. Domen RE. Adverse reactions associated with autologous blood transfusion: evaluation and incidence at a large academic hospital. Transfusion (Paris). 1998;38(3):296-300.
21. Takemura M, Osugi H, Higashino M, Takada N, Lee S, Kinoshita H. Effect of substituting allogenic blood transfusion with autologous blood transfusion on outcomes after radical oesophagectomy for cancer. Ann Thorac Cardiovasc Surg. 2005;11(5):293-300.
22. Carless PA, Henry DA, Moxey AJ, O'connell DL, Brown T, Fergusson DA. Cell salvage for minimising perioperative allogeneic blood transfusion. Cochrane Database Syst Rev. 2006;(4):CD001888.
23. Franchini M, Mengoli C, Cruciani M, Bergamini V, Presti F, Marano G, et al. Safety and efficacy of tranexamic acid for prevention of obstetric haemorrhage: an updated systematic review and meta-analysis. Blood Transfus. 2018;16(4):329-37.
24. CRASH-2 collaborators, Roberts I, Shakur H, Afolabi A, Brohi K, Coats T, et al. The importance of early treatment with tranexamic acid in bleeding trauma patients: an exploratory analysis of the CRASH-2 randomised controlled trial. Lancet. 2011;377(9771):1096-101, 1101.e1-2.
25. Barak M, Yoav L, Abu el-Naaj I. Hypotensive anesthesia versus normotensive anesthesia during major maxillofacial surgery: a review of the literature. Scientific World J. 2015;2015:480728.
26. Barile L, Fominskiy E, Di Tomasso N, Alpìzar Castro LE, Landoni G, De Luca M, et al. Acute Normovolemic Hemodilution Reduces Allogeneic Red Blood Cell Transfusion in Cardiac Surgery: A Systematic Review and Meta-analysis of Randomized Trials. Anesth Analg. 2017;124(3):743-52.
27. Bisbe E, Moltó L. Pillar 2: minimising bleeding and blood loss. Best Pract Res Clin Anaesthesiol. 2013;27(1):99-110.
28. Sharma S, Sharma P, Tyler LN. Transfusion of blood and blood products: indications and complications. Am Fam Physician. 2011;83(6):719-24.
29. Shi H, Shi B, Lu J, Wu L, Sun G. Application value of thromboelastography in perioperative clinical blood transfusion and its effect on the outcome of patient. Exp Ther Med. 2019;17(5):3483-8.
30. Goubran HA, Elemary M, Radosevich M, Seghatchian J, El-Ekiaby M, Burnouf T. Impact of transfusion on cancer growth and outcome. Cancer Growth Metastasis. 2016;9:1-8.
31. Vamvakas EC. Meta-analysis of randomized controlled trials investigating the risk of postoperative infection in association with white blood cell-containing allogeneic blood transfusion: the effects of the type of transfused red blood cell product and surgical setting. Transfus Med Rev. 2002;16(4):304-14.
32. Brander L, Reil A, Bux J, Taleghani BM, Regli B, Takala J. Severe transfusion-related acute lung injury. Anesth Analg. 2005;101(2):499-501.

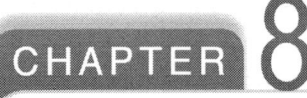

Newer Anticoagulants and Anesthesia

Bharti Wadhwa

INTRODUCTION

Anticoagulation is routinely used in many clinical settings and is a significant concern for the anesthesiologist managing such patients for routine or emergency surgery. The recently introduced direct acting oral anticoagulants overcome most of the limitations of warfarin and heparin use and have significant clinical benefits along with practical advantages of easier dosing schedules and no need for coagulation monitoring. The new oral anticoagulants (NOACs) available include dabigatran (antithrombin) and factor Xa inhibitors apixaban, edoxaban, and rivaroxaban.

Since the introduction of these NOACs into clinical practice, there has been increasing clinical evidence and studies published which has provided greater insight and numerous updates regarding their perioperative use. Not only the underlying pathology, but also the perioperative management of anticoagulant therapy is vital to management of anesthetic goals. NOACs have definite practical advantages of rapid onset of action, short elimination half-life, and predictable anticoagulant effects with no requirement for routine coagulation monitoring, but high individual variability in plasma levels makes the perioperative management challenging.

This chapter reviews the available literature and discusses the practical approach to perioperative management of NOACs in the perioperative settings.

UNDERSTANDING THE COAGULATION PATHWAY

Hemostasis is the result of complex interactions between the coagulation and the fibrinolytic system, the platelets and the vessel wall. The goal of coagulation is fibrin formation. The classic intrinsic and extrinsic pathways of coagulation cascade, both, converge on factor X activation. In combination with factor V, phospholipids and calcium, the activated factor X forms the prothrombinase complex that converts prothrombin to thrombin. Thrombin then converts the circulating inactive fibrinogen into insoluble fibrin and activates factor XIII, which covalently crosslinks fibrin polymers in the platelet plug. This creates a fibrin network, stabilizing the clot and forms a definitive secondary hemostatic plug. This creates a fibrin network, which stabilizes the clot and forms a definitive secondary hemostatic plug.[1]

The most important component of the coagulation cascade is thrombin. Thrombin not only converts fibrinogen to fibrin, but also amplifies its own generation by feedback activation of factors V, VIII, and XI and is a potent platelet agonist. Therefore, thrombin inhibition does not only attenuate fibrin formation but also reduces thrombin generation and platelet activation.

In vivo, the coagulation process is under the inhibitory control of several inhibitors that limit the clot formation and a balance is maintained between the hemostatic and hemorrhagic components. The naturally occurring anticoagulant mechanisms in the body include antithrombin, tissue factor plasminogen inhibitor (Protein S), Protein C pathway and Protein Z-dependent protease inhibitor/protein Z (PZI).

PHYSIOLOGY OF THERAPEUTIC ANTICOAGULATION

Therapeutic anticoagulation is based on inhibition of thrombin or factor Xa. Heparin binds to antithrombin III causing a conformational change and its activation. The activated antithrombin then inactivates thrombin, factor Xa and other proteases. The inactivation of thrombin prevents fibrin formation as well as inhibits the thrombin-induced activation of platelets and of factors V and VIII.[2] Vitamin K antagonists (VKAs), like warfarin exert their anticoagulant effect by inhibition of vitamin K-dependent synthesis of clotting factors II, VII, IX, and X, as well as the regulatory proteins C, S, and Z.[2] The newer direct acting oral anticoagulants are either reversible inhibitors of thrombin (dabigatran 2010) or factor Xa inhibitors (rivaroxaban 2011, apixaban 2012, and edoxaban 2015).[3]

LIMITATIONS OF TRADITIONALLY USED ANTICOAGULANTS

Low-molecular-weight Heparin and Fondaparinux

Introduction of low-molecular-weight heparin (LMWH) and fondaparinux simplified heparin therapy as they could be administered subcutaneously without coagulation monitoring and had lower risk of heparin-induced thrombocytopenia. However, certain limitations persist:
- The subcutaneous route of injection limits their long-term use in patients.
- The lack of antidote for fondaparinux, especially considering its long half-life is a serious concern.
- Protamine sulfate can only partly neutralize the anticoagulation of LMWH and has no effect on that of fondaparinux which can be problematic in an emergency situation or bleeding patient.[3]
- Routine coagulation monitoring is necessary to maintain the international normalized ratio (INR) in the therapeutic range that can be inconvenient for the patient as well as increase the healthcare burden.

Warfarin

Warfarin is a time-tested drug but has a narrow therapeutic window. So, its dose needs to be adjusted based on regular monitoring of INR. Quick reversibility of action in emergency situations is not feasible due to its long duration of action (2–5 days). Also, there is need for preoperative bridging therapy. Warfarin is primarily metabolized through the cytochrome P450 system. Drug interactions due to induction or inhibition of the enzyme system leading to alteration in metabolism which can increase the INR significantly.[2,4] Warfarin therapy also requires diet restriction for foods that are rich in vitamin K.

DIRECT ACTING ORAL ANTICOAGULANTS

The NOAC agents overcome most of the limitations of traditional anticoagulant therapy in that:[5]
- Rapid onset and offset of action obviate the need for preoperative bridging therapy.
- Predictable anticoagulant action precludes need for routine coagulation monitoring.
- They have specific enzyme action with low risk of side effects.
- There is no need for restriction of vitamin K rich foods (warfarin diet).
- There are fewer drug restrictions and low potential for drug interactions.
- They have practical advantages of oral dosing.

With these potential benefits and practical advantages, NOACs are being increasingly preferred in the treatment of venous thromboembolic disease (rivaroxaban) or the prevention of systematic embolism in atrial fibrillation (AF) (rivaroxaban, dabigatran) over warfarin.[3,6] Three large-scale randomized NOAC trials, the Randomized Evaluation of Long-Term Anticoagulant Therapy (RE-LY) trial which compared dabigatran etexilate with warfarin for stroke prevention in patients with AF. Rivaroxaban Once-daily oral direct Factor Xa Inhibition Compared with Vitamin K antagonism for prevention of stroke and Embolism Trial in AF (ROCKET-AF) trial and the Apixaban for Reduction In Stroke and Other Thromboembolic Events in AF (ARISTOTLE) trial have reported that in these patients the therapeutic action of NOACs was either superior to warfarin, or comparable with a similar rate of bleeding risk (rivaroxaban) or a lower risk of hemorrhage (dabigatran, apixaban).[7-9]

PHARMACOKINETICS OF NEWER ORAL ANTICOAGULANTS

The NOACs offer a suitable alternative and are fast gaining acceptance in clinical practice. Anesthesiologist may encounter patients on novel oral anticoagulants in different clinical situations: trauma, elective or emergent surgical procedures, spontaneous or postoperative bleeding, overdose, etc. The optimal management of anticoagulation in patients undergoing surgical procedures is challenging. Early interruption of anticoagulant therapy may transiently increase thromboembolism risk while a delayed discontinuation would increase the risk of bleeding and delay anticoagulant resumption.[10]

TABLE 1: Pharmacokinetics of NOACs

	Dabigatran	Rivaroxaban	Apixaban	Edoxaban
Action	Direct prothrombin inhibitor	Direct factor Xa inhibitor	Direct factor Xa inhibitor	Direct factor Xa inhibitor
Prodrug	Yes	No	No	No
Bioavailability	6%	60–80%	66%	58%
T_{Max} (peak plasma concentration)	1.5–3 hours	2.5–4 hours	3 hours	1.5 hours
Half life	12–17 hours	7–13 hours	8–15 hours	9–11 hours
Time to onset of action	0.5–2 hours	2–4 hours	1–3 hours	1–2 hours
Elimination	80% renal	70% renal (30% unchanged, 40% inactive, and 30% fecal)	25% renal	35% renal

(NOACs: newer oral anticoagulants; T_{Max}: time maximum)

It is, therefore, important to understand the pharmacodynamics of these drugs in order to fully understand their anesthetic implications **(Table 1)**.[11,12]

Dabigatran

Dabigatran is a direct acting reversible thrombin inhibitor that directly inhibits free and fibrin-bound thrombin without the need for antithrombin. It is a prodrug with a rapid onset of action and peak plasma concentration 1.5–3 hours after oral intake and a half-life of 12–17 hours in healthy volunteers.[4] The plasma protein binding of dabigatran is 35%, and 80% of the drug undergoes renal excretion in the unchanged form. The anticoagulant effect of dabigatran is prolonged in renal insufficiency. The protein binding of dabigatran is relatively low and thus, can be eliminated by hemodialysis in case of accidental over dosages. It can be safely administered in liver disorders and dose adjustment is not required.[5,6]

Factor Xa Inhibitors

Rivaroxaban is an oral, direct factor Xa inhibitor that has good bioavailability (80%), and is highly protein-bound with peak plasma concentrations occur within 2–4 hours of administration. Elimination of rivaroxaban is reduced only partially in renal impairment as 30% of the renal excretion is in active form.

Apixaban and edoxaban have good oral bioavailability, are highly protein bound with peak plasma concentrations within 2–3 hours and 1.5 hours after intake respectively.[6,12]

PRACTICAL CONCERNS WITH PERIOPERATIVE MANAGEMENT OF ANTICOAGULATION

The newer direct oral anticoagulants have a shorter half-life with a rapid onset (1-3 hours to peak action) and offset of action which has simplified discontinuation and resumption of treatment in the perioperative period. However, the practical concerns that need to be addressed include:
- Role of bridging therapy.
- Drug interactions.
- Optimal timing for the discontinuation and resumption of NOACs for surgery and neuraxial anesthesia.
- Preoperative coagulation monitoring with NOACs.
- Antidote for reversal of action.

Bridging Therapy and Newer Oral Anticoagulants

Traditionally used anticoagulants like warfarin take 2-5 days for reduction as well as restoration of anticoagulant effect. Bridging therapy with shorter acting anticoagulant heparin helps tide over the perioperative period but risks and benefits of "bridging" are unclear with NOACs. Most NOACs have a short elimination half-life of 8-14 hours and preoperative bridging therapy is not required and would not only be of questionable efficacy, but may even increase the risk of bleeding.[10,13]

Drug Interactions

Unrecognized drug-drug interactions can lead to inaccurate dosing and a higher risk of either thromboembolic and/or bleeding complications. It is important to look for co-medications with significant drug interactions in the preoperative evaluation. While the elimination of NOACs is primarily through renal route, P-glycoproteins (P-gp) transport proteins and cytochrome P450 enzymes play a partial role in the elimination of NOAC. Drugs that use similar pathways may lead to drug interactions resulting in over-or under-anticoagulation **(Table 2)**.[14]

Co-medication with amiodarone and fluconazole has been reported to be associated with elevated levels of dabigatran and rivaroxaban and increased risk for bleeding, especially in patients with reduced renal function. Administration of verapamil just before dabigatran leads to markedly elevated dabigatran drug levels, and should be avoided in patients with renal insufficiency; whereas, concurrent use of diltiazem can lead to raised rivaroxaban plasma levels. Food and Drug Administration (FDA) recommends avoiding concurrent use of rifampin, carbamazepine, phenytoin, and phenobarbital with both apixaban and rivaroxaban.[15] Surprisingly, higher bleeding risk with rifampicin and phenytoin in patients taking NOACs was observed, which is inexplicable as co-administration of rifampicin and phenytoin leads to lower NOAC plasma concentration.[15]

There are no reported interactions of NOACs with anesthetic drugs. Drug interactions with co-medications must be kept in mind during preoperative

TABLE 2: Drug interactions with NOACs (+ increased plasma levels)

Drug	Dabigatran	Apixaban	Edoxaban	Rivaroxaban
Amiodarone	++	No data	++	+
Digoxin	No effect	No effect	No effect	No effect
Diltiazem	No effect	++	No data	+
Quinidine	++	No data	+++	No data
Verapamil	+++	No data	++	+
Clarithromycin, erythromycin	+	No data	+++	++
Rifampicin	↓↓	↓↓	↓↓	↓↓
Carbamazepine, phenytoin, and phenobarbital	↓↓	↓↓	↓↓	↓↓
Fluconazole	No data	No data	No data	++
Antacids, PPI	↓	No effect	No effect	No effect

(PPI: proton pump inhibitor; NOACs: newer oral anticoagulants)

evaluation of a patient on NOACs to rule out supratherapeutic action and higher risk of bleeding.

Coagulation Tests/Monitoring

Presence of residual anticoagulant levels after discontinuation of NOAC therapy can be determined by preoperative coagulation monitoring. If residual anticoagulant activity is present in the preoperative period, the timing of the procedure may be delayed or the action reversed to reduce risk of bleeding.[16] However, NOAC specific coagulation tests are not widely available, reference ranges are lacking, and may not confer much benefit.[17] Patients on NOACs have a predictable anticoagulant effect by virtue of their pharmacodynamic and pharmacokinetic profiles and do not require routine coagulation monitoring. However, there are certain clinical situations when urgent assessment of the anticoagulant effect of NOACs is required.[18] These specific situations include:

- Before surgery or invasive procedure with last NOAC dose within 24 hours (or longer if creatinine clearance <50 mL/min).
- Bleeding patient on NOAC therapy.
- Newer oral anticoagulant overdose.
- Renal insufficiency.
- Thrombosis on treatment (to assess whether there is failure of therapy or lack of adherence).

Routine coagulation tests: Prothrombin time (PT), activated partial thromboplastin time (aPTT), and thrombin time (TT). The coagulation tests commonly used in clinical practice include PT, aPTT, and TT. Although PT is not the most conclusive of all tests available, it is commonly used in clinical practice for screening and coagulation studies.[19]

Dabigatran prolongs the aPTT and TT more than the PT. Out of these, TT is a more sensitive test and even low levels of dabigatran can prolong the TT. This means that a normal TT in dabigatran-treated patients can be safely taken

TABLE 3: Standard coagulation tests and NOAC

	Dabigatran	Apixaban	Edoxaban	Rivaroxaban
PT	–	↑	↑	↑
aPTT	↑↑	↑	↑	↑
TT	↑↑↑	–	–	–
Anti-F Xa	–	↑↑	↑↑	↑↑

(PT: prothrombin time; aPTT: activated partial thromboplastin time; TT: thrombin time; F Xa: factor Xa; NOAC: newer oral anticoagulant)

up for surgery even in the presence of high bleeding risk. A normal TT rules out any residual anticoagulant activity of dabigatran.[20] On the other hand, rivaroxaban and edoxaban prolong the PT more than the aPTT and they have no effect on the TT. Apixaban has little effect on either PT or aPTT.[21]

Normal values of PT do not exclude the presence of significant levels of factor Xa inhibitors and there exists a high variability in the interpretation of results. Consequently, PT is not recommended as a universal test for anticoagulant effect of NOACs.[12] Whereas, aPTT is a useful tool for assessment for dabigatran levels, normal values might still indicate presence of the drug.[22]

Antifactor Xa assay: The most reliable and accurate estimation of plasma levels of factor Xa inhibitors rivaroxaban, apixaban and edoxaban can be done with the antifactor Xa assay using the specific drug for calibration **(Table 3)**.

Point of care monitoring and other global assays: More specific and accurate monitoring for NOACs include Point-of-Care (POC) monitoring and assays like thromboelastography, thromboelastometry, thrombin generation assay, prothrombinase-induced clotting time, and activated clotting time. However, their application in clinical practice is limited as they are expensive, lack standardization and are not easily available.[23]

PERIOPERATIVE MANAGEMENT OF NEWER ORAL ANTICOAGULANT

The practical approach to perioperative management of NOAC is based on the estimation of the thromboembolic risk and bleeding risk as well as the elimination half-life of the NOAC. Interruption interval of NOAC therapy that is too long may increase the risk for thromboembolism, whereas an interruption interval that is too short may increase the risk for bleeding which, in turn, delays anticoagulant resumption. Thus, it is imperative that a balance is established between the risk of thromboembolism and prevention of excessive bleeding for each patient. To ensure minimal bleeding risk during surgery in a patient on NOACs, the timing of last dose and elimination half-life should be considered.

Estimation of Thromboembolic and Bleeding Risk

Thromboembolic risk: The risk of thromboembolism can be estimated from the duration since last episode of venous thromboembolism (VTE). The risk of thromboembolism is high if the last VTE episode occurred within the last 3 months. Whereas, the risk is low if the VTE episode was more than 12 months back. Between 3 and 12 months, the risk of thromboembolism was intermediate [American College of Chest Physicians (ACCP Guidelines)]. If surgery is planned within 3 months of VTE, NOAC discontinuation should be avoided and in case discontinuation is necessary, bridging therapy with heparin should be considered in consultation with a multidisciplinary team.[24]

Bleeding risk: The bleeding risk will depend on both, the bleeding risk of the patient and expected bleeding risk of the procedure. The bleeding risk of the patient can be determined by various factors and different scores such as the HAS-BLED score, the ORBIT bleeding risk score and the novel biomarker-based ABC–bleeding risk score can quantify the bleeding risk.[25]

The bleeding risk of invasive procedures can be classified into low risk, moderate risk and high risk procedures. Examples of procedure/surgery with low bleeding risk include superficial skin surgery such as abscess drainage, dermatologic procedures, cataract extraction, endoscopic surgery without biopsy, etc. Other procedures can be classified as low to moderate bleeding risk (e.g., laparoscopic cholecystectomy or hernia repair), or high bleeding risk (e.g., cardiovascular, intracranial or spine surgery, major cancer surgery, any surgery with spinal or epidural anesthesia). The CORDIA study recommended the time to discontinuation of NOACs prior to elective surgery based on the bleeding risk and pharmacokinetics of the drug.[26]

Elimination Half-life and Preoperative Interruption of Newer Oral Anticoagulant

The elimination half-life of the direct acting oral anticoagulant is an important consideration for discontinuation of the drug preoperatively. For surgery with low and intermediate bleeding risk, an interruption for the duration of 2 3 half-lives of the NOAC can safely reduce hemorrhagic risk. High bleeding risk surgery and neuraxial anesthesia requires an interruption for the duration of 4–5 half-lives of the drug. Renal insufficiency can prolong the elimination half-life and may require longer period of discontinuation in the preoperative period.[27]

The anticoagulant effect can be increased in the presence of severe liver insufficiency (factor Xa inhibitors), renal insufficiency (greatest with dabigatran followed by edoxaban, rivaroxaban and apixaban), and co-medications such as amiodarone and fluconazole. Older age and extreme low body weight (<50 kg) are other factors that can increase the half-life of NOAC **(Table 4)**.

Preoperative Anticoagulant Interruption
Elective Surgery

In a patient posted for elective surgery, preoperative discontinuation of NOACs is advised except in cases where the risk of bleeding is very low. A systemic review and meta-analysis by Hovaguimian et al. suggested that interrupting

TABLE 4: Discontinuation of NOAC prior to elective surgery (Sx: Surgery)

	Cr clearance	Low bleeding risk	High bleeding risk
Dabigatran	>50 mL/min	24–36 hours before Sx	48–72 hours before Sx
	<50 mL/min	48 hours before Sx	96 hours before Sx
Apixaban	>50 mL/min	24 hours before Sx	48 hours before Sx
	<50 mL/min	48 hours before Sx	48 hours before Sx
Edoxaban	>50 mL/min	24 hours before Sx	48 hours before Sx
	<50 mL/min	48 hours before Sx	72 hours before Sx
Rivaroxaban	>50 mL/min	24 hours before Sx	48 hours before Sx
	<50 mL/min	24–48 hours before Sx	48–72 hours before Sx

(NOAC: newer oral anticoagulant; Cr: creatinine)

anticoagulation in patients requiring invasive procedures did not seem to result in harm and protected against major bleeding.[28] During the duration of discontinuation of NOACs, bridging therapy has not been found to be useful as it does not reduce the risk of thromboembolic events but can further increase the risk of bleeding.[29]

Management protocol for interruption of newer oral anticoagulant therapy in elective surgery:
- For low bleeding risk elective surgery, discontinuation of NOACs is not required. To minimize the risk of bleeding further, the time of administration of the morning dose of anticoagulant may be adjusted to avoid peak plasma concentration during the procedure.[30]
- For a patient on a BD dosing schedule, the NOAC should be omitted after the morning dose of the day before surgery.
- For a patient on OD dosing schedule, the last dose should be on the morning of the day before the surgery.
- For a patient on OD dosing schedule with every evening intake, the last dose should be 2 days before the surgery.[30]

Time to Restart of Newer Oral Anticoagulant after Surgery

Spahn et al. suggested that in patients who undergo surgery with low bleeding risk, NOAC may be resumed 24 hours after surgery and in surgeries with high bleeding risk, the NOACs can be resumed 48–72 hours after surgery in the absence of ongoing bleeding and/or a surgical contraindication.[12] To simplify, NOAC administration can be resumed after the end of the invasive procedure as follows:
- *OD regimen with an evening intake*: Restart in the evening.
- *OD regimen with a morning intake*: Restart in the morning.
- *BD regimen*: Restart evening of the same day.

EMERGENCY SURGERY

Preoperative management will depend on time to last dose, NOAC plasma levels if feasible, specific coagulation tests and availability of antidote.

Time to Last Dose

The acceptable time to last dose of NOACs is >24 hours but very often in an emergency situation, it may not be possible to ascertain the time to last dose.

Newer Oral Anticoagulant Plasma Levels

In emergency situations, where the time to last oral intake cannot be ascertained and risk of bleeding is high, plasma level concentration may guide the preoperative management. Monitoring the plasma levels is especially useful in patients with renal insufficiency. For an emergency surgery with high bleeding risk, plasma levels should be less or equal to 30 ng/mL for dabigatran and rivaroxaban for safe conduct of surgery. Plasma concentration levels of more than 200 ng/mL are expected to have a significant risk of hemorrhage perioperatively.[6] In patients with plasma levels between 30 and 200 ng/mL, each case will need individual assessment, depending on the risk of bleeding.[31]

Coagulation Tests

The role of routine coagulation tests to assess the anticoagulant effect of NOACs is complex. The tests are not entirely reliable, as the responsiveness of these tests is to some extent, coagulometer and reagent dependent.[22] Furthermore, the NOACs have different responsiveness to the standard coagulation tests as discussed before and can be prolonged in many situations such as in traumatic coagulopathy **(Table 4)**. For reliable and accurate estimation of NOAC plasma concentrations, specific assays with the appropriate reagents and methods must be employed.

ADMINISTRATION OF ANTIDOTE

The specific antidote for dabigatran is idarucizumab (US FDA 2015). Idarucizumab is a humanized mouse Fab (monoclonal antibody fragment), which selectively binds to dabigatran and reverses dabigatran-induced anticoagulation. Idarucizumab can reverse the anticoagulant effects of dabigatran within 8 hours and can be used in patients with a major bleeding event, or requiring emergency surgery within 12–24 hours of intake of last oral dose. The reversal of anticoagulant effect is immediate and lasts up to 24 hours.[32] Standard coagulation tests are recommended 10 minutes after administration of idarucizumab to rule out other coagulation defects.[12]

For factor Xa inhibitors, the specific antidote is andexanet alfa which is a modified recombinant derivative of factor Xa and may soon be available (approved May 2018 in the US) for clinical practice. It is a reversal agent for not only factor Xa inhibitors but also LMWHs, and fondaparinux. However, andexanet-alfa has not been studied for reversal of anticoagulation in surgical patients to date.

Recently, a synthetic molecule ciraparantag (PER977, previously known as aripazine) that binds to factor Xa inhibitors, dabigatran, and heparins is under research as use as a reversal agent. It is being considered as a potential universal antidote for many anticoagulants.

The role of the antidotes is limited and not recommended for preoperative reversal as a routine. Wherever possible interventions should be delayed to enable anticoagulant clearance and all measures should be employed to stop bleeding with local hemostatic and supportive measures especially in patients with renal function.

Suggested Protocol for Management in a Patient for Emergency Surgery

The stepwise management includes assessment of the thromboembolic and bleeding risks and estimating half-life from the time to last intake of NOAC.

If last intake of NOAC > 24 hours, low bleeding risk: Proceed with surgery. Due to the short duration of action of NOACs, the discontinuation of the drug and supportive measures is in most cases sufficient to control the problem in low bleeding risk patients.

If last intake of NOAC within 12–24 hours and high bleeding risk procedure:
- Specific coagulation assay to assess anticoagulant activity.
- *Newer oral anticoagulant plasma levels*: Low risk if <30 ng/mL: proceed with surgery. High risk of hemorrhage with levels more than 200 ng/mL.
- Activated charcoal per oral to reduce bioavailability by reduction of intestinal absorption.
- Diuretics to increase in NOAC clearance, especially for patients taking dabigatran procedure needs to be rapidly planned.[31]
- Hemodialysis can be done for removal of dabigatran in high bleeding risk surgery.

In Patients with Severe Bleeding or High Bleeding Risk Emergency Surgery

- Use of tranexamic acid and desmopressin can help reduce bleeding.
- Blood transfusions and other supportive measures.
- Administration of prothrombin complex concentrates (PCCs) to provide coagulation factors. PCC contain lyophilized human plasma-derived vitamin K-dependent coagulation factors (clotting factors II, VII, IX, and X), anticoagulation proteins such as protein C, protein S, protein Z, antithrombin and heparin.[33] It can help control bleeding but should be considered only in patients on NOACs with life-threatening, severe bleeding.
- Specific antidotes are recommended for reversal of anticoagulation in patients requiring emergency surgery within 12–24 hours of intake of last oral dose of NOAC.

In a study with patients using rivaroxaban, majority of episodes of severe bleeding, could be controlled with supportive measures like local therapy or red blood cell transfusions and only 37% of patients required an intervention or surgery.[27]

For patients with high risk bleeding standard supportive measures, tranexamic acid, desmopressin blood transfusions and nonspecific reversal agents are recommended for controlling bleeding.[34] Pro-hemostatic agents such as PCCs, and activated factor VII have been tried for the NOAC-related bleeding with varying degrees of success.[35]

Hemodialysis can remove up to 60% of circulating dabigatran, while administration of activated charcoal may be useful to reduce absorption of dabigatran, if taken within 2 hours of ingestion, and rivaroxaban or apixaban if taken within 6 hours after overdose or accidental ingestion.[36]

NEURAXIAL BLOCK AND NEWER ORAL ANTICOAGULANT

The risk of neuraxial hematoma after administration of epidural or subarachnoid block is 1/220,000 and 1/320,000, respectively.[36] Although low, this incidence can increase by up to two times with multiple attempts, presence of spinal abnormalities, coexisting inherited or acquired coagulopathies, and coadministration of anticoagulant therapy. It is, thus, desirable that neuraxial block be administered in the presence of complete hemostatic function.

The American Society of Regional Anesthesia (ASRA) recommends an interval of five half-lives to allow complete elimination between discontinuation of NOAC and medium or high-risk pain procedures and neuraxial block.[37] Spahn et al. also make similar recommendations.[12] Due to the variability in NOAC metabolism and elimination, this period of five elimination half-lives corresponds to interruption of dabigatran for 4–5 days and rivaroxaban and apixaban for 3 days prior to the neuraxial block. The French Working Group on Perioperative Hemostasis proposes discontinuation of NOACs 5 days prior to neuraxial anesthesia.[30] Douketis et al. suggested that due to variability in NOAC plasma concentration, ideal timing of stopping NOAC treatment should be based on residual plasma concentration rather than based on elimination half-lives as per ASRA guidelines.[38] Both neuraxial puncture and the removal of a catheter are expected to have a comparable bleeding.

Restart of Newer Oral Anticoagulants after Neuraxial Block

After administration of a neuraxial block, formation of a stable clot takes 8 hours. For pain procedures, the recent ASRA guidelines suggest NOAC administration may be resumed after an interval of 24 hours, unless there is a high risk of VTE.[35] A longer delay is required, if there are multiple punctures or traumatic insertion of spinal or epidural catheter.[36] There is limited data on the safety of prophylactic dose NOAC, whilst a patient has an epidural catheter in situ, and therefore it is not recommended.

New oral anticoagulants may be resumed 6–8 hours after the end of a low bleeding-risk surgery. However, in the event of bleeding during needle puncture, bloody tap or catheter placement anticoagulant therapy should be delayed further by about 24 hours postsurgery.[37]

CONCLUSION

The perioperative management of NOACs needs careful consideration and a multidisciplinary approach. The preoperative evaluation must include assessment of thromboembolic and bleeding risk, time to last dose of NOAC, renal function as well as co-medications for potential drug interactions. With increasing clinical evidence, consensus is building on the timing of interruption of NOACs and resumption of therapy after the procedure. For an emergency surgery with high bleeding risk, NOAC plasma levels should be less or equal to 30 ng/mL for dabigatran and rivaroxaban for safe conduct of surgery. Accurate estimate of NOACs requires specific coagulation assays such as TT for dabigatran, anti-Xa levels for oral Xa inhibitors. However, standard coagulation screening tests such as PT for rivaroxaban and aPTT for dabigatran may provide a qualitative assessment of residual NOAC anticoagulant effect. Recently, antidote has been introduced for dabigatran but its role is limited and is not recommended for preoperative reversal as a routine. Wherever possible, interventions should be delayed to enable anticoagulant clearance and all measures should be employed to stop bleeding with local hemostatic and supportive measures especially in patients with impaired renal function.

KEY POINTS

- The newer oral anticoagulants (NOACs) overcome most limitations of warfarin and heparin and have significant clinical benefits along with practical advantages of easier dosing schedules and predictable coagulant action.
- A shorter half-life with a rapid onset and offset of action has simplified discontinuation and resumption of treatment in the perioperative period.
- Bridging therapy during NOAC interruption is of questionable efficacy and may even increase the risk of bleeding.
- Perioperative management involves assessment of thromboembolic and bleeding risk and elimination half-life of NOAC.
- Interruption of anticoagulation is not necessary for procedures with low risk of bleeding.
- Discontinuation of NOAC is recommended more than 24 hours preoperatively for low to moderate bleeding risk procedures and greater than 48 hours for high bleeding risk surgery.
- Renal insufficiency can prolong the elimination half-life depending on the specific NOAC and may require longer discontinuation of NOAC.
- For an emergency surgery with high bleeding risk, plasma levels should be less or equal to 30 ng/mL for dabigatran and rivaroxaban for safe conduct of surgery.
- Neuraxial procedures require interruption of dabigatran at least 5 days prior, and rivaroxaban and apixaban 3 days prior to the procedure.
- The role of the antidotes is limited and not recommended for preoperative reversal as a routine.

REFERENCES

1. Hall JE. Haemostasis and blood coagulation. In: Guyton and Hall Textbook of Medical Physiology: Enhanced E-Book, 11th edition. Philadelphia: Elsevier Health Sciences; 2010. pp. 457-9.
2. Harter K, Levine M, Henderson SO. Anticoagulation drug therapy: a review. West J Emerg Med. 2015;16(1):11-7.
3. Weitz JI, Hirsh J, Samama MM. New antithrombotic drugs: American College of Chest Physicians Evidence-Based Clinical Practice Guidelines (8th edition). Chest. 2008;133(6 Suppl):234S-56S.
4. Alquwaizani M, Buckley L, Adams C, Fanikos J. Anticoagulants: a review of pharmacology, dosing, and complications. Curr Emerg Hosp Med Rep. 2013;1(2):83-97.
5. Eikelboom JW, Weitz JI. New anticoagulants. Circulation. 2010;121(13):1523-32.
6. Levy JH, Key NS, Azran MS. Novel oral anticoagulants: implications in the perioperative setting. Anesthesiology. 2010;113(3):726-45.
7. Connolly SJ, Ezekowitz MD, Yusuf S, Eikelboom J, Oldgren J, Parekh A, et al. Dabigatran versus warfarin in patients with atrial fibrillation. N Engl J Med. 2009;361(12):1139-51.
8. Patel MR, Mahaffey KW, Garg J, Pan G, Singer DE, Hacke W, et al. Rivaroxaban versus warfarin in nonvalvular atrial fibrillation. N Engl J Med. 2011;365(10):883-91.
9. Lopes RD, Alexander JH, Al-Khatib SM, Ansell J, Diaz R, Easton JD, et al. Apixaban for reduction in stroke and other ThromboemboLic events in atrial fibrillation (ARISTOTLE) trial: design and rationale. Am Heart J. 2010;159(3):331-9.
10. Dunn AS, Spyropoulos AC, Turpie AG. Bridging therapy in patients on long-term oral anticoagulants who require surgery: the Prospective Peri-operative Enoxaparin Cohort Trial (PROSPECT). J Thromb Haemost. 2007;5(11):2211-8.
11. Mekaj YH, Mekaj AY, Duci SB, Miftari EI. New oral anticoagulants: their advantages and disadvantages compared with vitamin K antagonists in the prevention and treatment of patients with thromboembolic events. Ther Clin Risk Manag. 2015;11:967-77.
12. Spahn DR, Beer JH, Borgeat A, Chassot PG, Kern C, Mach F, et al. NOACs in Anesthesiology. Transfus Med Hemother. 2019;46(4):282-93.
13. Douketis JD, Healey JS, Brueckmann M, Eikelboom JW, Ezekowitz MD, Fraessdorf M, et al. Perioperative bridging anticoagulation during dabigatran or warfarin interruption among patients who had an elective surgery or procedure. Substudy of the RE-LY trial. Thromb Haemost. 2015;113(3):625-32.
14. Wessler JD, Grip LT, Mendell J, Giugliano RP. The P-glycoprotein transport system and cardiovascular drugs. J Am Coll Cardiol. 2013;61(25):2495-502.
15. Chang SH, Chou IJ, Yeh YH, Chiou MJ, Wen MS, Kuo CT, et al. Association between use of non-vitamin K oral anticoagulants with and without concurrent medications and risk of major bleeding in nonvalvular atrial fibrillation. JAMA. 2017;318(13):1250-9.
16. Tripodi A. To measure or not to measure direct oral anticoagulants before surgery or invasive procedures: reply. J Thromb Haemost. 2016;14(12):2559-61.
17. Spyropoulos AC, Al-Badri A, Sherwood MW, Douketis JD. To measure or not to measure direct oral anticoagulants before surgery or invasive procedures: comment. J Thromb Haemost. 2016;14(12):2556-9.
18. Baglin T, Keeling D, Kitchen S. Effects on routine coagulation screens and assessment of anticoagulant intensity in patients taking oral dabigatran or rivaroxaban: guidance from the British Committee for Standards in Haematology. Br J Haematol. 2012;159(4):427-9.

19. Salmonson T, Dogné JM, Janssen H, Garcia Burgos J, Blake P. Non-vitamin-K oral anticoagulants and laboratory testing: now and in the future: views from a workshop at the European Medicines Agency (EMA). Eur Heart J Cardiovasc Pharmacother. 2017;3(1):42-7.
20. Tran H, Joseph J, Young L, McRae S, Curnow J, Nandurkar H, et al. New oral anticoagulants: a practical guide on prescription, laboratory testing and periprocedural/bleeding management. Australasian Society of Thrombosis and Haemostasis. Intern Med J. 2014;44(6):525-36.
21. Cuker A, Siegal DM, Crowther MA, Garcia DA. Laboratory measurement of the anticoagulant activity of the non-vitamin K oral anticoagulants. J Am Coll Cardiol. 2014;64(11):1128-39.
22. Douxfils J, Mullier F, Robert S, Chatelain C, Chatelain B, Dogné JM. Impact of dabigatran on a large panel of routine or specific coagulation assays. Laboratory recommendations for monitoring of dabigatran etexilate. Thromb Haemost. 2012;107(5):985-97.
23. Weitz JI, Eikelboom JW. Urgent need to measure effects of direct oral anticoagulants. Circulation. 2016;134(3):186-8.
24. Douketis JD, Spyropoulos AC, Spencer FA, Mayr M, Jaffer AK, Eckman MH, et al. Perioperative management of antithrombotic therapy: Antithrombotic Therapy and Prevention of Thrombosis, 9th edition: American College of Chest Physicians Evidence-Based Clinical Practice Guidelines. Chest. 2012;141(2 Suppl):e326S-50S.
25. Dubois V, Dincq AS, Douxfils J, Ickx B, Samama CM, Dogné JM, et al. Perioperative management of patients on direct oral anticoagulants. Thromb J. 2017;15:14.
26. Godier A, Dincq A, Radu A, Leblanc I, Antona M, Vasse M, et al. Predictors of preprocedural concentrations of direct oral anticoagulants: a prospective multicentre study. Eur Heart J. 2017;38(31):2431-9.
27. Beyer-Westendorf J, Gelbricht V, Förster K, Ebertz F, Köhler C, Werth S, et al. Periinterventional management of novel oral anticoagulants in daily care: results from the prospective Dresden NOAC registry. Eur Heart J. 2014;35(28):1888-96.
28. Hovaguimian F, Köppel S, Spahn DR. Safety of anticoagulation interruption in patients undergoing surgery or invasive procedures: a systematic review and meta-analyses of randomized controlled trials and non-randomized studies. World J Surg. 2017;41(10):2444-56.
29. Raval AN, Cigarroa JE, Chung MK, Diaz-Sandoval LJ, Diercks D, Piccini JP, et al. Management of patients on non-vitamin K antagonist oral anticoagulants in the acute care and periprocedural setting: a scientific statement from the American Heart Association. Circulation. 2017;135(10):e604-33.
30. Levy JH, Verhamme P, Sellke FW, Reilly PA, Dubiel R, Eikelboom J, et al. Initial experience with idarucizumab in dabigatran-treated patients requiring emergency surgery or intervention: interim results from the RE-VERSE AD™ Study. London: European Society of Cardiology; 2015.
31. Grottke O, Aisenberg J, Bernstein R, Goldstein P, Huisman MV, Jamieson DG, et al. Efficacy of prothrombin complex concentrates for the emergency reversal of dabigatran-induced anticoagulation. Crit Care. 2016;20(1):115.
32. Weitz JI, Pollack CV Jr. Practical management of bleeding in patients receiving non-vitamin K antagonist oral anticoagulants. Thromb Haemost. 2015;114(6):1113-26.
33. Suryanarayan D, Schulman S. Potential antidotes for reversal of old and new oral anticoagulants. Thromb Res. 2014;133(Suppl 2):S158-66.

34. Dalal J, Bhave A, Chaudhry G, Rana P. Reversal agents for NOACs: connecting the dots. Indian Heart J. 2016;68(4):559-63.
35. Horlocker TT, Wedel DJ, Rowlingson JC, Enneking FK, Kopp SL, Benzon HT, et al. Regional anesthesia in the patient receiving antithrombotic or thrombolytic therapy: American Society of Regional Anesthesia and Pain Medicine evidence-based guidelines (third edition). Reg Anesth Pain Med. 2010;35(1):64-101.
36. Narouze S, Benzon HT, Provenzano DA, Buvanendran A, De Andres J, Deer TR, et al. Interventional spine and pain procedures in patients on antiplatelet and anticoagulant medications: guidelines from the American Society of Regional Anesthesia and Pain Medicine, the European Society of Regional Anaesthesia and Pain Therapy, the American Academy of Pain Medicine, the International Neuromodulation Society, the North American Neuromodulation Society, and the World Institute of Pain. Reg Anesth Pain Med. 2015;40(3):182-212.
37. Clinical Excellence Commission. Non-vitamin K Antagonist Oral Anticoagulant (NOAC) Guidelines. Sydney: CEC; 2017.
38. Douketis JD, Wang G, Chan N, Eikelboom JW, Syed S, Barty R, et al. Effect of standardized perioperative dabigatran interruption on the residual anticoagulation effect at the time of surgery or procedure. J Thromb Haemost. 2016;14(1): 89-97.

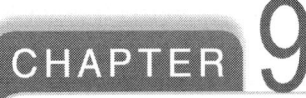

The Blood-Brain Barrier

Girija Prasad Rath, Vanitha Rajagopalan

INTRODUCTION

The blood-brain barrier (BBB) is a potent ostiary that prevents the free passage of substances between the blood and central nervous system (CNS). It is a dynamic organ that guarantees appropriate concentration of vital compounds such as oxygen and glucose within the brain. It also protects the brain from harmful substances present in the peripheral circulation. BBB transports nutrients such as glucose, amino acids, vitamins, and minerals, into the brain, and transports out of the brain toxins, electrolytes, and xenobiotics.[1] Thus, it plays protective, nutritive, homeostatic, and transmission roles inside the brain. Perturbations in its integrity result in a multitude of brain pathology.

HISTORICAL PERSPECTIVE

The concept of the BBB originated in the 19th century when, Paul Ehrlich, in 1885, noticed that intravenous (IV) administration of aniline dyes stained all organs except the brain and the spinal cord,[2] which made him conclude that the nervous system's uptake of the dye as compared to other tissues was poor. In 1913, Edwin Goldman, demonstrated that the dye trypan blue when injected intravenously was visualized in the choroid plexus and meninges but not in the brain,[2,3] and on direct cerebrospinal fluid (CSF) injection, it readily stained nervous tissue but not the other tissues in the body.[2] The term "blood-brain barrier" ("Barrie`re he´matoence´phalique") was coined by Stern in 1921, after she and her colleagues had performed a series of experiments which led to greater understanding of this barrier.[4] It was in 1960s that based on electron-microscopic studies, Reese along with his colleagues identified that this barrier is restricted to the capillary endothelial cells (ECs) within the brain.[5]

ANATOMY AND PHYSIOLOGY

The BBB is an extremely regulated interface that mediates the communication between the peripheral circulation and CNS. It is not just a physical barrier, but functions as a selective transport interface, a secretory body and a

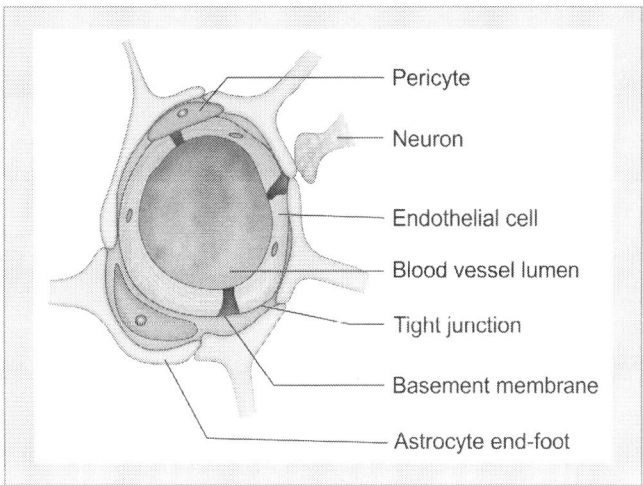

Fig. 1: Schematic structure of the blood-brain barrier.*
*The brain capillary endothelial cells are connected to each other by tight junctions and adherens junctions. Endothelial cells are surrounded by basal membrane, which covers the connecting pericytes. The astrocyte end-feet around the brain microvessels provide the barrier function. Additional supporting cell types are microglia cells and the connecting neurons.

metabolic barrier at the level of microvascular endothelium of the brain.[6] Although anatomically, the BBB consists of specialized ECs lining the intraluminal portion of brain capillaries, but physiologically it also includes the periendothelial accessory structures as its intrinsic functional components.[7,8] The astrocytes, pericytes, neurons, and the extracellular matrix along with ECs constitute the BBB. This established neurovascular unit (NVU) protects the brain cells and preserves the homeostasis of CNS which is essential for synchronized neuronal activities. The schematic structure of BBB is shown in **Figure 1**.

Brain Endothelial Cells

A monolayer of brain ECs lines the intraluminal surface of brain capillaries and are attached to one another by tight junctions (TJ) and adherens junctions (AJ). It is the first line of defense of the brain against circulating factors.[9] These ECs are morphologically different from peripheral ECs as they express TJ proteins, form a potent barrier, have reduced pinocytosis which restricts vesicle-mediated transcellular transport, and contain greater concentration of mitochondria to generate greater energy for the active transport of nutrients.[10] ECs have a luminal and abluminal side, with different polarity, differential receptor expression and density on each side, which influences the permeability of the barrier. The other cell types present in the NVU include neurons, astrocytes, and pericytes.

Neurons

Neurons are the elementary units of the CNS and have a role in signaling. They connect with astrocytic end-feet by being just 8–20 μm from a brain capillary at the BBB. The neurons regulate blood flow, capillary permeability, and release angiogenesis stimulating factors by interaction with the extracellular matrix, in response to the constantly changing local milieu. By aiding in TJ protein synthesis and localization, the neurons help tighten brain ECs. They also operate synergistically in the regulation of other cell types.[11]

Astrocytes

Astrocytes are the most plentiful cells in the brain and they reinforce barrier function and contact ECs on the abluminal side of the BBB endothelium.[12] They regulate BBB permeability and all the neuronal function such as survival, development, metabolism, and neurotransmission. They respond to changes in the local environment, by acting as metabolic sensors, and through unleash of several effector molecules, help in maintenance and repair function of BBB. They have a symbiotic relation with the ECs; by secreting a variety of chemical factors that induce the ECs while the ECs help in astrocytic differentiation.[13]

Pericytes

Pericytes are nondifferentiated contractile tissue cells that are present in capillary walls and regulate the growth of ECs and moderate the robustness of capillary cells.[14] They are lodged in the vascular basement membrane on the abluminal surface of the endothelial cell. Pericytes regulate angiogenesis and deposition of extracellular matrix, and thus, maintain and stabilize the ECs.[15] They are essential for development of TJs. The CNS has much greater endothelial: pericyte ratio, and the distinct properties of CNS pericytes compared to their peripheral counterparts is that they regulate blood flow in response to neural activity by controlling the vascular tone.

The pericytes help in the genesis of the BBB and regulate its structure and function, by communicating with one another through release of secretory factors and changes in movement of water through the channels.

Extracellular Matrix

The extracellular matrix provides physical integrity to the BBB, the disruption of which leads to impaired structural stability and compromised function. It functions as a binding site that imparts polarity at the EC-astrocyte interface. Various structural proteins, such as laminin, collagen type IV, and integrins interact with each other to maintain the structural robustness of the BBB.[16] The matrix proteins also play a role in upregulating TJ protein expression.[17]

Circumventricular Organs

There are niche zones of the brain situated on the surface of the 3rd and 4th ventricles, where the BBB being more permeable allows uninterrupted communication between the CNS and the vascular system. They include the neurohypophysis or posterior pituitary, median eminence, area postrema (vomiting center), subfornical organ, and vascular organ of the lamina terminalis; these are known as circumventricular organs.[18] Circumventricular organs are important peripheral chemosensors as they recognize changes in the concentration of different molecules in the circulation; they also secrete hormones, neurotransmitters, or cytokines into it.

DEVELOPMENT OF BLOOD-BRAIN BARRIER

Development of the BBB begins during the fetal-life, it is well-formed at birth but immature. At molecular level, Wnt/beta-catenin signaling controls the formation of the BBB.[19] Occludin and claudin-5 expression is noticed in the brain capillary endothelium of 14-week human fetus and the distribution observed is similar to the adult.[20] Postmortem studies in stillborn fetuses of 12-weeks' gestation and from perinatal deaths bear witness to presence of BBB to trypan blue, comparable to adults from the beginning of second trimester.[21]

REGULATION AND HOMEOSTASIS

The BBB is a dynamic system, which responds to changes in the local milieu and requirements, and is regulated via numerous mechanisms during both healthy and disease states. These regulations include changes in TJ function, and in expression and activity of many transporters and enzymes. The activities of the BBB are efficiently matched to the requirements of the brain, emphasizing the key role it plays in the day-to-day brain-functions. As we learn more about BBB regulation, it will emerge as a target for developing strategies for therapy to the brain to maintain homeostasis and to offer recovery from pathological conditions. The various agents, which cause modulation of the BBB, are shown in **Table 1.**

A network of small capillaries about 7 μm in diameter supply metabolic nutrients to the human brain. Each neuron is in close proximity of a capillary, within 20 μm. The brain requires a sound regulation of its local environment for its cells to function optimally. Maintenance of homeostasis and prevention of hindrance to signal initiation and transmission is a major challenge across the BBB.[22]

The BBB maintains cerebral homeostasis by regulation of its chemical milieu, immune cell transport, and entrance of xenobiotics. The concentrations of water, amino acids, ions, hormones, and neurotransmitters in the blood fluctuate at different time periods. If all these fluctuations were transmitted to the brain, it would result in local disruption of signal generation and uninhibited neural activity. Therefore, there is a need for a tightly regulated transport from the blood to the brain parenchyma. The transport of immune cells (e.g., leukocytes) is also regulated, as an uncontrolled inflammatory response could lead to increased intracranial pressure or cerebral edema, as the brain is enclosed within a rigid skull. The entry into the brain of toxins, and bacterial and viral pathogens circulating in the blood must also be prevented as it can lead to deleterious effects on neurons.

TRANSPORT ACROSS BLOOD-BRAIN BARRIER (FIG. 2)

The brain capillaries are around 100 times compact than peripheral microvessels as a result of the impenetrable TJs that critically restrict the

TABLE 1: Modulation of blood-brain barrier by various substances

Decreased blood-brain barrier permeability	Increased blood-brain barrier permeability
• Intracellular cyclic adenosine monophosphate (AMP) • Steroids • Adrenomedullin • Noradrenaline • Glial cell line-derived neurotrophic factor (GDNF) • Basic fibroblastic growth factor (bFGF) • Polyunsaturated fatty acids • Transforming growth factor-β (TGF-β)	• Bradykinin • Histamine • Serotonin (5-HT) • Thrombin • Glutamate • Purine nucleotides: adenosine triphosphate (ATP), adenosine diphosphate (ADP), AMP • Endothelin-1 • Adenosine • Platelet-activating factor • Phospholipase A2 • Arachidonic acid • Prostaglandins • Leukotrienes • Interleukins: IL-1α, IL-1β, IL-6 • Tumor necrosis factor-α (TNF-α) • Macrophage inhibitory proteins: MIP-1 and MIP-2 • Complement-derived polypeptide: C3a-desArg • Free radicals • Nitric oxide

Source: Modified from Abbott NJ. Dynamics of CNS barriers: evolution, differentiation, and modulation. Cell Mol Neurobiol. 2005;25:5-23.

paracellular movement of hydrophilic solutes. Tight regulation of solute gradients and molecular transport is mediated by four primary transport mechanisms.[23]

- *Paracellular aqueous diffusion*: Small water-soluble molecules (e.g., oxygen, carbon dioxide) diffuse freely along their concentration gradient across the endothelial lipid membranes through this extracellular pathway controlled by TJs.
- *Transcellular lipophilic diffusion*: In this transmembrane process, substances cross the BBB at a rate proportional to their molecular weight and lipid solubility. Highly lipophilic substances, easily diffuse across the BBB into the brain.
- *Adsorptive transcytosis*: This endocytotic process is mediated by clathrin-coated pits and, to a lesser extent, caveolae. It is generally selective for cationic molecules and is the predominant mechanism for passage of human immunodeficiency virus-1 (HIV-1) into the brain. This process is being investigated as a possible pathway for therapeutic drug delivery to the CNS.[24,25]
- Saturable transport:
    - *Receptor-mediated transcytosis*—is the transport of solutes through receptor-binding and subsequent endocytosis. The transport of

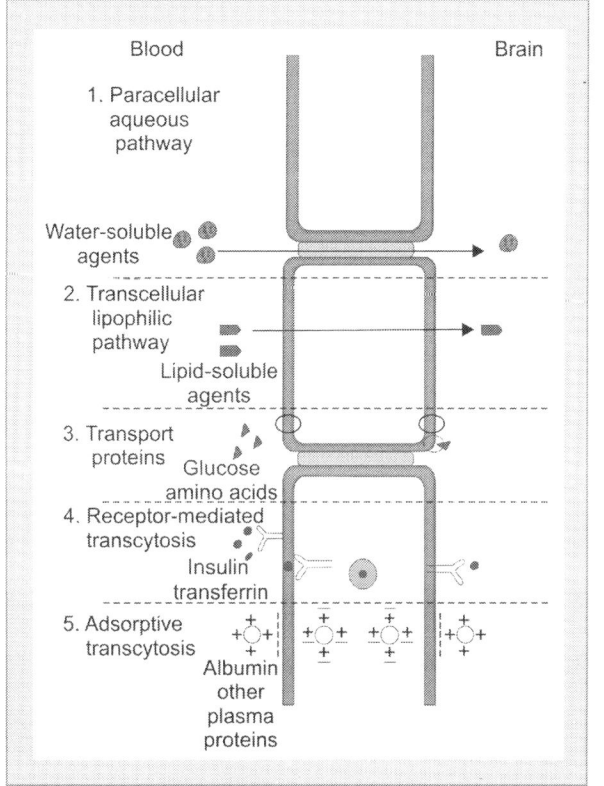

Fig. 2: Transport systems at the blood-brain barrier.

transferrin, insulin, and insulin-like growth factor, are examples of this energy-dependent type of transport.
- *Channel-mediated transport*—is a saturable mode of transit that mediates influx and efflux via transport proteins.

The BBB has various distinct transport systems, comprising of glucose-transporter 1 (GLUT-1), the L-system, and A-system amino acid carriers. BBB transporters ensure delivery of critical compounds that are essential for brain function.

Transportation of Drugs across Blood-Brain Barrier

The BBB prevents entry of a number of therapeutic agents which act on the CNS; it also prevents delivery of systemically administered drugs for the brain those require transportation through the BBB. The two most important factors which determine whether a given drug will penetrate the CNS are—its lipid solubility and molecular weight. Lipophilic drugs cross the BBB by solubilizing into lipid bilayer of the EC membrane or by passive diffusion. The lipophilicity of a drug determines its passage through the BBB, only when its molecular weight is ≤400–600 Dalton (Da). Drugs with larger molecular weight (>600 Da)

TABLE 2: Drug delivery and the blood-brain barrier (BBB)	
Drug delivery strategies	
Drug manipulation	• Lipophilic conjugation • Conjugation to bioactive molecules • Prodrugs
Exporter protein modulation	• Carrier-and receptor-mediated transport • Trojan horse liposome
Disruption of the BBB: Opening of endothelial tight junctions	• Chemical disruption • Hyperosmotic BBB disruption • Parasympathetic stimulation
Focused ultrasound disruption of BBB	
Alternative routes to CNS drug delivery	• Convection: Enhanced Delivery • Local delivery of polymer infused chemotherapy • Targeted toxin therapy

(CNS: central nervous system)

are not transported across the BBB even, if it is highly lipid soluble. The active drug efflux system present in the BBB is an additional obstacle for drug delivery to the CNS. P-glycoprotein (P-gp), located on the apical surface of the ECs, is an ATP-dependent 170 kDa phosphorylated glycoprotein-membrane transporter which actively removes drugs and potentially toxic metabolites from brain. P-gp in the BBB is a possible target for drug design.[26] Various drug delivery strategies[27] that have been developed for better CNS penetration of drugs are listed in **Table 2**.

BLOOD-BRAIN BARRIER AND DISEASE

A number of CNS pathologies are known to involve a facet of BBB affliction.[28-31] The disorders may range from transient TJ opening to chronic barrier failure; and there may even be the changes in transport systems and enzymes. Microglial activation is perceived as an early sign of CNS inflammation, even in disorders not hitherto regarded as inflammatory. In most cases, it is not possible to ascertain whether barrier compromise results in disease onset, but barrier disruption often promotes and aggravates the developing pathology (**Fig. 3**). It is important to develop superior diagnostic methods to recognize and reveal sites of barrier disturbance, as timely intervention reduces long-term disease evolution and dysfunction.

Traumatic Brain Injury

The pathology after traumatic brain injury (TBI) is mainly due to two different processes. The primary damage, which occurs at the time of injury, results in mechanical distortion of the BBB. The heightened cerebrovascular

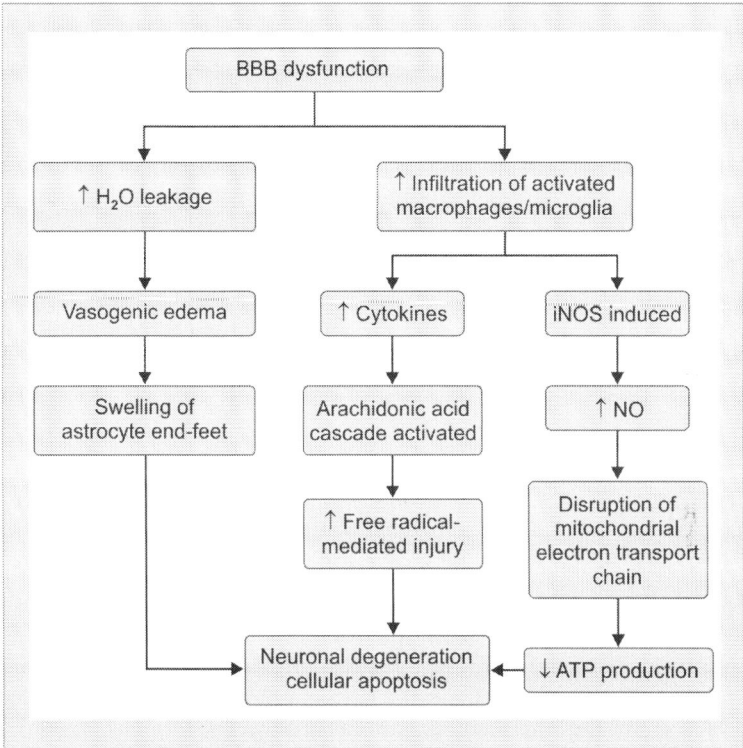

Fig. 3: Consequences of blood-brain barrier (BBB) dysfunction.

permeability and ensuing vasogenic edema leads to increased brain tissue water after TBI.

Secondary, insult is predominantly due to ischemia and prompts a cytotoxic edema formation, mainly due to disruption of the BBB resulting from disarray of TJ proteins, release of inflammatory mediators, such as inter-cellular adhesion molecule (ICAM-1) and vascular endothelial growth factor (VEGF), and mitochondrial dysfunction. Matrix metalloproteinases (MMP) activation causes proteolysis of the basal lamina causing further tissue damage.[32]

The transmembrane water transport also results in cerebral edema. There is up-regulation of AQP4 in reactive astrocytes after TBI. Early neurosurgeries such as decompressive craniectomy and contusionectomy, causes a reduction in MMP levels and limits the breakdown of BBB.[33]

Ischemic Stroke

Ischemic stroke-related cerebral ischemia commences sequence of events that leads to increased permeability of BBB. The main factors include cytokines, VEGF, and nitric oxide. VEGF release induces fenestration formation in ECs and augments BBB capillary permeability, leading to cerebral edema formation with ongoing ischemia and further infarction of the penumbra. VEGF antagonism can limit postischemic brain injury.[32]

Brain Tumor

The microvasculature of brain tumors is inadequately developed, lacks a BBB, and is leaky that results in cerebral edema and attendant mass effect that is usually, greater than that corresponding to the tumor itself. Ultrastructure examination of human gliomas and metastatic adenocarcinoma have established opening of interendothelial TJs, which is related with an increase in paracellular permeability and perimicrovessel edema. Neoplastic astrocytes fail to provide the requisite factors for the maintenance of BBB integrity in peritumoral areas, and further secrete permeability factors that annul normal barrier function. Even though, the exact mechanism of action is unclear, the mainstay of therapy of brain tumor-related edema is corticosteroids as they appear to reduce endothelial permeability.[34]

Epilepsy

Osmotic BBB disruption is commonly complicated with seizures. Present-day research strives to demonstrate an association between the occurrence of seizures and the level of BBB disruption.[35]

The role of neuroinflammation in seizures is supported by evidence of autoantibodies in several seizure disorders, by the ability of infection and autoimmunity disease to induce seizures, and by similarities between the immunologic dysfunction seen in the CNS of animal models of both MS and epilepsy. A well-documented consequence of seizures is opening of the BBB. This may be accompanied by increased EC selectin expression, increased VEGF signaling, and induction of autoantibodies. Furthermore, although the mechanisms underlying post-traumatic epilepsy remain poorly characterized, elevated immune tone, vascular remodeling, and potential development of autoantibodies may lead to long-term BBB disruption.

Septic Encephalopathy

Septic encephalopathy is frequently seen in intensive care units and is associated with adverse patient outcomes. It causes diffuse brain dysfunction related to dysfunction of BBB and cerebral edema. Septic encephalopathy-related BBB disruption incorporates increased pinocytosis in cerebral microvessel endothelium and disorganized interendothelial junctional proteins leading to a "leaky" TJ. These changes occur due to effects of inflammatory mediators in circulation on the brain endothelium, neurotransmitter-composition of the reticular activating system, dysfunction of the astrocytes, and direct neuronal injuries.[34]

Infectious or Inflammatory Processes

Infectious agents can cross the BBB through a number of mechanisms, including transcytosis, direct BBB disruption, reverse neuronal transport, and several others.[36] The brain is protected from direct infection because brain ECs lack CD4 and galactosylceramide receptors. HIV-1 enters the brain by adsorptive endocytosis. HIV-infected white blood cells enter the CNS with greater efficiency than noninfected cells, and the virus continues to grow rapidly in glial cells. The presence of the BBB prevents effective delivery of antiviral therapeutics.[37]

Clostridium perfringens has high affinity for TJ laudin proteins, and its binding leads to increased BBB permeability, prompting investigation into claudin as a target for enhanced CNS drug delivery. Pneumococci bind to ECs at receptors for platelet-activating factor, crossing the BBB through transcellular transport. On the other hand, *Neisseria meningitidis* binds to ECs, causing phosphorylation of EC-binding proteins, inhibiting transportation of leukocyte, and suppresses inflammation. Concurrent use of steroids with antibiotics in patients with bacterial meningitis, minimizes inflammation in the brain. In the setting of meningitis, dexamethasone, a synthetic glucocorticoid, reinforces the BBB and may block antibiotic permeability. Herpes virus enters the CNS through olfactory nerves, whereas rabies enters through spinal nerves. Bacterial perturbation of the BBB tends to be greater than that induced by viral infection.

IMAGING THE BLOOD-BRAIN BARRIER

Evolution in the techniques of neuroimaging provides insights into the effect of cerebral neoplasms on BBB. The technology helps clinicians to understand invasiveness of the tumor and its effect on the permeability of BBB.[38] These developments have expedited evaluation of the efficacy of various treatment strategies. Breakdown of BBB by tumors can be seen with the help of contrast-enhanced computed tomography (CT) and magnetic resonance imaging (MRI) scans.[39] Drug delivery can be monitored by MRI of brain which also, helps assessing the treatment outcomes of CNS neoplasms.

For imaging of tumors, iron-oxide nanoparticles are being used. Compared with gadolinium contrast, nanoparticles display better intravascular retention and may more precisely characterize brain tumor perfusion. Advances in positron emission tomography (PET) may help distinguish tumor regrowth from radiation necrosis and even aid in tumor staging.

MARKERS OF DAMAGED BLOOD-BRAIN BARRIER

With the opening of the BBB, molecules present in blood usually egress into the CNS. This does not work in just one direction, unless specific transporters are involved. Proteins normally present in blood are free to diffuse into the CNS while proteins present in high concentration in the CNS freely diffuse down concentration gradients into blood. These peripheral BBB markers that can be detected in blood help in estimating the permeability properties of the BBB at any given time. Marchi and associates[40] reviewed the ideal characteristics of a peripheral marker of BBB disruption. Such proteins should have infinitesimal plasma levels in normal subjects, be normally present in CSF, and have higher CSF to plasma concentration. Furthermore, the CSF concentration of the marker should increase in response to insults. The marker should be normally blocked by the BBB and shift across the BBB during barrier disruption.

Various proteins, including S100B, ubiquitin carboxyl-terminal esterase L1, neuron-specific enolase, and glial fibrillary acidic protein, have been analyzed for this purpose.

S100B: A Peripheral Marker of Damaged Blood-Brain Barrier

Plasma levels of S100B are generally one-third of CSF levels. Several diseases cause a rise in S100B levels in plasma. Plasma S100B levels increase in cases of cerebral ischemia, peaking around day 3 after infarction. These levels have practical utility in evaluating both infarct size and long-term clinical outcome. TBI has also been shown to increase plasma S100B, with the extent of damage after head injury being directly proportional to the elevation of S100B.

Plasma levels of S100B are elevated in patients with hemorrhagic shock, aneurysmal subarachnoid hemorrhage, hypoxia resulting from cardiac arrest, and brain damage postcardiopulmonary resuscitation due to nervous tissue damage. The peripheral S100B levels rise even in the diseases causing disruption of the BBB without brain tissue damage.[41,42]

Shifting Paradigms

The white matter (WM) and gray matter (GM) in different brain regions show differences in morphology, cellular content, and microvascular density. However, extensive functional differences have been seen in GM and WM astrocytes as suggested by differential expression of transporters such as glutamate-transporters and GLUT-1 subtypes. RNA-seq studies of populations of brain cells showed high heterogeneity in the morphology of astrocytes, glia, ECs and pericytes, and also, in the physiologic and metabolic functions. Understanding the regional heterogeneity of the brain microvasculature, and its implications in health and disease is relatively newer aspect for brain vascular research.[43]

FUTURE PERSPECTIVES

Central nervous system drug delivery is a major impediment for treatment of several neurological disorders. Headway in our comprehension of the structure and function of the BBB and development of innovative techniques for evading this barrier will be needed to vanquish the limited access to CNS.[44] There is a growing recognition that BBB disruption causes CNS diseases to rapidly progress. A prime obstacle is in understanding how the barrier elements respond to focal disruptions and in developing tactics to stimulate repair.

While there is apparent cognizance about the formation of the BBB during development, very little is known age-related changes in barrier function. This is important, as aging is a significant risk factor for neurodegenerative disorders. Understanding of the properties and dynamic behavior of ECs with aging, and functional interactions with other cell types in the NVU will be required to identify its role in both age-dependent cognitive decline, and the progression of neurodegenerative diseases.

Indispensable to advances in our scientific knowledge of the BBB will be better models for scientific and translational research. Deducing how these attributes of the microvasculature interrelate will help in the inception of BBB models in tune with high output screening methods that are likely to be pivotal to the development of innovative therapeutics.

CONCLUSION

The BBB which is a constituent of the NVU acts as the blood-brain interface. The BBB in addition to being a physical barrier, also acts as a transport interface, a secretory body, and a metabolic barrier. The anatomy and physiology of the BBB is a basis for understanding neurologic disorders and for strategies to deliver therapeutics to the brain. Various transporter systems in the BBB play a pivotal role in the exchange of different nutrients and could be useful for delivery of drugs.

Conflict of Interest: Nil.

KEY POINTS

- The BBB is an important passage for nutrients and cells from the blood to brain.
- It protects the brain from the entry of deleterious substances.
- Understanding the damage of the BBB and its permeability in various neurologic disorders is important for mastering the pathophysiologic mechanisms, and formulating plan for management.
- Permeability of the BBB is maneuvered for delivery of drugs to the brain.

REFERENCES

1. Abbott NJ, Romero IA. Transporting therapeutics across the blood-brain barrier. Mol Med Today. 1996;2(3):106-13.
2. Ribatti D, Nico B, Crivellato E, Artico M. Development of the blood-brain barrier: a historical point of view. Anat Rec B New Anat. 2006;289(1):3-8.
3. Liddelow SA. Fluids and barriers of the CNS: a historical viewpoint. Fluids Barriers CNS. 2011;8(1):2.
4. Vein AA. Science and fate: Lina Stern (1878-1968), a neurophysiologist and biochemist. J Hist Neurosci 2008;17(2):195-206.
5. Bradbury MW. The blood- brain barrier. Exp. Physiol. 1993;78(4):453-72.
6. Abbott NJ, Ronnback L, Hansson E. Astrocyte-endothelial interactions at the blood-brain barrier. Nat Rev Neurosci. 2006;7(1):41-53.
7. Abbott NJ, Patabendige AA, Dolman DE, Yusof SR, Begley DJ. Structure and function of the blood- brain barrier. Neurobiol Dis. 2010;37(1):13-25.
8. Hawkins BT, Davis TP. The blood-brain barrier/neurovascular unit in health and disease. Pharmacol Rev. 2005;57(2):173-85.
9. Tietz S, Engelhardt B. Brain barriers: crosstalk between complex tight juntionsTJs and adherens junctions. J Cell Biol. 2015;209(4):493-506.
10. Reese TS, Karnovsky MJ. Fine structural localization of a blood-brain barrier to exogenous peroxidase. J Cell Biol. 1967;34(1):207-17.
11. Savettieri G, Di Liegro I, Catania C, Licata L, Pitarresi GL, D'Agostino S, et al. Neurons and ECM regulate occluding localization in brain endothelial cells. Neuroreport. 2000;11(5):1081-4.

12. Tao-Cheng JH, Brightman MW. Development of membrane interactions between brain endothelial cells and astrocytes in vitro. Int J Dev Neurosci. 1988;6(1):25-37.
13. Mi H, Haeberle H, Barres BA. Induction of astrocyte differentiation by endothelial cells. J Neurosci. 2001;21(5):1538-47.
14. Miller FN, Sims DE. Contractile elements in the regulation of macromolecular permeability. Fed Proc. 1986;45(2):84-8.
15. Armulik A, Genové G, Mäe M, Nisancioglu MH, Wallgard E, Niaudet C, et al. Pericytes regulate the blood-brain barrier. Nature. 2010;468(7323):557-61.
16. del Zoppo GJ, Hallenbeck JM. Advances in the vascular pathophysiology of ischemic stroke. Thromb Res. 2000;98(3):73-81.
17. Tilling T, Engelbertz C, Decker S, Korte D, Huwel S, Galla HJ. Expression and adhesive properties of basement membrane proteins in cerebral capillary endothelial cell cultures. Cell Tissue Res. 2002;310(1):19-29.
18. Ballabh P, Braun A, Nedergaard M. The blood-brain barrier: an overview structure, regulation, and clinical implications. Neurobiol Dis. 2004;16(1):1-13.
19. Liebner S, Corada M, Bangsow T, Babbage J, Taddei A, Czupalla CJ, et al. Wnt/beta-catenin signalling controls development of the blood–brain barrier. J. Cell Biol. 2008;183(3):409-17.
20. Virgintino D, Errede M, Robertson D, Capobianco C, Girolamo F, Vimercati A, et al. Immunolocalization of tight junction proteins in the adult and developing human brain. Histochem. Cell Biol. 2004;122(1):51-9.
21. GRONTOFT O. Intracranial haemorrhage and blood-brain barrier problems in the new-born: a pathologico-anatomical and experimental investigation. Acta Pathol Microbiol Scand Suppl. 1954;100:8-109.
22. Wong AD, Ye M, Levy AF, Rothstein JD, Bergles DE, Searson PC. The blood-brain barrier: an engineering perspective. Front Neuroeng. 2013;6:7.
23. Banks WA. Characteristics of compounds that cross the blood-brain barrier. BMC Neurol. 2009;9(Suppl 1):S3.
24. Herve F, Ghinea N, Scherrmann JM. CNS delivery via adsorptive transcytosis. AAPS J. 2008;10(3):455-72.
25. Pardridge WM. Drug transport across the blood-brain barrier. J Cereb Blood Flow Metab. 2012;32(11):1959-72.
26. Schinkel AH. P-Glycoprotein, a gatekeeper in the blood-brain barrier. Adv Drug Del Rev. 1999;36(2-3):179-94.
27. Lawther BK, Kumar S, Krovvidi H. Blood–brain barrier. Cont Edu Anaesth Crit Care Pain. 2011;11(4):128-32.
28. Kaur C, Ling EA. Blood brain barrier in hypoxic-ischemic conditions. Curr. Neurovasc Res. 2008;5(1):71-81.
29. Rosenberg GA, Yang Y. Vasogenic edema due to tight junction disruption by matrix metalloproteinases in cerebral ischemia. Neurosurg Focus. 2007;22(5):E4.
30. Remy S, Beck H. Molecular and cellular mechanisms of pharmacoresistance in epilepsy. Brain. 2006;129(Pt 1):18-35.
31. Bronger H, König J, Kopplow K, Steiner HH, Ahmadi R, Herold-Mende C, et al. ABCC drug efflux pumps and organic anion uptake transporters in human gliomas and the blood-tumor barrier. Cancer Res. 2005;65(24):11419-28.
32. Marmarou A. A review of progress in understanding the pathophysiology and treatment of brain edema. Neurosurg Focus. 2007;22(5):E1.
33. Vajtri D, Benada O, Kukacka J, Prusa R, Houstava L, Toupalik P, et al. Correlation of ultrastructural changes of endothelial cells and astrocytes occurring during blood brain barrier damage after traumatic brain injury with biochemical markers of BBB leakage and inflammatory response. Physiol Res. 2009;58(2):263-8.

34. Davies DC. Blood-brain Barrier breakdown in septic encephalopathy and brain tumours. J Anat. 2002;200(6):639-46.
35. Marchi N, Angelov L, Masaryk T, Fazio V, Granata T, Hernandez N, et al. Seizure-promoting effect of blood-brain barrier disruption. Epilepsia. 2007;48(4):732-42.
36. Ivey NS, MacLean AG, Lackner AA. Acquired immunodeficiency syndrome and the blood-brain barrier. J Neurovirol. 2009;15(2):111-22.
37. Strelow LI, Janigro D, Nelson JA. The blood-brain barrier and AIDS. Adv Virus Res. 2001;56:355-88.
38. Prager BC, Nimjee SM, Grant GA, Ghosh C, Janigro D. The blood-brain barrier. In Winn HR (Ed). Youmans and Winn Neurological Surgery, 7th edition. Philadelphia, PA: Elsevier; 2017. pp. 372.
39. Provenzale JM, Mukundan S, Dewhirst M. The role of blood-brain barrier permeability in brain tumor imaging and therapeutics. Am J Roentgenol. 2005;185(3):763-7.
40. Marchi N, Rasmussen PA, Kapural M, Fazio V, Kight K, Mayberg MR, et al. Peripheral markers of brain damage and blood-brain barrier dysfunction. Restor Neurol Neurosci. 2003;21(3-4):109-21.
41. Marchi N, Cavaglia M, Fazio V, Bhudia S, Hallene K, Janigro D. Peripheral markers of blood-brain barrier damage. Clin Chim Acta. 2004;342(1-2):1-12.
42. Kanner AA, Marchi N, Fazio V, Mayberg MR, Koltz MT, Siomin V, et al. Serum S100beta: a noninvasive marker of blood-brain barrier function and brain lesions. Cancer. 2003;97(11):2806-13.
43. Villabona-Rueda A, Erice C, Pardo CA, Stins MF. The evolving concept of the blood brain barrier (BBB): from a single static barrier to a heterogeneous and dynamic relay center. Front Cell Neurosci. 2019;13:405.
44. Wong AD, Ye M, Levy AF, Rothstein JD, Bergles DE, Searson PC. The blood-brain barrier: an engineering perspective. Front Neuroeng. 2013;6:7.

CHAPTER 10

Pediatric Difficult Airway

Neerja Bhardwaj, Anudeep Jafra

INTRODUCTION

The possibility of encountering a situation of difficult airway in a child is a rare but significant cause of morbidity and mortality.[1] On the other hand, the presence of anatomical and physiological differences, even in a normal pediatric airway makes airway management difficult in inexperienced hands especially so in an infant and neonate leading to poor decision making.[2] A delayed response to hypoxia and management of airway obstruction can lead to serious life-threatening complications in children due to shorter apnea tolerance time. Also, the long-term effect of prolonged hypoxemia on cognitive function and motor development is not known.[3]

The reported incidence of difficult airway in children is less as compared to adults. The closed claims studies suggest that the most common cause of morbidity and mortality in children arises due to failure to ventilate and oxygenate rather than intubate.[4] The incidence of difficult face mask (FM) ventilation is 0.15%, difficult laryngoscopy (DL) around 1.35% (4.7% in infants and 3.2% in neonates) and that of difficult intubation (DI) ranges from 0.05 to 0.57%.[5,6] In a pediatric closed claim analysis, respiratory events accounted for 43% of adverse respiratory events, of these 20% were due to inadequate ventilation and 14% accounted for esophageal intubation, airway obstruction and DI. The Pediatric Perioperative Cardiac Arrest (POCA) registry, related 20% of cardiac arrests in children to respiratory events, of these 27% were due to airway obstruction and 13% due to DI.[7] Neonates and infants remain at a high risk especially those with cardiopulmonary comorbidities and those undergoing emergency procedures.

At present there are very few specifically designed difficult airway guidelines for pediatric patients. The reason being unavailability of high-quality studies and lack of best quality of evidence. This has led to formation of guidelines on the basis of consensus by the experts.[8-10]

PRINCIPLE APPROACH TO A DIFFICULT PEDIATRIC AIRWAY

The key differences between the anatomy and physiology of pediatric and adult airway as well as of respiratory system have major implications for airway

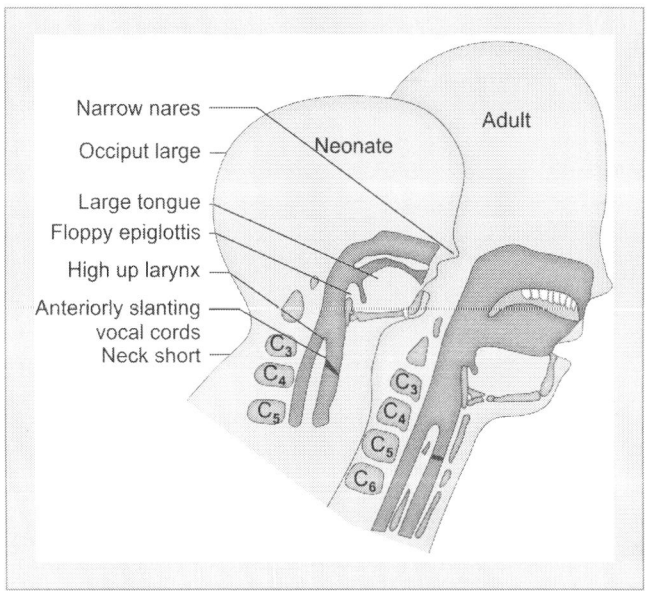

Fig. 1: Anatomical differences between adults and children.

management in children **(Fig. 1)**. Due to a wide range of ages, pediatric airway comes in different sizes, shapes, position and composition which make it more prone to airway obstruction. Some of the important features implicated for difficult airway are large head, prominent occiput, large tongue, high up larynx, angulated vocal cords and a large and floppy epiglottis.[5] Children have high oxygen consumption, lower residual capacity, greater closing capacity and smaller airway diameter making them desaturate fast.

An immature nervous system, immature brain, underdeveloped respiratory system and higher basal parasympathetic tone predispose a pediatric airway to complications. Failure to oxygenate and ventilate a child results in hypoxia. This leads to bradycardia in a child whose cardiac output (CO) is heart rate dependent, hence decreased CO further leads to reduced oxygen delivery resulting in a vicious triad of worsening hypoxia, increasing hypercarbia, acidosis eventually resulting into cardiac arrest.

PREDICTORS OF DIFFICULT AIRWAY IN CHILDREN

In a retrospective study including 11,219 children, authors reported young age below 1-year, higher American Society of Anesthesiologists (ASA) grades III and IV, low body mass index, higher Mallampati grades (III, IV) and faciomaxillary and cardiac surgery to be some of the predictors of DL.[6] The risk of DI is greater in neonates, those undergoing emergency procedures and those with cardiopulmonary compromise as well as those with congenital syndromes and history of (H/O) obstructive sleep apnea (OSA). The most common causes of difficult airway in children are anticipated and include congenital syndromes. Other causes such as temporomandibular (TM) joint ankylosis, retropharyngeal abscess, Ludwig's angina and airway trauma may also be the reasons of difficulty in securing the airway **(Table 1)**.

TABLE 1: Causes of difficult airway in children

Congenital disorders

Difficult mask ventilation	Difficult intubation mandibular hypoplasia (micrognathia)	Macroglossia
Midface hypoplasia	Pierre Robin sequence	Mucopolysaccharidosis
Apert syndrome	Treacher Collins syndrome	Beckwith-Wiedemann syndrome
Crouzon's syndrome	Goldenhar syndrome	Down's syndrome
Pfeiffer syndrome		

Acquired causes

Tonsillar hypertrophy Adenoid hypertrophy	Acute obstruction	
Glottic web Subglottic stenosis	Infection	
Burns	Inflammation	
Thyromental joint disorders	Trauma	
Hemangioma	Foreign body	

PREOPERATIVE ASSESSMENT OF THE AIRWAY

A low incidence of difficult airway in children should not prevent one from a thorough preoperative assessment, which includes a complete medical and surgical history, airway and systemic examination, and certain investigations which can point toward an anticipated difficult airway.

A complete and detailed history including birth history, history of any stridor or sounds during breathing, cyanosis, feeding difficulties, mouth breathing, snoring, history of previous anesthesia exposure and any previous problems encountered during anesthesia, any history of previous surgery on face or neck and presence or history of recent upper respiratory tract infection is required.

Routine airway examination should be done from both front and lateral profile, the latter helps to identify presence of any micrognathia or retrognathia.[11] Any syndromic appearance and facial asymmetry should also be noticed. The bedside tests for airway examination like mouth opening, modified Mallampati (MMP) grading, size of the tongue, neck movements, ear and teeth problems, thryomental and sternomental distance and dentition are dependent on the co-operation of the child. Till date there are no valid scoring systems, neither any defined values of the above mentioned tests to delineate a difficult airway in a child. Studies in children have suggested that MMP grading also does not accurately predict poor glottic views.[12] The airway assessment can be divided into assessment of problems encountered during FM ventilation such as abnormal facies, any extraoral pathology or presence of tonsillar or adenoid hypertrophy as well as assessment of problems during intubation, like short mandible, retrognathia, midfacial deformities, presence of any intraoral pathology, etc. **(Figs. 2A to F)**.

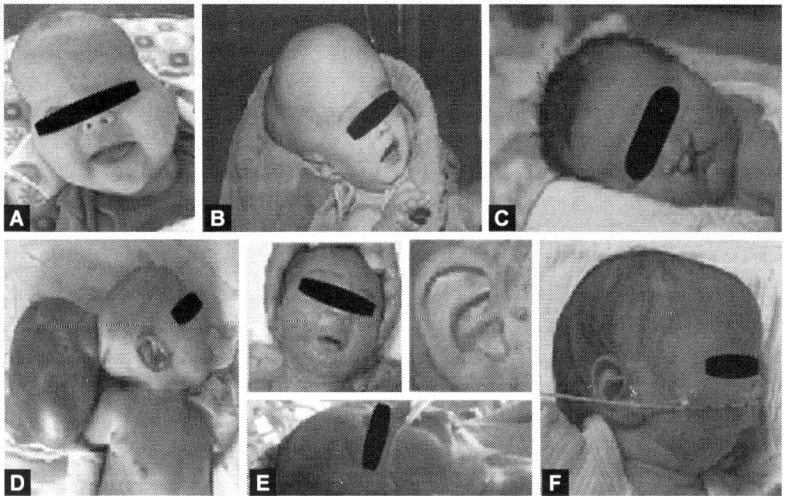

Figs. 2A to F: Predictors of difficult airway in children.

Systemic examination especially pertaining to respiratory system such as respiratory distress, stridor, use of accessory muscles, chest sounds on auscultation should also be performed. Most importantly the fasting status of the child should be confirmed.

A number of factors contribute to the difficulty arising during pediatric airway management. These include poor assessment of the airway, poor planning, lack of expertise, lack of appropriate monitoring equipment, medication errors, failure to formulate plan A, B and C, failure to respond emergently to falling saturation and early use of rescue techniques. During management of airway related complications in children, National Audit Project 4 recommended, seeking expert help, changing the approach to airway management and avoiding multiple attempts at intubation.[13]

INVESTIGATIONS

Apart from routine investigations required for the surgical procedure to be performed, certain investigations could help in delineating the airway related problems. These can range from basic investigations like a pulse oximeter reading, arterial blood gas analysis to pulmonary function test which could help to differentiate between intra and extra thoracic obstruction and severity of obstruction. A chest roentgenogram or X-ray of neck in anterior posterior view and lateral view for airway patency, collapse or adenoid hypertrophy may be helpful, whereas advanced imaging like computed roentgenogram and magnetic resonance imaging of neck can help in identifying the site and size of airway obstruction in tracheal and bronchial lumen. There is not much role of nasoendoscopy, as children are not cooperative enough for the procedure and sleep studies also lack significance as these are difficult to conduct and decipher in children.

ANESTHETIC MANAGEMENT

Preparation and Planning

The key to successful airway management is meticulous preparation and planning. It can be divided into preparation of equipment and patient, monitoring techniques available and choice of anesthesia. No best technique or instrument or airway device is available, what is required is presence of good basic airway skills and the knowledge and clear idea that oxygenation and ventilation take priority over intubation.[5]

Equipment

The key to success in securing airway is availability of appropriate size equipment like FM with adequate seal and minimal leak, nasopharyngeal and oropharyngeal airways and correct size of endotracheal tube (ETT) preferably a cuffed tube. Basic monitoring equipment like five lead electrocardiogram, pulse oximetry, end tidal carbon dioxide and noninvasive blood pressure should be available.

Difficult Airway Cart

A dedicated pediatric difficult airway cart should be readily available and on floor during induction of patients with anticipated difficult airway. The cart should be regularly checked. It should be well-organized with proper labeling so as to provide utmost help in time of crisis. The cart can be organized in a step wise approach, with different drawers with labeled instruments **(Table 2)**.

Expected or Anticipated Difficult Airway

First and foremost, it is important to discuss with the surgeon about the need and urgency of surgery to outweigh the risk of anesthesia exposure. In case of lack of expertise or equipment the child should be referred to a higher center. It is pertinent to discuss all possible scenarios and the anesthesia plan with the parents. Once decision has been made to proceed with the surgery, the whole plan should be discussed not only with the surgeon but the entire operation theater staff and all the equipment should be checked prior. A clear plan A, B and C should be formulated and clear to all. A pediatric otolaryngologist should

TABLE 2: Difficult airway cart	
Drawer 1	Different size face mask, oral and nasopharyngeal airway, endotracheal tubes cuffed and uncuffed, airway adjuncts such as stylet, bougie
Drawer 2	Different types of supraglottic airways with different pediatric sizes, different sizes and types of laryngoscope blades, videolaryngoscope, airway exchange catheter
Drawer 3	Fiberoptic bronchoscope
Drawer 4	Material for surgical or needle cricothyrotomy

be informed and present in the operation theater in case of a worse scenario where the need for surgical airway access arises.

Premedication

Use of premedication in presence of a potential airway problem is controversial. The use of sedative drugs to produce anxiolysis should be balanced against the risk of exacerbating airway obstruction. The problems are highlighted especially in a syndromic child or child with an anticipated difficult airway wherein sedative medication can lead to over sedation or a drowsy child. On the other hand, a crying or howling child can produce a lot of secretions, increasing risk of laryngospasm, inability to secure an IV line or place monitoring, or even do inhalational induction. Hence, a small dose of 0.3–0.5 mg/kg of oral/nasal midazolam can be administered under strict vigilance and monitoring. Use of anticholinergic agents like glycopyrrolate or atropine for antisialagogue action and prevention of bradycardia can be given preoperatively in a dose of 10 and 20 µg/kg respectively. In children at high risk of aspiration, consider using H_2 receptor blockers and metoclopramide.

Intravenous Cannulation

In older children an intravenous (IV) cannula can be applied preoperatively using a eutectic mixture of local anesthetics (EMLA). For infants or neonates, aim should be to apply an IV cannula before any airway instrumentation, hence, it rests on the anesthetist's discretion to apply cannula preinduction or after inhalational induction.

Preoxygenation

Prior to anesthetizing the child, preoxygenation is desirable especially so in small infants and children to avoid rapid desaturation. However, preoxygenating a child is difficult owing to lack of cooperation. The onset of desaturation in apneic children occurs much faster than in adults and is known to be age dependent. Children have a smaller functional residual capacity (FRC) than adults, have a greater metabolic demand, generating a higher carbon dioxide output, and have a greater tendency for airway collapse. Therefore, the time frame to establish a safe airway in infants and children is much shorter than in adults.

Use of supplemental oxygen during preoxygenation and induction of anesthesia is recommended either passively or actively with 100% oxygen to achieve an end expired oxygen target of 99%. Preoxygenation in children especially infants, plays an important role in denitrogenation, filling the oxygen reserves and providing sufficient time for airway instrumentation without desaturation episodes.

Use of nasal prongs or nasal cannula or nasopharyngeal airway or modified nasal trumpet in the other nostril can be used at low oxygen flows of 2–4 L/min. Recently, transnasal humidified rapid insufflation ventilatory exchange (THRIVE) has been shown to be more useful in children by doubling the apnea time compared to passive oxygenation thereby, increasing the margin of safety during intubation attempts.[14,15] However, it has not been shown to improve carbon dioxide accumulation rates.

Technique of Induction

Awake intubation in children with anticipated difficult airway is not feasible and is practically impossible especially, in younger children and infants. Hence, children need to be anesthetized for intubation with the aim being to maintain spontaneous ventilation. Inhalational induction with titrated sevoflurane is the ideal modality for induction but under expert hands total intravenous anesthesia using propofol in titrated doses could also be utilized. The use of muscle relaxants in situations of difficult mechanical ventilation (MV), unless the cause is laryngospasm is controversial.[16,17] If the cause is an airway or mediastinal mass or mucopolysaccharidosis, paralysis will worsen the situation. Once the child has been anesthetized, one should assess the possibility of ventilation by mask and optimize it by use of oropharyngeal airway, chin lift and jaw thrust maneuver, two hand ventilation, roll under shoulders, etc. It should be confirmed that the child is adequately anesthetized otherwise anesthesia should be deepened. One should look out for gastric distension which may be interfering with mask ventilation. If still there is a problem with mask ventilation then a supraglottic airway (SGA) device should be introduced.

In older children who are cooperative, literature suggests use of awake fiberoptic intubation (FOI) under sedation utilizing an alpha-2 agonist such as dexmedetomidine. This agent has been recommended as a bolus dose of 1 µg/kg over 10 minutes followed by 0.5 µg/kg/h infusion. It is recommended to titrate the drug in such a way that spontaneous ventilation is intact but the depth of anesthesia is deep enough to allow for laryngoscopy.[18]

Intubation Technique

In situations of anticipated difficulty in securing the airway, intubation techniques with high first pass success rate are advisable to reduce severe complications and it is important to assess whether DL or videolaryngoscopy or fiberoptic bronchoscopy (FOB) will be successful. Most of the scientific literature available to identify approaches of high first pass success rate in children with difficult airway are single center data. Therefore, it is essential to identify the clinical usefulness of these techniques in difficult situations.

Videolaryngoscopy produces a better laryngoscopic view and greater intubation success in difficult airway scenarios. However, in certain anomalies like Hunter's, the first technique of choice may be an FOB-guided intubation. It has been recommended that FOB through an SGA device is a good alternative to secure a difficult airway in children with advantages like ensuring continuous oxygenation and ventilation as well as working as a conduit for FOI since hypoxemia is the most common reason for intubation related adverse events.[19] It also relieves upper airway obstruction in syndromes such as Pierre Robin sequence and Treacher Collins syndrome. Presently, SGA devices most suitable for FO intubation seem to be Air-Q and Ambu AuraGain.[20,21] Information about the size of ETT and FOB which can pass through the SGA device is important if they are being used as a conduit **(Table 3 and Fig. 3)**. In certain situations, a hybrid technique utilizing VL as well as FOB may be successful.

Burjek et al.[19] compared the success rates of FOI via SGA to VL in children with difficult airways with the secondary aim to compare the complication rates of these techniques from the pediatric difficult intubation (PeDI) registry. The authors found that FOI through a SGA and VL have similar first-attempt success rates in children with difficult airways. However, the overall success rate was better with FOI-SGA. The number of attempts required to secure the airway were also similar. In children <1 year of age, FOI-SGA was associated with significantly higher rates of first-attempt success. Selecting FOI-SGA as the first technique was associated with significantly fewer intubation attempts and changes in airway management strategies. Hypoxemia was significantly less common during the FOI-SGA technique when continuous ventilation was used throughout the intubation attempt. Based on this large study, use of

TABLE 3: Size of endotracheal tube (ETT) for passage through supraglottic airway device (SGA) and over fiberoptic bronchoscopy (FOB)

External diameter of scope (mm)	2.0	2.5	2.8	3.5	3.5	4.1	5
Internal diameter of endotracheal tube (mm)	2.5	3	3.5	4	4.5	5	6
Classic LMA size	1	1	1.5	2	2	2.5	3
Airway exchange catheter size (F)	7	8	8	11	11	11	14

(LMA: laryngeal mask airway)

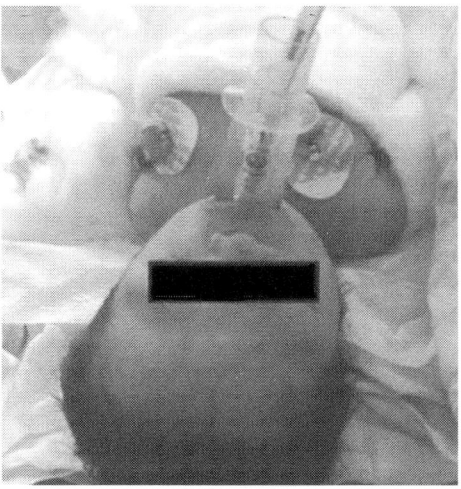

Fig. 3: Supraglottic airway device used as a conduit for FOB-guided endotracheal intubation.

SGA device as a conduit for FOI looks a suitable technique for intubation in children with difficult airway.

UNEXPECTED DIFFICULT INTUBATION

During an unanticipated DI it is required to limit the number of attempts at intubation, keeping the initial attempt limit to 2–3, and further attempts should be made by an expert in pediatric difficult airway. Multiple attempts lead to airway edema which could further worsen the patency of airway.[1,22] With every new attempt at intubation, a change in technique should be made like change in head position, change in laryngoscope blade, size of ETT, use of airway adjuncts such as bougie, stylet or videolaryngoscopes, change in personnel, use of external laryngeal manipulation or increasing the depth of anesthesia. Still, if it is impossible to visualize the larynx, insertion of an SGA is recommended to maintain oxygenation and ventilation and this can be further utilized as a conduit for endotracheal intubation.

Cannot Intubate–Cannot Oxygenate

This is one of the most dreaded complications of airway management for a difficult airway. In case of cannot intubate–cannot oxygenate (CICO), early use of rescue techniques (front of neck access) is desired to prevent lethal hypoxemia and cardiac arrest. The use of muscle relaxation is desirable in situations of CICO proceeding to surgical or needle cricothyrotomy or tracheostomy. The techniques include surgical or needle cricothyroidotomy, of which limited evidence is available in pediatrics. At present there are no randomized controlled trials to compare the two techniques in children during CICO.

Technically both the techniques are challenging in children due to limited evidence, small, elastic, mobile and flaccid trachea which is more prone to collapse but needle cricothyrotomy is not considered to be feasible in children less than 8 years old. Also, identification of cricothyroid membrane (CTM) is difficult in children especially, infants due to presence of abundant adipose tissue and prominent hyoid bone. The size of CTM is 2.6 × 3 mm in neonates which limits the size of tracheal tube passing through it with chances of injury to laryngeal cartilages.[23] In children, compared to CTM it is easier to identify the tracheal rings therefore, surgical tracheostomy could be a better option with less morbidity.[8] The overall incidence of complications in pediatric tracheostomies is around 30% with mortality of 1–2%. The complications range from trauma, bleeding, pneumothorax, pneumomediastinum, subacute emphysema, accidental decannulation and displacement and blockage of tracheostomy tube.[24]

The pediatric difficult airway registry mentions that in 2% of children with anticipated and unexpected DI and CICO, emergency front of neck access (FONA) was initiated, but it was found to have high morbidity and mortality.[1] In such a situation, presence of an ENT specialist and a rigid bronchoscope could play a valuable role for maintaining oxygenation. The PeDI collaborative committee recommended use of a difficult airway bundle checklist including:

(1) use of supplemental oxygen while attempting intubation; (2) after two attempts at intubation, reserve the next attempt for an expert; and (3) call for early help.

DIFFICULT AIRWAY ALGORITHMS

Several pediatric anesthesia societies have given different algorithms for difficult airway management both anticipated and unanticipated in children such as All India Difficult Airway Association (AIDAA) Management Guidelines for children, Pediatric modification of American Society of Anesthesiologists' difficult airway algorithm and Difficult Airway Society/Association of Paediatric Anaesthetists of Great Britain and Ireland[8-10] These guidelines cater to children above infancy and there are no guidelines for neonates with difficult airway still, hence a need for universal simple framework still exists. The framework should be simple, applicable to children of all age groups, easy to learn and memorize and practice.

EXTUBATION

Pediatric patients who have had difficulty in intubation should be considered as difficult for extubation also. APRICOT study mentioned that tracheal extubation following general anesthesia is associated with greater risk of complications as compared to intubation.[22] Hence, adequate preparation and formulation of a plan should be done at the time of extubation.

An awake extubation should be considered, in case of suspected airway trauma and edema and dexamethasone in a dose range of 0.1–0.2 mg/kg body weight IV is recommended. The best time to extubate is when child is hemodynamically stable and there is no hypothermia. Before extubation 100% oxygen should be given, for at least 10 minutes to increase the lung volume and oxygen reserves and the reversal of neuromuscular blockade should be adequate with a "train of four" >0.9 along with clinical signs of recovery.[25,26] Use of airway exchange catheters or guidewire in case of infants and neonates is recommended, which can act as a guide and conduit if reintubation is required. In some scenarios postextubation stridor can develop, which can be dealt with use of continuous positive airway pressure (CPAP), nebulization with adrenaline (400 µg/kg), use of steroids and helium in 30–50% oxygen.

ROLE OF ULTRASOUND IN AIRWAY MANAGEMENT IN CHILDREN

Point-of-care ultrasound (POCUS) of the airway in children is becoming a first line noninvasive adjunct for airway assessment in children. This requires a lot of expertise, high learning curve and a greater and thorough knowledge of the airway anatomy. Use of ultrasound can help in assessment of vocal cord dysfunction, calculating the size of airway and ETT, identification of CTM and tracheal rings as well as in assessing dynamic airway collapsibility and air column width **(Figs. 4A to C)**.[27-30]

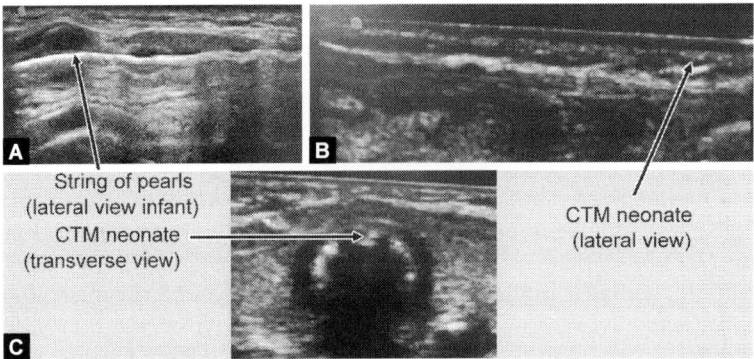

Figs. 4A to C: Ultrasound image of trachea in a child; showing string of pearls appearance. (CTM: cricothyroid membrane)

CONCLUSION

Management of a difficult airway may be challenging even for a pediatric anesthetist. FOB-SGA-guided technique appears to be a good choice for securing the pediatric airway in the 1st attempt. Muscle relaxants should be avoided in anticipated difficult airway till the airway is secured. USG appears to be a promising tool to perform cricothyrotomy in complete ventilation failure situations.

KEY POINTS

- The normal airway of small children is "difficult" because of anatomic and physiological differences compared to adults.
- There is no validated scoring system or anthropometric values which can predict airway difficulty.
- Congenital malformations are the most common causes of difficult airway in children.
- Children cannot undergo awake intubation and require deep sedation or general anesthesia for securing the airway.
- Supraglottic device guided fiberoptic intubation as well as videolaryngoscopy is the best technique for a management of difficult airway in children.
- Front of neck access in CI-CV situation is challenging in infants and includes surgical or needle cricothyrotomy or tracheostomy. However, no randomized controlled trials have been conducted to prove superiority of one over other.

REFERENCES

1. Fiadjoe JE, Nishisaki A, Jagannathan N, Hunyady AI, Greenberg RS, Reynolds PI, et al. Airway management complications in children with difficult tracheal intubation from the Pediatric Difficult Intubation (PeDI) registry: a prospective cohort analysis. Lancet Respir Med. 2016;4(1):37-48.
2. Eich C, Timmermann A, Russo SG, Cremer S, Nickut A, Strack M, et al. A controlled rapid-sequence induction technique for infants may reduce unsafe actions and stress. Acta Anaesthesiol Scand. 2009;53(9):1167-72.

3. Poets CF, Roberts RS, Schmidt B, Whyte RK, Asztalos EV, Bader D, et al. Association between intermittent hypoxemia or bradycardia and late death or disability in extremely preterm infants. JAMA. 2015;314(6):595-603.
4. Jimenez N, Posner KL, Cheney FW, Caplan RA, Lee LA, Domino KB. An update on pediatric anesthesia liability: a closed claims analysis. Anesth Analg. 2007;104(1):147-53.
5. Weiss M, Engelhardt T. Proposal for the management of the unexpected difficult pediatric airway. Paediatr Anaesth. 2010;20(5):454-64.
6. Heinrich S, Birkholz T, Ihmsen H, Irouschek A, Ackermann A, Schmidt J. Incidence and predictors of difficult laryngoscopy in 11,219 pediatric anesthesia procedures. Paediatr Anaesth. 2012;22(8):729-36.
7. Morray JP, Geiduschek JM, Ramamoorthy C, Haberkern CM, Hackel A, Caplan RA, et al. Anesthesia-related cardiac arrest in children: initial findings of the Pediatric Perioperative Cardiac Arrest (POCA) Registry. Anesthesiology. 2000;93(1):6-14.
8. Pawar DK, Doctor JR, Raveendra US, Ramesh S, Shetty SR, Divatia JV, et al. All India Difficult Airway Association 2016 guidelines for the management of unanticipated difficult tracheal intubation in paediatrics. Indian J Anaesth. 2016;60(12):906-14.
9. Apfelbaum JL, Hagberg CA, Caplan RA, Blitt CD, Connis RT, Nickinovich DG, et al. Practice guidelines for management of the difficult airway: an updated report by the American Society of Anesthesiologists Task Force on Management of the Difficult Airway. Anesthesiology. 2013;118(2):251-70.
10. The Association of Paediatric Anaesthetists (APA). Guidelines for difficult airway management in children 2012. [online] Available from http://www.apagbi.org.uk/publications/apa-guidelines. [Last accessed October, 2020].
11. Gupta S, Sharma R, Jain D. Airway assessment: predictors of difficult airways. Indian J Anaesth. 2005;49:257-62.
12. Rafique NB, Khan FA. Comparison of Mallampatti test, thyromental distance and distance from tragus to nares for predicting difficult intubation in pediatric patients. Open J Anesthesiol. 2014;4:104-9.
13. Cook TM, Woodall N, Frerk C; Fourth National Audit Project. Major complications of airway management in the UK: results of Fourth National Audit Project of the Royal College of Anaesthetists and the Difficult Airway Society. Part 1: anaesthesia. Br J Anaesth. 2011;106(5):617-31.
14. Humphreys S, Lee-Archer P, Reyne G, Long D, Williams T, Schibler A. Transnasal humidified rapid-insufflation ventilatory exchange (THRIVE) in children: a randomized controlled trial. Br J Anaesth. 2017;118(2):232-8.
15. Riva T, Pedersen TH, Seiler S, Kasper N, Theiler L, Greif R, et al. Transnasal humidified rapid insufflation ventilatory exchange for oxygenation of children during apnoea: a prospective randomised controlled trial. Br J Anaesth. 2018;120(3):592-9.
16. Julien-Marsollier F, Michelet D, Bellon M, Horlin AL, Devys JM, Dahmani S. Muscle relaxation for tracheal intubation during paediatric anaesthesia: a meta-analysis and trial sequential analysis. Eur J Anaesthesiol. 2017;34(8):550-61.
17. Meakin GH. Role of muscle relaxants in pediatric anesthesia. Curr Opin Anaesthesiol. 2007;20(3):227-31.
18. Jooste EH, Ohkawa S, Sun LS. Fiberoptic intubation with dexmedetomidine in two children with spinal cord impingements. Anesth Analg. 2005;101(4):1248.
19. Burjek NE, Nishisaki A, Fiadjoe JE, Adams HD, Peeples KN, Raman VT, et al. Videolaryngoscopy versus Fiber-optic Intubation through a Supraglottic Airway in Children with a Difficult Airway: an Analysis from the Multicenter Pediatric Difficult Intubation Registry. Anesthesiology. 2017;127(3):432-40.

20. Jagannathan N, Kozlowski RJ, Sohn LE, Langen KE, Roth AG, Mukherji II, et al. A clinical evaluation of the intubating laryngeal airway as a conduit for tracheal intubation in children. Anesth Analg. 2011;112(1):176-82.
21. Kim HJ, Park HS, Kim SY, Ro YJ, Yang HS, Koh WU. A Randomized Controlled Trial Comparing Ambu AuraGain and i-gel in Young Pediatric Patients. J Clin Med. 2019;8(8):1235.
22. Engelhardt T, Virag K, Veyckemans F, Habre; WAPRICOT Group of the European Society of Anaesthesiology Clinical Trial Network. Airway management in paediatric anaesthesia in Europe-insights from APRICOT (Anaesthesia Practice In Children Observational Trial): a prospective multicentre observational study in 261 hospitals in Europe. Br J Anaesth. 2018;121(1):66-75.
23. Navsa N, Tossel G, Boon JM. Dimensions of the neonatal cricothyroid membrane: how feasible is a surgical cricothyroidotomy? Paediatr Anaesth. 2005;15(5):402-6.
24. D'Souza JN, Levi JR, Park D, Shah UK. Complications following pediatric tracheotomy. JAMA Otolaryngol Head Neck Surg. 2016;142(5):484-8.
25. Grandville B, Petak F, Albu G, Bayat S, Pichon I, Habre W. High inspired oxygen fraction impairs lung volume and ventilation heterogeneity in healthy children: a double-blind randomized controlled trial. Br J Anaesth. 2019;122(5):682-91.
26. Meretoja OA. Neuromuscular block and current treatment strategies for its reversal in children. Paediatr Anaesth. 2010;20(7):591-604.
27. Wang LM, Zhu Q, Ma T, Li JP, Hu R, Rong XY, et al. Value of ultrasonography in diagnosis of pediatric vocal fold paralysis. Int J Pediatr Otorhinolaryngol. 2011;75(9):1186-90.
28. Kim EJ, Kim SY, Kim WO, Kim H, Kil HK. Ultrasound measurement of subglottic diameter and an empirical formula for proper endotracheal tube fitting in children. Acta Anaesthesiol Scand. 2013;57(9):1124-30.
29. Sheth M, Jaeel P, Nguyen J. Ultrasonography for verification of endotracheal tube position in neonates and infants. Am J Perinatol. 2017;34(7):627-32.
30. Walsh B, Fennessy P, Ni Mhuircheartaigh R, Snow A, McCarthy KF, McCaul CL. Accuracy of ultrasound in measurement of the pediatric cricothyroid membrane. Paediatr Anaesth. 2019;29(7):744-52.

CHAPTER 11

Peripheral Analgesic Effect of Opioids

Manpreet Kaur

INTRODUCTION

Opioids are considered the prototype drugs of centrally acting analgesics. However, over the last decade there is vast upcoming literature upon assessing its clinical utility as peripherally acting analgesics. Peripheral opioids analgesia occurs by activation of opioid receptors on the peripheral nerve terminals of primary sensory nerves. Local peripheral application of opioids provides high concentration of the active ingredient at the pain site and limits the central side-effects which occur with systemically administered opioids. The peripheral analgesic effect of opioids is dose related, stereospecific and blocked by opioid antagonists. Under inflammatory conditions, there is migration of opioid cells to the injured tissues, thus finding its scope in postsurgical pain and chronic arthritic pains like shoulder arthralgia, knee arthroscopies, etc. In this review we focus on various clinical applications of "peripheral opioid analgesia".

NEED FOR PERIPHERAL ADMINISTRATION OF OPIOIDS

Systemic administration of opioids carries high risk of systemic complications like sedation, respiratory depression, nausea, vomiting, pruritus, constipation and miosis. There is increased risk of over sedation and respiratory depression with systemic opioids in elderly patients, obese, sleep apneic patients, and smokers. Local peripheral application of opioids offers advantage of providing high concentration of opioid without increasing systemic adverse effects and abuse potential.

PERIPHERAL OPIOID RECEPTORS

The three common opioid receptors are: (1) mu (μ), (2) kappa (κ) and (3) delta (δ) receptors which are expressed throughout the central nervous system (CNS) and modulate pain. Animal and human studies have shown that these receptors are present in non-nervous tissues as well.[1] Peripheral structures with opioid receptors include peripheral neurons, postganglionic sympathetic neurons, neuroendocrine organs (pituitary, adrenals), ectodermal, and immune cells.[2]

Flowchart 1: Mechanism of analgesia at cellular level.

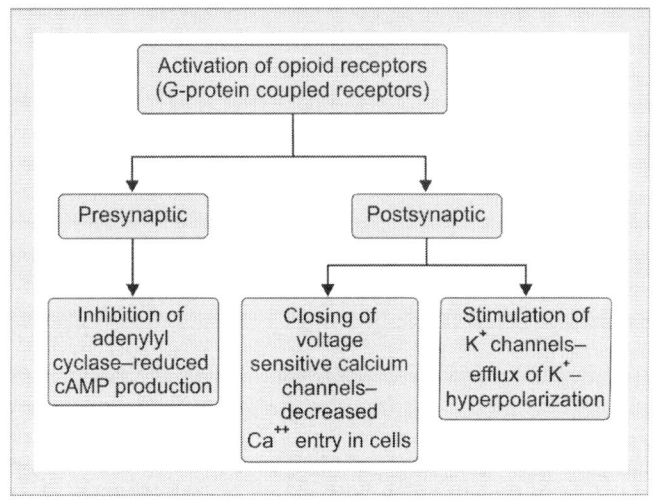

(cAMP: cyclic adenosine monophosphate)

Within the damaged peripheral tissues (like skin, muscles, joints, viscera) there is migration of immune cells which contain opioid peptides. These peripheral receptors modulate pain and inflammation. Inflammation results in sprouting of opioid receptor bearing peripheral sensory nerve terminals. Disrupted perineural barrier due to inflammation along with low pH facilitates binding of the opioids to the receptors.[3] Activation of opioid receptors results in reduction of cyclic adenosine monophosphate (cAMP) production, closes the voltage sensitive calcium channels thereby, decreasing Ca^{++} entry into the cells and hyperpolarizes the membrane by efflux of K^+ **(Flowchart 1)** thereby producing analgesia.

The (κ) receptors are sited on visceral and somatic afferent neurons, hence κ-agonists are used for relief of visceral and neuropathic pain.[4] For δ-agonists to be effective a state of inflammation is needed wherein, delta opioid receptors migrate to the neuronal cell surface increasing accessibility to delta opioid agonists, hence are effective in inflammatory pain.

INFLAMMATION AND PERIPHERAL OPIOID RECEPTOR

Cell bodies of dorsal root ganglion (DRG) express mRNA and proteins of μ, δ, and κ receptors which are then transported along intra-axonal microtubules to peripheral (and central) terminals of sensory neurons. Inflammation augments the synthesis of opioid receptors in DRG and increases expression, transport, and accumulation of opioid receptors in the sensory neurons. There is migration of opioid containing immunocytes into the injured tissues which release endogenous opioid peptides facilitating binding and activation of peripheral opioid receptors thereby producing potent analgesic effect.[1] Mechanisms responsible for enhanced antinociceptive efficacy of opioids in inflamed tissue are **(Fig. 1)**:

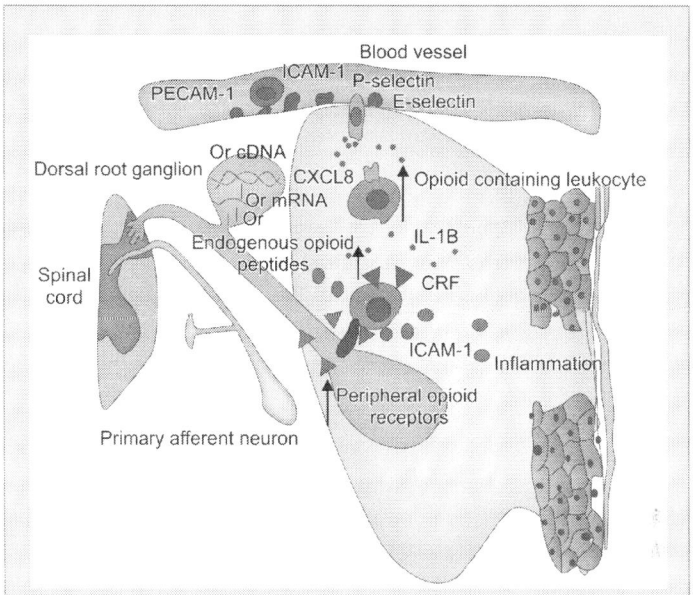

Fig. 1: Inflammation and correlation of peripheral opioid receptors. (ICAM-1: intercellular adhesion molecule-1; PECAM-1: platelet-endothelial cell adhesion molecule-1; CRF: corticotrophin-releasing factor)

- Opioid receptors are upregulated in DRG.
- Increased peripherally directed axonal transport of opioid receptors.
- Enhanced stimulation from cytokines and nerve growth factor (such as corticotrophin releasing factor (CRF), chemokines or noradrenaline (NA) of the inflamed tissue.
- Infiltrating immune cells within inflamed tissue express, contain and release opioid peptides.[5]
- Excitatory ion channels (e.g., TRPV1, Ca^{2+}) and substance P inhibition.
- Endogenously released opioid peptides from inflamed tissues (like leukocyte-derived beta-endorphin and its precursor pro-opiomelanocortin (POMC).

At an early stage (6 hours) of inflammation, there is contribution from both the peripheral and central opioid mechanisms, but at later stages (several days) analgesia is mediated principally by peripheral opioid receptors.[6] Hence, peripheral opioid mechanisms of analgesia become more relevant with the chronicity and with the severity of inflammation.[7]

ROUTES OF ADMINISTRATION

Prerequisites for good peripheral analgesic effects of opioids are good approachability of the painful site, local inflammation at the site, absence of fast systemic absorption at the site, presence of clinically significant pain and use of potent opioid analgesics. Different peripheral sites wherein opioids have been administered are subcutaneous tissue, perineurium, intra-articular, and other sites (tooth socket, wound, intraperitoneal, intrapleural, etc.)

Perineural

Opioids can be used as adjuvants to local anesthetics. Coadministration of opioids with local anesthetic agents may improve the speed of onset and duration of analgesia and counteract disadvantages of high dose of local anesthetics.[8] Opioids potentiate local anesthetics analgesic effects through hyperpolarization of afferent sensory neurons. This "Combination Wisdom", i.e., use of opioids as adjuvants to local anesthetics can be used perineurally in major orthopedic surgeries. Opioids being used are either lipophilic (fentanyl and sufentanyl) or hydrophilic (morphine). Many studies have evaluated utility of morphine in peripheral nerve blocks, but it is limited due to its systemic adverse effects. Besides, it is no way better than intramuscular or intravenous use. Fentanyl and sufentanyl when used in peripheral nerve blocks has shown inconclusive evidence for their benefit.[9] Buprenorphine consistently increased the duration of regional blockade compared to other opioid[10] but increased the incidence of nausea and vomiting. Buprenorphine has been used as adjuvants in nerve blocks in upper extremity peripheral (interscalene or axillary perivascular brachial plexus) blocks and sciatic nerve block.[3,11]

Subcutaneous

Wound infiltrative techniques with or without catheters have been widely used in almost all type of surgical procedures. It is now recommended as a part of multimodal regimens by several societies such as American Society of Anesthesiologists[12] and Australian and New Zealand College of Anesthetists. Subcutaneous infusion of M6G has been found to be clinically useful for advanced cancer pain.[13]

Inflammatory Arthropathy/Intra-articular

Opioids have great effect upon inflammatory pain compared to neuropathic pain as inflammation enhances the migration of opioid receptors.[3] Research in animal models in inflamed knee suggest that activation of mu (μ), and kappa (κ) opioid receptors and not delta (δ) receptors blocked autonomic response to pain at the inflamed tissues.[14] Kappa opioids have powerful anti-inflammatory effect to attenuate arthritis pain (up to 80%) by exerting multiple anti-inflammatory actions.[15] They reduce expression of the adhesion molecules, hamper cell trafficking, decrease release and expression of tumor necrosis factor (TNF), and alter mRNA expression and levels of neuropeptides in the joint tissue. Kappa opioids are therapeutic during disease onset while mu-and delta (δ) agonists have therapeutic anti-inflammatory activity at near toxic doses.[15] Kappa opioid receptor agonist (CR845) found positive results for hip osteoarthritis,[16] while delta opioid receptor agonist (ADL5859, ADL5747) and oxycodone controlled release showed no difference from placebo in a Phase 2a trial in patients with osteoarthritis.[17] There are conflicting results of pain relief with intra-articular injection of morphine after arthroscopic surgeries.[18] Intra-articular μ-agonist has been found to provide effective analgesia in knee surgery, chronic rheumatoid arthritis and osteoarthritis, spinal fusion surgery due to morphine's anti-inflammatory action and decreased number of synovial inflammatory cells. However, need of repeated injection in chronic inflammatory condition limits its use due to risk of infection and it cannot be applied to more than one joint.[19] Periarticular analgesia using local anesthetics with opioids have been injected into the hip joint or periarticular tissues and is gaining popularity recently.

Other Sites (Tooth Socket, Skin, Wound, Intraperitoneal, Intrapleural)

Tooth socket: Administration of low doses (0.4–3.6 mg) of morphine into the inflamed hyperalgesic tooth's ligamental space locally results in significant relief of spontaneous endodontic pain which did not occur with systemic administration of similar morphine dose in multiple randomized control trials.[20]

Painful skin conditions: Topical analgesics are especially beneficial for pediatric patients with painful skin lesions, like burns or postsurgical wounds. Topical morphine gel has been used to treat pain of epidermolysis bullosa without adverse effects.[21] Other agents tried for local application are diamorphine fentanyl and loperamide.

Pain from cutaneous ulcers (both malignant and nonmalignant) have been successfully treated with low dose local morphine without increasing the systemic adverse effects. Intrasite gel, a ready-mixed hydrogel has water, propylene glycol, and carboxymethyl cellulose and is widely used in the palliative care setting for treating skin ulcers. When intrasite gel is placed in contact with the wound, it absorbs excess exudates and produces a moist environment at the wound surface. These fluid handling properties effect the pharmacokinetics of opioids when they are mixed with intrasite gel and applied to skin ulcers.[22]

Neuropathic pain: Local application of mu (μ), kappa (κ) and delta (δ) opioid agonists produce antihyperalgesic effects in animal models. The effective dose (ED) range of μ, κ agonists as analgesic for neuropathic pain is much higher than ED as anti-inflammatory. But, (δ) opioid agonists had same effective dose range as analgesic and anti-inflammatory suggesting its utility in treating chronic pain.[3]

RECENT ADVANCES

Development of novel opioid ligands with exclusive peripheral action and lacking untoward central adverse effects are under clinical trials. A common approach is to develop exogenous opioid receptor ligands which are hydrophilic compounds and do not cross the blood–brain barrier. Agents such as μ-agonist loperamide and the κ-agonist asimadoline have been tried. Novel strategies for development of agents that selectively attract opioid-producing cells, augment opioid peptide production or increase peripheral opioid receptors in inflamed tissues should be further evaluated.[7]

CONCLUSION

Peripheral analgesic effects of opioids have attracted great interest recently, and it has been incorporated into clinical practice widely. Peripheral opioid analgesia is a safer alternative to central opioids or nonsteroidal anti-inflammatory drugs which carry adverse effects (sedation, respiratory depression, nausea, vomiting, dysphoria, addiction, tolerance) and (gastrointestinal bleeding, ulcers, thromboembolic complications) respectively. Future studies may be directed toward assessment of its clinical utility in inflammatory pain and evaluating extended duration opioid formulations.

KEY POINTS

- Peripheral opioids analgesia occurs by activation of opioid receptors on the peripheral nerve terminals of primary sensory nerves.
- Peripheral opioids limit the central side-effects and abuse potential which occur with systemically administered opioids.
- Within the damaged inflamed peripheral tissues like skin, muscles, joints, viscera, there are multifactorial mechanisms of pain relief which include increased opioid receptors and increased immune cells which contain opioid peptides.
- Different peripheral sites wherein opioids have been administered are subcutaneous tissue, perineurium, intra-articular, and other sites (tooth socket, wound, intraperitoneal, intrapleural, etc.).

REFERENCES

1. Sehgal N, Smith HS, Manchikanti L. Peripherally acting opioids and clinical implications for pain control. Pain Physician. 2011;14(3):249-58.
2. Zöllner C, Stein C. Opioids. Handb Exp Pharmacol. 2007;177:31-63.
3. Obara I, Parkitna JR, Korostynski M, Makuch W, Kaminska D, Przewlocka B, et al. Local peripheral opioid effects and expression of opioid genes in the spinal cord and dorsal root ganglia in neuropathic and inflammatory pain. Pain. 2009;141(3):283-91.
4. Vanderah TW. Delta and kappa opioid receptors as suitable drug targets for pain. Clin J Pain. 2010;26(Suppl 10):S10-15.
5. Cabot PJ. Immune-derived opioids and peripheral antinociception. Clin Exp Pharmacol Physiol. 2001;28(3):230-2.
6. Machelska H, Schopohl JK, Mousa SA, Labuz D, Schäfer M, Stein C. Different mechanisms of intrinsic pain inhibition in early and late inflammation. J Neuroimmunol. 2003;141(1-2):30-9.
7. Stein C, Lang LJ. Peripheral mechanisms of opioid analgesia. Curr Opin Pharmacol. 2009;9(1):3-8.
8. Kaur M. Adjuvants to local anesthetics: a combination wisdom. Anesth Essays Res. 2010;4(2):122-3.
9. Emelife PI, Eng MR, Menard BL, Myers AS, Cornett EM, Urman RD, et al. Adjunct medications for peripheral and neuraxial anesthesia. Best Pract Res Clin Anaesthesiol. 2018;32(2):83-99.
10. Koyyalamudi V, Sen S, Patil S, Creel JB, Cornett EM, Fox CJ, et al. Adjuvant Agents in Regional Anesthesia in the Ambulatory Setting. Curr Pain Headache Rep. 2017;21(1):6.
11. Candido KD, Hennes J, Gonzalez S, Mikat-Stevens M, Pinzur M, Vasic V, et al. Buprenorphine enhances and prolongs the postoperative analgesic effect of

bupivacaine in patients receiving infragluteal sciatic nerve block. Anesthesiology. 2010;113(6):1419-26.
12. American Society of Anesthesiologists Task Force on Acute Pain Management. Practice guidelines for acute pain management in the perioperative setting: an updated report by the American Society of Anesthesiologists Task Force on Acute Pain Management. Anesthesiology. 2012;116(2):248-73.
13. Penson RT, Joel SP, Roberts M, Gloyne A, Beckwith S, Slevin ML. The bioavailability and pharmacokinetics of subcutaneous, nebulized and oral morphine-6-glucuronide. Br J Clin Pharmacol. 2002;53(4):347-54.
14. Nagasaka H, Awad H, Yaksh TL. Peripheral and spinal actions of opioids in the blockade of the autonomic response evoked by compression of the inflamed knee joint. Anesthesiology. 1996;85(4):808-16.
15. Walker JS. Anti-inflammatory effects of opioids. Adv Exp Med Biol. 2003;521:148-60.
16. Cara Therapeutics. Top-line Results From Phase 2b Trial of Oral CR845 in Chronic Pain Patients With Osteoarthritis of the Hip or Knee. [online] Available from http://ir.caratherapeutics.com/news-releases/news-release-details/cara-therapeutics-announces-top-line-results-phase-2b-trial-oral. [Last accessed October, 2020].
17. Fierce Biotech. Adolor Corporation Provides Clinical Update; Will Host Conference Call. [online]. Available from https://www.fiercebiotech.com/biotech/adolor-corporation-provides-clinical-update-will-host-conference-call. [Last accessed October, 2020].
18. Heard SO, Edwards WT, Ferrari D, Hanna D, Wong PD, Liland A, et al. Analgesic effect of intraarticular bupivacaine or morphine after arthroscopic knee surgery: a randomized, prospective, double-blind study. Anesth Analg. 1992;74(6):822-6.
19. Stein C, Schäfer M, Machelska H. Attacking pain at its source: new perspectives on opioids. Nat Med. 2003;9(8):1003-8.
20. Dionne RA, Lepinski AM, Gordon SM, Jaber L, Brahim JS, Hargreaves KM. Analgesic effects of peripherally administered opioids in clinical models of acute and chronic inflammation. Clin Pharmacol Ther. 2001;70(1):66-73.
21. Watterson G, Howard R, Goldman A. Peripheral opioids in inflammatory pain. Arch Dis Child. 2004;89(7):679-81.
22. Ribeiro MD, Joel SP, Zeppetella G. The bioavailability of morphine applied topically to cutaneous ulcers. J Pain Symptom Manage. 2004;27(5):434-9.

CHAPTER 12

Maternal Morbidity and Mortality: An Anesthesiologist's Role and Perspective

Medha Mohta

INTRODUCTION

Health care in India has been consistently improving over last few decades. A lot has been done to improve maternal health, which may be considered one of the determinants of a healthy society. However, the maternal mortality and morbidity in India still remains very high compared to developed nations. Anesthesiologists are the key members of the team managing pregnant and postpartum patients, and thus bear a great responsibility in improving overall maternal outcome.

DEFINITIONS

World Health Organization (WHO) defines *maternal mortality* as "the death of a woman while pregnant or within 42 days of termination of pregnancy, irrespective of the duration and site of the pregnancy, from any cause related to or aggravated by the pregnancy or its management but not from accidental or incidental causes".[1]

The *maternal mortality ratio (MMR)* is defined as "the number of maternal deaths during a given time period per 100,000 live births during the same time period".

Maternal morbidity is defined as "any health condition attributed to and/or aggravated by pregnancy and childbirth that has a negative impact on the woman's wellbeing".[2]

The WHO definition of *severe maternal morbidity (SMM)* is "a woman who nearly died but survived a complication that occurred during pregnancy, birth or within 42 days of termination of pregnancy". "Maternal near miss" (MNM) is another term described for similar condition, which is diagnosed by a set of clinical, laboratory-based and management-based criteria.[3]

THE CURRENT SITUATION

The Millennium Development Goals had set a target of 75% decrease in the global MMR by 2015. However, the world was able to achieve a reduction in

MMR by only 44% between 1990 and 2015. The new Sustainable Development Goal now aims to reduce global MMR to less than 70 per 100,000 live births by 2030.[4] As MMR varies largely across the world, it should not be more than 140 per 100,000 in any country in the world.

For every woman dying due to pregnancy-related causes, a much larger number have SMM and suffer life-threatening complications, which may lead to massive blood transfusion, hysterectomy, other surgical or medical interventions, or prolonged hospital stay.[5] Besides endangering the maternal life, SMM also has serious consequences for fetal or neonatal outcome.[6]

Although United States of America (USA) has comparatively a very low MMR (26.4 per 100,000 live births in 2015), it witnessed a 50% increase in MMR over previous 25 years;[7] whereas SMM increased by 75% from 1998 to 2009.[5]

India's MMR during the years 2014–16 was 130 per 100,000 live births, which came down to 122 during 2015–17.[8] However, maternal mortality in India is still quite high and it accounted for about 15% of global maternal deaths in 2015.[9] A pilot program conducted in six institutions in India found an incidence of MNM to be 0.96%, with hemorrhage being the leading cause.[10]

CAUSES OF MATERNAL MORBIDITY AND MORTALITY

It is extremely important to make all possible efforts to reduce maternal morbidity and mortality. To achieve this goal, it is essential to understand various factors responsible for maternal morbidity and mortality. During perioperative period, the causes can be anesthesia-related adverse events or nonanesthetic perioperative complications **(Table 1)**.

The risk of anesthesia-related adverse events as well as nonanesthetic complications has been seen to be higher during cesarean section than during vaginal delivery, especially during emergency cesareans, procedures performed under general anesthesia (GA), and in patients with comorbidities.[11]

TABLE 1: Causes of maternal morbidity and mortality during perioperative period

Anesthesia-related complications	Nonanesthetic complications
General anesthesia-related: • Difficult or failed intubation • Pulmonary aspiration • Intracranial hemorrhage (hypertensive response to intubation in pre-eclampsia) *Neuraxial anesthesia-related:* • Postdural puncture headache • High or total spinal anesthesia • Intravascular injection of local anesthetic drug • Epidural hematoma • Infectious complications (epidural abscess, meningitis)	• Hemorrhage • Hypertensive disorders of pregnancy • Venous thromboembolism • Severe anemia • Cardiovascular disease • Coagulopathy • Sepsis • Respiratory failure • Renal failure • Amniotic fluid embolism

> **BOX 1: Risk factors for maternal mortality.**
> - Pre-existing medical illness
> - Problems/complications in previous pregnancy
> - Advanced maternal age
> - Multiple gestation
> - Inadequate antenatal care
> - Obesity
> - Abnormal placentation, especially placenta accreta
> - Low socioeconomic status

The factors which increase the risk for adverse maternal outcome are listed in **Box 1**.

Amongst nonanesthetic causes, hemorrhage and hypertensive disorders of pregnancy account for approximately half of overall maternal mortality. Hemorrhage was found to be responsible for one third of deaths in the Serious Complications Repository (SCORE) by Society for Obstetric Anesthesia and Perinatology (SOAP) in 2014.[12]

ROLE OF ANESTHESIOLOGIST IN MANAGEMENT OF PARTURIENTS

Anesthesiologists play multiple roles in management of obstetric patients. They provide labor analgesia, and anesthesia for cesarean section and other obstetric and nonobstetric surgical procedures. Besides these, they manage critically ill obstetric patients in intensive care unit (ICU). They are also frequently called to help in management of almost all types of obstetric crises.

Obstetric patients may require oxygen therapy, tracheal intubation and mechanical ventilation in labor room or wards. Hemodynamically unstable patients also may require interventions by anesthesiologists for securing vascular access, invasive monitoring, management of vasoactive infusions, and massive transfusion.[13]

Recent studies have shown that the incidence of anesthesia-related adverse events is decreasing; whereas nonanesthetic perioperative complications are increasing.[11] According to Mhyre and Bateman, anesthesiologists can play an important role in reducing both types of complications.[14]

ANESTHESIA-RELATED COMPLICATIONS

General Anesthesia-related Complications

Although neuraxial anesthesia, especially spinal anesthesia, is the technique of choice for most cesarean sections; administration of GA may be required for many maternal or fetal indications, e.g., severe thrombocytopenia, coagulopathy, infection at the site of injection, sepsis, neurological abnormalities, severe uncorrected hypovolemia, pulmonary edema, evidence of raised intracranial pressure, severe anemia, maternal refusal, umbilical cord prolapse, severe fetal distress, and failure of neuraxial block.

In modern anesthesia, administration of GA has become very safe. However, special attention must be paid, and adequate precautions taken to avoid the following complications:

Difficult or Failed Intubation

Obstetric airway is considered to be more difficult than nonobstetric. The main reasons are airway edema due to vascular engorgement, weight gain, enlarged breasts and full dentition in parturient.[15] Airway edema may be further exacerbated in pre-eclampsia, patients having upper respiratory tract infection or those in prolonged second stage of labor. The Mallampati class deteriorates during advanced pregnancy, especially during labor. The mother tends to desaturate faster due to reduced functional residual capacity and increased oxygen requirements. In addition, very often the surgery is conducted on emergency basis. All these factors lead to a higher risk of failed intubation.

The best option to avoid failed intubation is to avoid GA. American Society of Anesthesiologists (ASA) has recommended insertion of early epidural catheter to reduce the need for administration of GA if an emergency surgery is required in patients having anesthetic indications, i.e., anticipated difficult airway or obesity; or obstetric indications, i.e., pre-eclampsia or twin pregnancy.[16] Rapid sequence spinal anesthesia has also been described for category I urgent cesarean sections.[17]

If it is not possible to avoid GA and airway examination suggests anticipated difficult airway, awake intubation or intubation using difficult airway adjuncts may be planned. An experienced anesthesiologist must be present to manage anticipated difficult airway. One must always remember that even in cases with fetal distress, maintenance of maternal oxygenation and ventilation remains the topmost priority.

In case of unanticipated difficulty with airway management, the difficult airway algorithm must be followed.[18,19] The algorithm by the Obstetric Anesthetists' Association and Difficult Airway Society[18] emphasizes the need for adequate preinduction planning and preparation for provision of safe obstetric GA. During rapid sequence induction, proper positioning with 20–30° head up or ramping with left uterine displacement are important. Preoxygenation should be done to achieve an end-point of end-tidal oxygen fraction ($F_{ET}O_2$) $\geq$ 0.9 to ensure adequate denitrogenation; nasal oxygenation should be continued during intubation. Another important change in the traditional viewpoint is that gentle facemask ventilation should be considered during rapid sequence induction, keeping the maximum inflation pressure less than 20 cmH$_2$O. If two intubation attempts fail, failed intubation must be declared. A second generation supraglottic device, or facemask with or without an oropharyngeal airway should be used to maintain oxygenation. Cricoid pressure should be removed during insertion of supraglottic device. Even during difficulty with intubation or mask ventilation, one should have a low threshold for removal of cricoid pressure. If despite all these attempts, maintenance of adequate oxygenation is not possible, front-of-neck airway access must be performed. The All India Difficult Airway Association has also formulated guidelines to manage unanticipated difficult intubation in obstetric patients.[19]

Aspiration of Gastric Contents

Obstetric patients are at a high risk of aspiration due to reduced lower esophageal sphincter tone and increased intragastric pressure. Gastric emptying is usually not altered; however, it may be delayed in the presence of labor pains or opioid intake.

To minimize this risk, the mother should fast for 6–8 hours for solids and 2 hours for clear liquids.[16] Ranitidine, an H_2 receptor antagonist, is administered to reduce gastric acidity and volume, in a dose of 50 mg intravenous (IV) 30–45 minutes or 150 mg oral 60–90 minutes before induction. Metoclopramide 10 mg increases lower esophageal sphincter tone, decreases gastric volume by increasing gastric peristalsis and also has an antiemetic action. Oral 0.3 M sodium citrate 30 mL, when given within 30 minutes of induction, reduces acidity. Finally, cricoid pressure must be applied at the time of induction of anesthesia.

Nowadays, risk of pulmonary aspiration has drastically reduced due to availability and awareness of clear guidelines related to fasting, aspiration prophylaxis and safe rapid sequence intubation; and increased use of neuraxial techniques.[13] The serious complication repository project did not find even a single instance of aspiration of gastric contents among 5000 general anesthetics.[12]

Intracranial Hemorrhage (Hypertensive Response to Intubation in Pre-eclampsia)

In severely pre-eclamptic patients, hypertensive response to laryngoscopy and intubation/extubation can lead to complications such as cerebral hemorrhage or pulmonary edema. Therefore, it is essential to attenuate this response to reduce the risk of these serious complications. The goal should be to reduce blood pressure to approximately 140/90 mm Hg before induction, and then to maintain systolic blood pressure of 140–160 mm Hg and diastolic blood pressure at 90–100 mm Hg during laryngoscopy and intubation.[20] According to the latest American College of Obstetricians and Gynecologists (ACOG) Committee Opinion,[21] "induction of GA and intubation should never be undertaken without first taking steps to eliminate or minimize hypertensive response to intubation".

Neuraxial Anesthesia-related Complications

According to the SCORE, the incidence of most of the complications was very low, with epidural hematoma occurring in 1:250,000 patients, epidural abscess/meningitis in 1:60,000, and serious neurological injury in 1:35,000 cases. However, 1 in 4,000 patients had high spinal blockade.[12]

High Spinal Blockade

High spinal block is said to occur when the block level ascends more than intended. With total spinal, the block height is usually higher than T1 dermatomal level and there is loss of consciousness due to hypoperfusion of brain stem. This can result in respiratory and cardiovascular collapse. The initial symptoms are usually nausea and anxiety due to cerebral hypoperfusion.

The most common cause is inadvertent placement or migration of epidural catheter into intrathecal or subdural space. Other common causes include administration of excessively high doses of spinal local anesthetic (LA) or spinal injection after recently administered epidural bolus.[22]

Conversion of an epidural placed for labor analgesia to surgical anesthesia demands extreme caution as the risk of high spinal block due to administration of large and frequent doses of LA or boluses through unidentified intrathecal catheter is high during this period.[13]

Postdural Puncture Headache

Postdural puncture headache (PDPH) is a frontal-occipital headache which is aggravated in sitting or standing position and is relieved on lying down. It occurs because of leakage of cerebrospinal fluid following dural puncture, which in turn, results in intracranial hypotension. It may be associated with symptoms such as neck stiffness, nausea/vomiting, photophobia, tinnitus or diplopia. The management involves aggressive hydration, rest, pharmacologic measures including caffeine and paracetamol, and epidural blood patch if the headache does not respond to conservative measures.[22]

The risk of development of PDPH following dural puncture with epidural needle is quite high (approximately 52%).[23] During spinal anesthesia, incidence of PDPH depends on size and shape of spinal needle; smaller gauge pencil point needles having the minimum risk.

Although the overall incidence of PDPH in obstetric patients is 1-2%,[13] it accounts for 96% of neuraxial anesthesia related adverse events.[11] Therefore, it is very important to take precautionary measures to prevent its occurrence; and to diagnose and treat it properly, if it occurs.

Intravascular Injection of Local Anesthetic

This is a very serious complication of neuraxial anesthesia and analgesia, and leads to local anesthetic systemic toxicity (LAST). It presents with central nervous symptoms, e.g., perioral numbness, agitation, confusion, tinnitus, loss of consciousness and seizures; followed by cardiovascular symptoms such as hypotension, arrhythmias, and finally cardiac arrest.

Pregnant patients are at a higher risk of developing LAST as they have decreased plasma levels of α_1-acid glycoprotein and increased cardiac output, leading to enhanced perfusion and rapid LA absorption. Drug absorption and possibility of migration of epidural catheter are also higher due to epidural venous engorgement.[24]

Immediate management of LAST includes stopping of LA injection and management of airway, breathing and circulation. Oxygen must be started, and airway secured to prevent hypoxia, hypercapnia and acidosis. According to the third American Society of Regional Anesthesia and Pain Medicine practice advisory on LAST,[25] 20% lipid emulsion 100 mL (1.5 mL/kg in patients weighing less than 70 kg) should be administered intravenously over 2–3 minutes. This is followed by an infusion of 200–250 mL over 15–20 minutes (0.25 mL/kg/min if body weight <70 kg). If required, another bolus may be administered, or the rate of infusion may be increased to 0.5 mL/kg/min. The infusion should be continued for 10 minutes after achieving circulatory stability. Seizures should be treated with benzodiazepines; if these are not effective, small doses of neuromuscular blockers may be considered. If cardiac arrest occurs, advanced cardiac life support algorithm must be followed. Amiodarone is the preferred antiarrhythmic, if ventricular arrhythmias develop. Calcium channel blockers, β-adrenergic receptor blockers and lignocaine are not recommended.

Epidural Hematoma

Epidural hematoma is a rare but serious complication, with a lower incidence in parturient than in general surgical patients.[26] The risk factors for development of this complication include thrombocytopenia, coagulopathy, iatrogenic administration of anticoagulants, and multiple or traumatic attempts at catheter placement.[13]

Platelet count >80,000/mm^3 in the absence of other coagulation abnormalities is considered adequate for epidural catheter insertion as well as removal; whereas a count <50,000/mm^3 contraindicates neuraxial procedure.[20] Between 50,000 and 80,000/mm^3, one must weigh risk and benefit of the technique. If decided in favor of neuraxial technique, spinal is preferred, that too by a skilled anesthesiologist and with careful neurologic monitoring after the procedure. If required, immediate neurosurgical consultation must be taken. If hematoma develops, it must be surgically evacuated at the earliest.

The SOAP have published a consensus statement on the anesthetic management of women receiving antepartum or postpartum thromboprophylaxis with unfractionated heparin (UFH) or low molecular weight heparin (LMWH).[27] With UFH, the dose of anticoagulant, the time elapsed after the last dose and coagulation profile determine the safety of neuraxial procedure. In case of low dose LMWH, neuraxial procedure can be safely performed at least 12 hours after the last dose administration; whereas one should wait for at least 24 hours if the patient is receiving high dose LMWH. The SOAP guidelines also provide detailed guidance on catheter management while receiving thromboprophylaxis, the timing of catheter removal and initiating/restarting of thromboprophylaxis in the postpartum period.

Infectious Complications

American Society of Anesthesiologists, in 2017, developed an advisory for prevention, diagnosis, and management of neuraxial procedures-related infectious complications.[28] Neuraxial procedures should be avoided in patients suspected to have bacteremia. If still decided to select these techniques, antibiotics must be administered before the procedure. Strict aseptic precautions are mandatory in all cases. Chlorhexidine with alcohol, with adequate drying time, should be used for skin preparation. Use of sterile occlusive dressings, bacterial filters, and limiting disconnection and reconnection of delivery systems further reduce the risk of infection. Catheters found disconnected must be removed.

For early diagnosis, patients must be regularly monitored for signs and symptoms of infection. In case of suspected infection, appropriate cultures, blood tests, imaging and specialist consultation must be obtained. If an infectious complication develops, appropriate antibiotics must be administered and consultation for the surgical management must be taken.

NONANESTHETIC PERIOPERATIVE COMPLICATIONS

Hemorrhage

Obstetric hemorrhage is a major cause of maternal mortality and severe morbidity; and majority of these deaths are preventable.[29] A consensus bundle on obstetric hemorrhage was developed by National Partnership on Maternal Safety in 2015.[30] It involved representatives from multiple organizations including SOAP. This bundle has four components: (1) readiness, (2) recognition and prevention, (3) response, and (4) reporting and systems learning. Each maternity unit must be ready with a hemorrhage cart having required supplies, uterotonic medications, a response team and a well-defined protocol for massive and emergency transfusion. Recognition and prevention involve hemorrhage risk assessment for every patient, accurate blood loss measurement and oxytocin administration after delivery. For proper and timely response to hemorrhage, every unit must have an emergency management plan with checklists; and support system for patients, their families, and staff. Reporting and systems learning include debriefs, multidisciplinary review and outcome monitoring.

The important components of massive transfusion protocols include fixed ratio transfusions of red blood cells, plasma and platelets; early coagulation testing and serial monitoring; and cryoprecipitate transfusion if fibrinogen levels fall.[30] Hypofibrinogenemia occurs early in severe obstetric hemorrhage. Therefore, fibrinogen levels must be measured, with values less than 200 mg/dL requiring aggressive monitoring and management in the setting of postpartum hemorrhage (PPH).[31] Administration of tranexamic acid within 3 hours of delivery has also been seen to be effective in reducing maternal mortality by 31%.[32]

In the safety bundle on obstetric hemorrhage, anesthesiologist has been identified as an important member of the core response team.[30] Presence of an anesthesiologist has been shown to have a positive effect on quality of care during obstetric hemorrhage.[33] Delay in calling anesthesiologist for help was also associated with greater severity of PPH.[34] Thus, anesthesiologists have a definite role to play in improving outcome of a bleeding mother.

Hypertensive Disorders of Pregnancy

Anesthesiologists have significant involvement almost at every step in management of pre-eclamptic patients.

Treatment of Hypertension

Systolic blood pressure >160 mm Hg or diastolic blood pressure >110 mm Hg must be treated expeditiously to prevent maternal complications such as myocardial ischemia, hypertensive encephalopathy or cerebrovascular hemorrhage.[20] The first-line drugs used for this are labetalol, hydralazine, and immediate release oral nifedipine, if IV access is not available. Second-line therapy includes nicardipine, esmolol and sodium nitroprusside. Although initial management is started by the obstetricians, anesthesiologists are quite often requested to help manage patients with refractory hypertension.

Seizure Prophylaxis and Control

Magnesium sulfate is administered as continuous IV infusion or intermittent intramuscular (IM) injections for prophylaxis of seizures in severe pre-eclampsia or treatment of seizures in eclampsia. The patient must be watched for signs of magnesium toxicity by monitoring respiration, urine output and deep tendon reflexes. Treatment of toxicity involves discontinuation of magnesium, IV calcium gluconate 1 g over 10 minutes, oxygen administration and mechanical ventilation, if required.[20] Anesthesiologists are involved in management of most of these patients, either to provide anesthesia or to manage them in ICU.

Appropriate Fluid Management

Pre-eclamptic patients are very prone to have pulmonary edema. Therefore, maintenance fluids should be limited to 80 mL/h unless the patient is having ongoing fluid losses, e.g., hemorrhage.[35]

Management of Pulmonary Edema

The incidence of pulmonary edema in pre-eclampsia is 3%, with only 30% cases occurring before delivery. The causes predisposing pre-eclamptic patients to develop pulmonary edema are low colloid osmotic pressure due to proteinuria, increased intravascular hydrostatic pressure and increased pulmonary capillary permeability. All these patients are admitted to ICU. The treatment principles remain same as in nonobstetric population.

Venous Thromboembolism

Pregnancy is a hypercoagulable state and therefore, risk of venous thromboembolism is four times higher in pregnant and postpartum women than nonpregnant.[36] The risk is higher in parturient with anemia, hyperemesis, fluid/electrolyte/acid-base imbalance, pre-eclampsia, antepartum hemorrhage, PPH, multiple gestation, those receiving transfusion or women undergoing cesarean delivery.[37]

Thromboprophylaxis in the form of mechanical and/or pharmacological intervention has been recommended for high-risk patients. Mechanical thromboprophylaxis can be provided with pneumatic compression devices. Pharmacological prophylaxis involves use of LMWH or UFH, which have implications for safety of neuraxial techniques and risk of PPH.[38] Provision of safe anesthesia in patients receiving LMWH or UFH has already been discussed under the heading of "Epidural hematoma".

Severe Anemia

Anemia is a very common problem during pregnancy in India. A recent single center study from South India reported an overall prevalence of 33.9%, with 2.1% pregnant women having severe anemia.[39] Although incidence in developed high-income countries is much lower than in low and middle-income countries, anemia has been recognized as a preventable risk factor for maternal morbidity even in these developed countries.[40]

Anemia adds to maternal morbidity due to an association with pre-eclampsia, antepartum and postpartum hemorrhage, higher rates of induction of labor and cesarean delivery, requirements of blood transfusion, infectious complications including sepsis, higher antibiotic use and longer hospital stay.[41]

Anemia is also a direct and indirect contributor to maternal deaths.[41] Severely anemic patients can have cardiac decompensation leading to heart failure. Risk of hypotension leading to shock and death is also higher in these patients even with moderate bleeding during third stage of labor. A multilevel analysis was carried out in 359 hospitals in 29 countries, including India, to study the independent association between severe anemia and maternal mortality.[42] The odds of mortality in severely anemic patients were found to be twice as high than in those without severe anemia.

Amniotic Fluid Embolism

Amniotic fluid embolism is another nonanesthetic complication which can cause high maternal and fetal mortality. It occurs in 1.2–6.6 women per 100,000 deliveries.[43] Eclampsia, placenta previa, placental abruption, cesarean delivery, cervical laceration or uterine rupture, instrumental vaginal delivery, diabetes, pre-eclampsia, medical induction of labor, amniocentesis, premature rupture of membranes, multiparity and advanced maternal age are considered risk factors for occurrence of amniotic fluid embolism. Women usually present with hypotension, hypoxia, respiratory distress, cardiopulmonary collapse, disseminated intravascular coagulopathy (DIC) or atonic bleeding. Management requires resuscitation with oxygenation; cardiovascular support; transfusion of large volumes of blood products, including plasma, platelets, and cryoprecipitate to manage hemorrhage and coagulopathy; and delivery of fetus.[43] Advanced cardiac life support is required in case of cardiac arrest.

Cardiac Diseases

Cardiac diseases such as cardiomyopathy, congenital heart diseases and coronary artery disease are frequent causes of death during pregnancy in United States;[38] whereas in India, rheumatic heart disease still remains the most frequent cardiac cause of maternal mortality and morbidity.[44] It accounts for 69% of the cardiac cases during pregnancy, with mixed mitral valve lesions being the most common.[45] Many of these patients develop cardiac failure and require multidisciplinary critical care management. Anesthesiologists have an important role in ICU management as well as in providing labor analgesia and anesthesia for cesarean delivery to these high-risk patients. Both GA and neuraxial techniques have been safely used. Understanding pathophysiology of the disease, appropriate patient selection and cautious anesthetic management results in an improved outcome.

Sepsis

Sepsis is a cause for significant number of maternal deaths all over the world. Besides maternal mortality, it also results in a poor fetal outcome, with a high incidence of abortions, stillbirths and preterm births.[46] In India, the sepsis related maternal mortality has been reported as 128/100,000 live births in a single center study.[47] Genital tract, respiratory system, urinary tract, and surgical site are the common sources of infection leading to sepsis during pregnancy. WHO has reported prevalence of puerperal sepsis as 4% of live births.[48] Gram-negative bacteria are the most common organisms responsible for maternal sepsis.

During pregnancy and puerperium, the mother's defenses to fight infection are impaired due to physiological and immunological changes. In addition, diagnosis of early sepsis becomes difficult as the early signs may be confused with physiological changes of pregnancy.[46] This contributes to progression of many cases to severe sepsis and septic shock. Most of these critically ill patients are managed in ICU and hence require involvement of an anesthesiologist.

Royal College of Obstetricians and Gynaecologists (RCOG) have defined indications for transfer of these patients to ICU.[49,50] These include hypotension or raised serum lactate refractory to fluid resuscitation and requiring inotropic support, need for mechanical ventilation, pulmonary edema, airway protection, decreased consciousness, need for dialysis, multiorgan failure, hypothermia and uncorrected acidosis.

The two main aspects of management are initial resuscitation and control of source of infection. For initial resuscitation in presence of hypotension and/or blood lactate level >4 mmoL/L, RCOG has recommended IV fluid resuscitation with 20 mL/kg crystalloid, with a target to achieve mean arterial pressure of 65 mm Hg.[49,50] Source control involves early administration of broad-spectrum antibiotics, with de-escalation once the culture reports are available; and surgical removal of infectious material such as abscess drainage, if required.

MEASURES TO BE TAKEN TO REDUCE SEVERE MATERNAL MORBIDITY AND MORTALITY

To reduce overall maternal mortality and morbidity, both anesthesia-related and nonanesthetic complications must be minimized. The incidence of anesthesia-related complications is much lower than the nonanesthetic complications. It is the direct responsibility of anesthesiologists to further improve the safety of anesthesia and analgesia provided to obstetric patients, especially in rare and emergency situations. For this, adequate preparedness and improved skills can be achieved by team training and use of protocols.[11]

At the same time, there is an urgent need to take multidisciplinary measures to implement protocols to reduce nonanesthetic maternal complications. Some examples are hemorrhage protocols, universal thromboembolism prophylaxis protocols and rapid antihypertensive administration protocols for pre-eclamptic patients.[14] Efficacy of such measures has already been proven. Implementation of pneumatic compression device application in all patients undergoing cesarean section, rapid antihypertensive therapy protocols in pre-eclamptic patients, and maternal hemorrhage protocols resulted in seven-fold decrease in deaths due to pulmonary embolism,[51] no deaths due to intracranial hemorrhage[51] and 26% decrease in blood consumption[52] respectively.

The most common causes leading to SMM have been identified as failure to timely detect high-risk patients with resultant delays in diagnosis and proper management.[6] Early recognition of maternal morbidity and timely action can improve outcome. It has been suggested to formulate and implement maternal early warning criteria.[53] These include vital signs, e.g., heart rate, blood pressure, respiratory rate, oxygen saturation, urine output, neurologic response, etc.; and also suggest differential diagnosis of hemorrhage, hypertensive crisis, thromboembolism, heart failure or sepsis. Anesthesiologists are experts in interpreting the changes in these vital signs and thus can efficiently contribute toward implementing these systems.[31]

Simulation of obstetric critical events, multidisciplinary communication and educational activities can also greatly help in enhancing patient safety.[54]

Low Dose Oxytocin

High dose oxytocin may be associated with number of side-effects. Low doses have been found to be effective and safe and thus improve maternal outcome. Anesthesiologists' contribution has been significant in this field as most of the studies establishing efficacy of low dose oxytocin have been conducted by anesthesiologists.

ANESTHESIOLOGISTS AS PERIDELIVERY PHYSICIANS

Anesthesiologists are important members of multidisciplinary work groups in USA for formulation of practice guidelines and safety bundles to reduce maternal morbidity and mortality.[31] Their training provides them the ability to significantly improve maternal outcome by their contributions in management of most of the conditions associated with a high morbidity and mortality such as obstetric hemorrhage, hypertensive disease, pulmonary embolism, amniotic fluid embolism, sepsis, peripartum cardiomyopathy and other comorbid conditions.[29] They should utilize their expertise in the field of anesthesia and critical care to contribute to improved management of high risk, unstable and critically ill pregnant patients; and thus take up the role of "peridelivery physicians".[55]

CONCLUSION

The causes of perioperative maternal morbidity and mortality may be anesthesia-related adverse events, or nonanesthetic perioperative complications. The incidence of anesthesia-related complications has decreased due to increased safety of anesthetic techniques and agents. On the other hand, nonanesthetic complications are rising. The anesthesiologists can play an important role in reducing both types of complications. They must strive hard to further improve the safety of anesthesia and analgesia, especially in rare and emergency situations. At the same time, they must realize their responsibility and potential to make significant contributions to the multidisciplinary measures needed for improvement of overall maternal outcome.

KEY POINTS

- The maternal morbidity and mortality in India have significantly decreased; however, these still remain high compared to developed nations.
- Perioperative maternal mortality and morbidity can be due to anesthesia-related adverse events or nonanesthetic perioperative complications.
- Common general anesthesia-related complications include difficult/failed intubation, pulmonary aspiration and intracranial hemorrhage due to hypertensive response to intubation in pre-eclamptic patients.
- Neuraxial anesthesia-related complications may be postdural puncture headache, high/total spinal, intravascular injection of local anesthetic, epidural hematoma or infectious complications such as epidural abscess or meningitis.
- The causes of nonanesthetic complications may be hemorrhage, hypertensive disorders of pregnancy, venous thromboembolism, severe anemia, cardiovascular disease, sepsis, coagulopathy, amniotic fluid embolism, etc.
- Hemorrhage and hypertensive disorders of pregnancy account for approximately half of overall maternal mortality.
- The incidence of anesthesia-related adverse events is decreasing; whereas nonanesthetic perioperative complications are increasing.
- In the safety bundle on obstetric hemorrhage, anesthesiologist has been identified as an important member of the core response team.
- Anesthesiologists have significant involvement, almost at every step, in management of pre-eclamptic patients in labor room, operating room and intensive care unit.
- Pharmacological prophylaxis for venous thromboembolism has implications for safety and timing of neuraxial techniques and the anesthesiologist must be cautious with neuraxial block in these patients.
- There is an urgent need to implement protocols to reduce nonanesthetic maternal complications, e.g., hemorrhage protocols, universal thromboembolism prophylaxis protocols and rapid antihypertensive administration protocols for pre-eclamptic patients.
- Maternal early warning criteria may help in early detection of high-risk patients, enabling timely action to improve outcome.
- Anesthesiologists, with their expertise in the field of anesthesia and critical care, can contribute to improved management of high risk, unstable and critically ill pregnant and postpartum patients.

REFERENCES

1. World Health Organization. Health statistics and information systems. [online] Available from https://www.who.int/healthinfo/statistics/indmaternalmortality/en/. [Last accessed November, 2020].
2. Firoz T, Chou D, von Dadelszen P, Agrawal P, Vanderkruik R, Tuncalp O, et al. Measuring maternal health: focus on maternal morbidity. Bull World Health Organ. 2013;91(10):794-6.
3. Say L, Souza JP, Pattinson RC, WHO working group on Maternal Mortality and Morbidity classifications. Maternal near miss—towards a standard tool for monitoring quality of maternal health care. Best Pract Res Clin Obstet Gynaecol. 2009;23(3):287-96.
4. Maternal Health Task Force at the Harvard Chan School. Center of Excellence in Maternal and Child Health. The Sustainable Development Goals and maternal mortality. [online] Available from https://www.mhtf.org/topics/the-sustainable-development-goals-and-maternal-mortality/. [Last accessed November, 2020].
5. Callaghan WM, Creanga AA, Kuklina EV. Severe maternal morbidity among delivery and postpartum hospitalizations in the United States. Obstet Gynecol. 2012;120(5):1029-36.
6. Geller SE, Koch AR, Garland CE, MacDonald EJ, Storey F, Lawton B. A global view of severe maternal morbidity: moving beyond maternal mortality. Reprod Health. 2018;15(Suppl 1):98.
7. GBD 2015 Maternal Mortality Collaborators. Global, regional, and national levels of maternal mortality, 1990-2015: a systematic analysis for the Global Burden of Disease Study 2015. Lancet. 2016;388(10053):1775-812.
8. UNICEF. Maternal health: UNICEF's concerted action to increase access to quality maternal health services. [online] Available from https://www.unicef.org/india/what-we-do/maternal-health#. [Last accessed November, 2020].
9. World Health Organization. Trends in maternal mortality: 1990-2015: estimated by WHO, UNICEF, UNFPA, World Bank Group and the United Nations population division. 2015. [online] Available from https://www.who.int/reproductivehealth/publications/monitoring/maternal-mortality-2015/en/. [Last accessed November, 2020].
10. Purandare C, Bhardwaj A, Malhotra M, Bhushan H, Chhabra S, Shivkumar P. Maternal near-miss reviews: lessons from a pilot programme in India. BJOG. 2014;121(Suppl 4):105-11.
11. Guglielminotti J, Wong CA, Landau R, Li G. Temporal trends in anesthesia-related adverse events in cesarean deliveries, New York State, 2003-2012. Anesthesiology. 2015;123(5):1013-23.
12. D'Angelo R, Smiley RM, Riley ET, Segal S. Serious complications related to obstetric anesthesia: the serious complication repository project of the Society of Obstetric Anesthesia and Perinatology. Anesthesiology. 2014;120(6):1505-12.
13. McQuaid E, Leffert LR, Bateman BT. The role of the anesthesiologist in preventing severe maternal morbidity and mortality. Clin Obstet Gynecol. 2018;61(2):372-86.
14. Mhyre JM, Bateman BT. Stemming the tide of obstetric morbidity: An opportunity for the anesthesiologist to embrace the role of peridelivery physician. Anesthesiology. 2015;123(5):986-9.
15. Russell R, Popat M. The difficult airway: risk, assessment, prophylaxis, and management. In: Chestnut DH, Wong CA, Tsen LC, Ngan Kee WD, Beilin Y, Mhyre JM (Eds). Chestnut's Obstetric Anesthesia: Principles and Practice, 5th edition. Philadelphia: Elsevier; 2014. pp. 684-712.

16. Practice guidelines for obstetric anesthesia: an updated report by the American Society of Anesthesiologists task force on obstetric anesthesia and the Society for Obstetric Anesthesia and Perinatology. Anesthesiology. 2016;124(2):270-300.
17. Kinsella SM, Girgirah K, Scrutton MJ. Rapid sequence spinal anaesthesia for category-1 urgency caesarean section: a case series. Anaesthesia. 2010;65(7):664-9.
18. Mushambi MC, Kinsella SM, Popat M, Swales H, Ramaswamy KK, Winton AL, et al. Obstetric Anaesthetists' Association and Difficult Airway Society guidelines for the management of difficult and failed tracheal intubation in obstetrics. Anaesthesia. 2015;70(11):1286-306.
19. Ramkumar V, Dinesh E, Shetty SR, Shah A, Kundra P, Das S, et al. All India Difficult Airway Association 2016 guidelines for the management of unanticipated difficult tracheal intubation in obstetrics. Indian J Anaesth. 2016;60(12):899-905.
20. Bateman BT, Polley LS. Hypertensive disorders. In: Chestnut DH, Wong CA, Tsen LC, Ngan Kee WD, Beilin Y, Mhyre JM (Eds). Chestnut's Obstetric Anesthesia: Principles and Practice, 5th edition. Philadelphia: Elsevier; 2014. pp. 825-59.
21. American College of Obstetricians and Gynecologists. Emergent therapy for acute-onset, severe hypertension during pregnancy and the postpartum period. ACOG Committee Opinion No. 767. Obstet Gynecol. 2019;133:e174-80.
22. Hoefnagel A, Yu A, Kaminski A. Anesthetic complications in pregnancy. Crit Care Clin. 2016;32(1):1-28.
23. Choi PT, Galinski SE, Takeuchi L, Lucas S, Tamayo C, Jadad AR. PDPH is a common complication of neuraxial blockade in parturients: a meta-analysis of obstetrical studies. Can J Anaesth. 2003;50(5):460-9.
24. El-Boghdadly K, Pawa A, Chin KJ. Local anesthetic systemic toxicity: current perspectives. Local Reg Anesth. 2018;11:35-44.
25. Neal JM, Barrington MJ, Fettiplace MR, Gitman M, Memtsoudis SG, Mörwald EE, et al. The Third American Society of Regional Anesthesia and Pain Medicine Practice Advisory on Local Anesthetic Systemic Toxicity: executive summary 2017. Reg Anesth Pain Med. 2018;43(2):113-23.
26. Bateman BT, Mhyre JM, Ehrenfeld J, Kheterpal S, Abbey KR, Argalious M, et al. The risk and outcomes of epidural hematomas after perioperative and obstetric epidural catheterization: a report from the Multicenter Perioperative Outcomes Group Research Consortium. Anesth Analg. 2013;116(6):1380-5.
27. Leffert L, Butwick A, Carvalho B, Arendt K, Bates SM, Friedman A, et al. The Society for Obstetric Anesthesia and Perinatology Consensus Statement on the Anesthetic Management of Pregnant and Postpartum Women Receiving Thromboprophylaxis or Higher Dose Anticoagulants. Anesth Analg. 2018;126(3):928-44.
28. Practice Advisory for the Prevention, Diagnosis, and Management of Infectious Complications Associated with Neuraxial Techniques: an updated report by the American Society of Anesthesiologists Task Force on Infectious Complications Associated with Neuraxial Techniques and the American Society of Regional Anesthesia and Pain Medicine. Anesthesiology. 2017;126(4):585-601.
29. Scavone BM, Main EK. The National Partnership for maternal safety: a call to action for anesthesiologists. Anesth Analg. 2015;121(1):14-6.
30. Main EK, Goffman D, Scavone BM, Low LK, Bingham D, Fontaine PL, et al. National Partnership for Maternal Safety: consensus bundle on obstetric hemorrhage. Obstet Gynecol. 2015;126(1):155-62.
31. Lim G, Facco FL, Nathan N, Waters JH, Wong CA, Eltzschig HK. A review of the impact of obstetric anesthesia on maternal and neonatal outcomes. Anesthesiology. 2018;129(1):192-215.

32. WOMAN Trial Collaborators. Effect of early tranexamic acid administration on mortality, hysterectomy, and other morbidities in women with post-partum haemorrhage (WOMAN): an international, randomised, double-blind, placebo-controlled trial. Lancet. 2017;389(10084):2105-16.
33. Bouvier-Colle MH, Ould El Joud D, Varnoux N, Goffinet F, Alexander S, Bayoumeu F, et al. Evaluation of the quality of care for severe obstetrical haemorrhage in three French regions. BJOG. 2001;108(9):898-903.
34. Driessen M, Bouvier-Colle MH, Dupont C, Khoshnood B, Rudigoz RC, Deneux-Tharaux C, et al. Postpartum hemorrhage resulting from uterine atony after vaginal delivery: factors associated with severity. Obstet Gynecol. 2011;117(1):21-31.
35. NICE. Hypertension in pregnancy: diagnosis and management. NICE guideline [NG133] Published date: 25 June 2019. [online] Available from https://www.nice.org.uk/guidance/ng133/chapter/Recommendations#management-of-pre-eclampsia. [Last accessed November, 2020].
36. Heit JA, Kobbervig CE, James AH, Petterson TM, Bailey KR, Melton LJ 3rd. Trends in the incidence of venous thromboembolism during pregnancy or postpartum: a 30-year population-based study. Ann Intern Med. 2005;143(10):697-706.
37. James AH, Jamison MG, Brancazio LR, Myers ER. Venous thromboembolism during pregnancy and the postpartum period: incidence, risk factors, and mortality. Am J Obstet Gynecol. 2006;194(5):1311-5.
38. Abir G, Mhyre J. Maternal mortality and the role of the obstetric anesthesiologist. Best Pract Res Clin Anaesthesiol. 2017;31(1):91-105.
39. Vindhya J, Nath A, Murthy GVS, Metgud C, Sheeba B, Shubhashree V, et al. Prevalence and risk factors of anemia among pregnant women attending a public-sector hospital in Bangalore, South India. J Family Med Prim Care. 2019;8(1):37-43.
40. Smith C, Teng F, Branch E, Chu S, Joseph KS. Maternal and perinatal morbidity and mortality associated with anemia in pregnancy. Obstet Gynecol. 2019;134(6):1234-44.
41. Iyengar K. Early postpartum maternal morbidity among rural women of Rajasthan, India: a community-based study. J Health Popul Nutr. 2012;30(2):213-25.
42. Daru J, Zamora J, Fernández-Félix BM, Vogel J, Oladapo OT, Morisaki N, et al. Risk of maternal mortality in women with severe anaemia during pregnancy and postpartum: a multilevel analysis. Lancet Glob Health. 2018;6(5):e548-54.
43. Sultan P, Seligman K, Carvalho B. Amniotic fluid embolism: update and review. Curr Opin Anaesthesiol. 2016;29(3):288-96.
44. Agrawal S, Agrawal A, Bhandari M, Siddiqui SS, Koonwar S. Critical analysis of all pregnancies with heart disease, misses and near misses over 1-year period along with expert group so as to optimize outcome and improve patient care—Need-based analysis. Heart India. 2019;7(2):55-62.
45. Konar H, Chaudhuri S. Pregnancy complicated by maternal heart disease: a review of 281 women. J Obstet Gynaecol India. 2012;62(3):301-6.
46. Greer O, Shah NM, Johnson MR. Maternal sepsis update: current management and controversies. Obstet Gynaecol. 2020;22:45-55.
47. Kumari A, Suri J, Mittal P. Descriptive audit of maternal sepsis in a tertiary care centre of North India. Int J Reprod Contracept Obstet Gynecol. 2018;7(1):124-7.
48. Bonet M, Oladapo OT, Khan DN, Mathai M, Gulmezoglu AM. New WHO guidance on prevention and treatment of maternal peripartum infections. Lancet Glob Health. 2015;3(11):e667-8.
49. Royal College of Obstetricians and Gynaecologists. Bacterial sepsis in pregnancy. Green-top Guideline No.64a. London: RCOG; 2012. [online] Available from https://www.rcog.org.uk/en/guidelines-research-services/guidelines/gtg64a/.[Last accessed November, 2020].

50. Royal College of Obstetricians and Gynaecologists. Bacterial sepsis following pregnancy. Green-top Guideline No.64b. London: RCOG; 2012. [online] Available from https://www.rcog.org.uk/en/guidelines-research-services/guidelines/gtg64b/. [Last accessed November, 2020].
51. Clark SL, Christmas JT, Frye DR, Meyers JA, Perlin JB. Maternal mortality in the United States: predictability and the impact of protocols on fatal postcesarean pulmonary embolism and hypertension-related intracranial hemorrhage. Am J Obstet Gynecol. 2014;211(1):32. e1-9.
52. Shields LE, Wiesner S, Fulton J, Pelletreau B. Comprehensive maternal hemorrhage protocols reduce the use of blood products and improve patient safety. Am J Obstet Gynecol. 2015;212(3):272-80.
53. Mhyre JM, D'Oria R, Hameed AB, Lappen JR, Holley SL, Hunter SK, et al. The maternal early warning criteria: a proposal from the national partnership for maternal safety. Obstet Gynecol. 2014;124(4):782-6.
54. Kacmar RM. Safety interventions on the labor and delivery unit. Curr Opin Anaesthesiol. 2017;30(3):287-93.
55. Bateman BT, Tsen LC. Anesthesiologist as epidemiologist: insights from registry studies of obstetric anesthesia-related complications. Anesthesiology. 2014;120(6):1311-2.

CHAPTER 13

Opioid-free Anesthesia and Analgesia

Sukanya Mitra, Subodh Kumar

INTRODUCTION

Traditionally, general anesthesia is accomplished by three clinical endpoints: (1) unconsciousness, (2) immobility and (3) analgesia. The above triad is fulfilled by a combination of drugs along with the maintenance of homeostasis which is termed as balanced anesthesia.[1] Opioids remain the cornerstone of balanced anesthesia by managing the intraoperative nociception and postoperative analgesia. This overdependence on intraoperative opioids has been implicated to cause increased incidence of postoperative pain and increased chronization of postoperative pain.[2] The above adverse effects of opioid-based balanced anesthesia has caused the anesthesiologist to think beyond the opioid μ receptor for intraoperative hemodynamic stability and postoperative pain.[3] This paradigm shift in balanced anesthesia led to development of a new concept, which is called opioid-free anesthesia (OFA) where opioids are used only as a rescue analgesic when other nonopioid measures fail. The aim of this chapter is to familiarize the anesthesiologist to understand the concept of OFA and how to use OFA technique in perioperative management of different surgeries.

DEFINITION

Opioid-free anesthesia is defined as the perioperative utilization of opioid-sparing techniques for intraoperative homeostasis leading to complete avoidance of intraoperative opioids without causing any patient discomfort.[4,5] OFA includes combination of various nonopioid adjuvants with/without locoregional techniques for intraoperative nociception and postoperative pain management.[4,6]

WHY IS OPIOID-FREE ANESTHESIA NECESSARY?

Opioids, which were once considered indispensable for general anesthesia, now have come to disrepute because of their side effects which can cause poor recovery in the surgical patients.[7] These side effects are respiratory depression, hypoxemia, nausea and vomiting, paralytic ileus, urinary retention, confusion and delirium, opioid paradox, iatrogenic addiction, immunosuppression, and chronization of pain.[8,9] Many of these typically occur in the acute phase of administration and are very well known. Some of the side effects and concerns are seen in the longer term and are relatively less appreciated. These are discussed in some details here.

Opioid-induced Hyperalgesia

It is a phenomenon in which there is increased perception of postoperative pain in spite of adequate supplementation of intraoperative opioids.[10] It is caused by neurobiological adaptation of μ receptor and concomitant activation of pronociceptive process.[11,12] OFA can be a solution to opioid-induced hyperalgesia (OIH).[13]

Opioid Paradox

Acute tolerance of opioid along with OIH results in opioid paradox, which result in acute increase in opioid dosing in postoperative period. It should be noted here that acute tolerance and OIH can be easily differentiated by repetitive assessment of pain following serial increase in opioid dosage.[14]

Iatrogenic Addiction

It is observed that approximately 6–10% of postsurgical opioid naive patients become chronic opioid users due to intraoperative use of opioid.[15] It may be one of the causes of the opioid epidemic in the developed world.[16]

Opioid-induced Immunosuppression

Pain can cause immunosuppression resulting in delayed wound healing. Traditionally, opioids are used for intraoperative and postoperative pain, but they themselves have been implicated to cause immunosuppression.[14] Studies have shown decreased activity of natural killer (NK) cells and increased apoptosis of B and T cells following opioid administration. Most of the opioids have been shown to have immunosuppressive activity except tramadol.

Cancer Recurrence

The use of perioperative opioids and its linkage with cancer recurrence remains controversial.[17] Most of the studies which have tried to establish the role of opioid in cancer recurrence are in vitro studies whose results cannot be extrapolated to humans.[5] Although, there is inconclusive evidence that associates opioid with cancer recurrence, it is advisable to use OFA technique whenever feasible.[17,18]

COMPONENTS

Opioid-free anesthesia has components that target multiple pain receptors and pain pathways. This list includes many agents with some having proven potential to replace opioids. This includes:[16,19]
- Alpha-2 adrenergic receptor agonists.
- Ketamine.
- Lidocaine.
- Gabapentinoids.
- Magnesium.
- Acetaminophen.
- Nonsteroidal anti-inflammatory drugs (NSAIDs).
- Locoregional anesthetics.

GOAL

The ultimate goal of OFA is to avoid opioid without compromising intraoperative hemodynamic stability, nociception and postsurgical pain.[5] The other goals include:[6]
- Prevention of opioid related adverse effects.
- Early recovery after surgery (ERAS).
- Prevention of iatrogenic addiction.
- Prevention of development chronic postsurgical pain (CPSP).

INDICATIONS

As the surgeons are moving more toward ERAS protocols for every surgery, anesthesiologists are adopting OFA technique to achieve the goals of above protocols.[20] Although, any patient can be given OFA, there are certain specific groups of patients for whom OFA may be more appropriate. These include:[21]
- Patients with obstructive sleep apnea (OSA).
- Complex regional pain syndrome (CRPS) patients.
- Patients addicted to, or otherwise dependent on, opioids.
- Geriatric patients.
- Patients with respiratory insufficiency.
- Oncosurgery and bariatric surgery.

ADVANTAGES AND DISADVANTAGES

Opioid-free anesthesia offers several advantages over opioid-based anesthesia, which include reduced postoperative pain, better hemodynamic stability, less intraoperative bleeding, reduction in postoperative nausea vomiting (PONV), better quality of recovery, shorter duration of intensive care unit (ICU) stay, and prevention of OIH.

Nevertheless, there are certain disadvantages of OFA that should be kept in mind. Drugs involved in OFA may cause hypotension and bradycardia, ideal intubating condition may not be achieved, and intraoperative awareness may occur if proper institutional protocol is not in place.

NONOPIOID ADJUNCTS

It is imperative to understand the difference between nociception and pain before discussing the mechanism of action of nonopioid adjuvants. As we know, pain is defined as an "unpleasant sensory and emotional experience", which requires a conscious mind to describe it. In general anesthesia, patients are unconscious, so it is better to use the term nociception.[22] Surgical insult results in activation of nociceptive pathways, which consist of receptors, ascending and descending tracts. Simultaneous and synergistic action of these nonopioid adjuncts on the multitude target of the above pathways laid the foundation of OFA.[3] The role of each adjunct is overlapping and a protocolized approach is needed to provide maximum benefits to patients. Various nonopioid adjuncts with their mechanism of action, dose, side effects and usage are listed in **Table 1**.

Alpha-2 Adrenergic Receptor Agonists

Clonidine and dexmedetomidine are the two alpha-2 receptor agonists used to provide OFA, with the latter preferred to the former because of better efficacy and safety.[23] They appear to have both central and peripheral antinociceptive action.[6] The stimulation of alpha-2 receptor at substantia gelatinosa decreases the release of nociceptive neurotransmitter which appears to be main mechanism of antinociception.[24] The other antinociceptive effect takes place through locus ceruleus and adrenergic nuclei present in thalamus, hypothalamus, basal forebrain and cortex. It causes hyperpolarization of adrenergic neurons of the locus ceruleus resulting in decreased arousal and consequently antinociception.[3] Dexmedetomidine has 8 times more affinity for alpha-2 receptor than clonidine making it better choice as an adjuvant in neuraxial and peripheral nerve blocks.[25,26] Perioperative use of dexmedetomidine along with other nonopioid adjuvant decreases postoperative pain and surpasses opioids in terms of hemodynamic stability and quality of recovery.[7,27] The effect of dexmedetomidine on chronic pain and OIH are indeterminate. Dexmedetomidine is given in the dose of 0.5–1 µg/kg over 10 minutes before induction and followed by an infusion of 0.2–0.8 µg/kg/h after intubation. The common side effects are bradycardia, hypotension and dry mouth.[26] Dexmedetomidine has now become an integral part of ERAS protocol but its efficacy as a sole analgesic in place of opioids remains to be determined.[16]

Ketamine

Ketamine, an old drug, has recently generated a lot of interest in the context of OFA. The cause of renewed interest in this anesthetic is its proven opioid sparing effect in both opioid naive and tolerant patients. Ketamine, a phencyclidine derivative, primarily antagonizes the spinal N-methyl

TABLE 1: Nonopioid adjuvants

Drugs	Antinociceptive mechanism of action	Dose	Side-effects	Recommended surgeries
Dexmedetomidine[27]	Stimulation of alpha-2 receptor	• Loading dose 0.5–1 μg/kg over 10 minutes • Maintenance dose 0.2–0.8 μg/h	Brady-cardia, hypotension	• Laparoscopic surgery • Bariatric surgery • Abdominal hysterectomy
Ketamine[29]	Decreases nociceptive inputs and inflammatory mediators by antagonizing NMDA receptor	• Bolus dose 0.25–0.5 mg/kg • Intraoperative infusion dose 50–500 μg/kg/h	• Salivation • Hallucinations • Psychotomimetic effects	• Abdominal surgery • Thoracic surgery • Orthopedic surgery • Spine surgery
Lidocaine[51]	Inhibit the release of proinflammatory cytokines and NMDA receptor postsynaptic depolarization	• Bolus dose 1–2 mg/kg • Continuous infusion 0.5–3 mg/kg/h	LAST	• Abdominal surgery (both open and laparoscopic) • Spine surgery • Trauma and burn
Magnesium[38]	NMDA antagonism and inhibit catecholamine release during surgery	• Bolus dose 30–50 mg/kg • Continuous infusion 8–25 mg/kg/h	• Sedation • Sudden AV block	Cardiac and thoracic surgery
Gabapentinoids[44] • Gabapentin (GP) • Pregabalin (PGL)	Blocks the nociceptive transmission by blocking the voltage gated calcium channel	Preoperatively GP: 600–900 mg PO PGL: 150–300 mg PO Postoperatively GP: 600 mg TDS PGL: 150–300 mg BD	• Somnolence • Dizziness • Visual disturbances	• Spine surgery • Thoracic surgery • Orthopedic surgery • Abdominal hysterectomy
Acetaminophen	Inhibit COX enzyme	15 mg/kg IV QID	Hepatic toxicity	All surgeries
NSAIDs[16,43] • Ketorolac (KL) • Celecoxib (CB)	• KL: Nonselective COX inhibitor • CB: COX-2 inhibitor	• KL: 30 mg IV • CB: 200–400 mg PO	• KL: Gastrointestinal bleeding, peptic ulceration • CB: Thrombotic and cardiovascular effects	All surgeries

(NMDA: N-methyl d-aspartate; LAST: local anesthetic systemic toxicity; NSAIDs: nonsteroidal anti-inflammatory drugs; COX: cyclooxygenase) d-aspartate (NMDA) receptor noncompetitively to block the nociceptive inputs.[28] The other mechanisms of antinociception are modulation of production of inflammatory cytokines, altering opioid receptors, augmentation of endogenous antinociceptive symptoms.[23] Ketamine can be administered intravenously, neuraxially, subcutaneously and orally.[29] Perioperative use of a subanesthetic dose of intravenous ketamine results in better quality of recovery in terms of pain, PONV, and opioid consumption.[30] In a recent randomized controlled trial on 48 patients surgical site infiltration of ketamine was found superior to levobupivacaine for postoperative analgesia.[31] Although beneficial, the neuraxial use of ketamine remains controversial because of worries linked to its neurotoxicity.[29] Off-label oral administration of ketamine in the dose of 1 mg/kg thrice daily was found to be effective for analgesia.[32] Though its horizon has expanded now from being just an anesthetic, there are certain side effects that are needed to be kept in mind. These include increased salivation, psychotomimetic behavior, iatrogenic addiction potential and neurotoxicity.[33]

Lidocaine (Lignocaine)

Lidocaine, an amide local anesthetic, has traditionally been used intravenously to blunt the hemodynamic response to endotracheal intubation or as an antiarrhythmic.[34] It has been proposed that its perioperative use decreases postoperative pain along with opioid requirement and hasten the recovery of bowel habit. The requirement of volatile anesthetic was found to be decreased by 30% with the concurrent use of intravenously lignocaine while maintaining the depth. The above finding favors its use as a component of OFA. Lidocaine has analgesic and anti-inflammatory properties. The analgesic effect has not been attributed to its customary sodium channel blockade action. The proposed mechanisms of its analgesic action are modulation of the descending inhibitory pain pathway, NMDA receptor antagonism, and decreasing excitability of pain receptors. Low dose lignocaine causes inhibition of priming of polymorphonuclear granulocytes (PMNs) thus suppressing the release of inflammatory cytokines during surgery.[35] It should be given in a loading dose of 1-2 mg/kg to be followed by intravenous infusion of 1-2 mg/kg/h.[16] It is advisable to stop infusion within 1 hour at the end of surgery as it did not provide any additional benefit.[36] The plasma concentration of lidocaine is estimated to remain well below the toxic plasma concentration during the above infusion thus, negating local anesthetic systemic toxicity (LAST).[34] Perioperative use of intravenously lidocaine is found beneficial in abdominal surgery and spine surgery but remains controversial in other surgeries.[37] A recent Cochrane review remains uncertain about the perioperative benefit of lidocaine and its utility when compared to regional anesthesia.[35] Further high quality studies are needed for the same.

Magnesium

Magnesium sulfate has been used because of its diversified actions. It is used as a bronchodilator, antiarrhythmic, antihypertensive and neuroprotective in pre-eclamptic. It has been suggested that perioperative use of magnesium as an adjuvant attenuate intraoperative hemodynamic responses, decrease anesthetic requirement and postoperative pain.[38] Magnesium exerts its antinociceptive effect by blocking NMDA receptors thus preventing central sensitization.[39] Magnesium antinociceptive effect is not limited to perioperative period but it also prevents the development of postsurgical chronic pain.[40] Along with antinociception, it also reduces catecholamine release during surgical stress.[38] Magnesium is given in the loading dose of 30–50 mg/kg over 10–15 minutes followed by infusion of 6–25 mg/kg/h.[38] It is imperative to reduce the dose of neuromuscular blocking agent and anesthetic during perioperative use of magnesium.[16] Close monitoring of magnesium toxicity through clinical signs and symptoms, electrocardiogram (ECG) changes help in prevent atrioventricular block, and sudden cardiac arrest.[41] Although, it has proven its role as an anesthetic adjuvant we await the results of future studies to see if it can replace opioids from general anesthesia.

Gabapentinoids

Gabapentinoids, in addition to their approved role as antiepileptic agents, are also used for treatment of postherpetic neuralgia, neuropathic pain, and anxiety disorder. They are structurally similar to gamma-aminobutyric acid (GABA) but their mechanism is devoid of any GABA receptor activity.[42] Recently, the two gabapentinoids (gabapentin and pregabalin) have been recommended by American Pain Society (APS) and American Society of Anesthesiologists (ASA) for the multimodal management of postoperative pain.[43] They bind to alpha-2 delta subunit of presynaptic voltage gated calcium channels and inhibit the nociceptive transmission by modulating the release of excitatory neurotransmitters in the dorsal horn. They also activate the antinociceptive descending inhibitory norepinephrine pathway.[44] Perioperative administration of above two is thought to have opioid sparing potential. Gabapentin appears to be superior to pregabalin for perioperative use.[42] However, their postoperative analgesic potential as a part of multimodal nonopioid analgesia has recently been challenged by two well-conducted meta-analysis.[45,46] Increased incidence of postoperative respiratory depression forbids the perioperative use of gabapentinoids as a part of ERAS protocol.[47] Sedation, dizziness, somnolence, visual disturbances and neurocognitive dysfunction are some of the side effects that need to be taken care of.[48] The use of gabapentinoids might not decrease the acute and CPSP but they are found to lessen postoperative opioid usage thereby preventing iatrogenic addiction of opioids.[49] The dilemma for perioperative gabapentinoids for postoperative pain appears to continue till the results of ongoing meta-analyses are made available.

Acetaminophen (Paracetamol)

Acetaminophen is a potent antipyretic with moderate analgesic potential. It is recommended for both children and adults to control mild to moderate pain.[43] It can be administered intravenously, orally, or rectally. It is a centrally acting analgesic, which antagonizes the cyclooxygenase (COX) enzyme responsible for prostaglandin synthesis. These prostaglandins are involved in sensitization of nociceptive receptors to noxious stimulus.[25] However, it is unclear if its anti-COX properties are responsible for its analgesic action or there may be other mechanisms of action as well. Its use with other nonopioid adjuvants reduces the need of opioids in the postoperative period even for major surgery, an effect known as the "opioid-sparing effect".[50] The maximum dose of acetaminophen is 4 g/day, which is decreased to 2 g/day in case of liver disease. Intravenous administration bypasses the first pass metabolism in the liver and therefore, appears to be safe.[25] It has become an integral part of ERAS protocols irrespective of whether given preoperatively, intraoperatively and postoperatively. Further, it has an added advantage over NSAIDs as it does not have negative influence on platelet counts and gastrointestinal tract.

Nonsteroidal Anti-inflammatory Drugs

These are the strongly recommended analgesics for postsurgical pain along with acetaminophen.[43] Their anti-inflammatory action inhibits the release of inflammatory mediators in response to surgical insults.[3] Various NSAIDs act selectively and nonselectively on COX isoenzymes to inhibit the release of prostaglandin thereby exerting their antinociceptive effects. Nonselective NSAIDs such as ketorolac have been found to be associated with increased risk of bleeding with respect to selective COX-2 inhibitors.[16] Nevertheless, selective COX-2 inhibitors like celecoxib are strongly recommended to be given preoperatively; they are found to be associated with life-threatening thrombotic and cardiovascular events.[43] They are also contraindicated in grade 3 and above chronic kidney disease patients.[28] When used along with acetaminophen, it increases the opioid sparing potential and decreases side effects. It should be noted here that they have no role in management of neuropathic pain.[28]

MEASUREMENT OF NOCICEPTION

Monitoring constitutes an integral part of general anesthesia. There are validated monitoring tools for assessing hypnosis and immobility but nonavailability of an authentic analgesia monitor is a bane for anesthesiologist.[51] Analgesia under general anesthesia is assessed in terms of nociception. Nociception is the pathophysiological response to noxious stimuli. OFA components control these pathophysiological responses; they themselves have some unwarranted hemodynamic effects leading to inadvertent judgment.[13] Various quantitative monitoring tools that have been developed to assess various nociceptive responses are heart rate variability, skin conductance changes, withdrawal reflexes, pupillary responses and neurophysiological changes. These changes are measured either individually or simultaneously using a multiparameter monitor. These monitors include:[52]

Single Parameter Monitor

- *Skin conductance tests.*
- *Pupillometry tests.*
- *Analgesia nociception index (ANI) (MDoloris Medical Systems, France)*: It is a measure of heart rate variability; higher ANI scores reflect higher parasympathetic activity, and hence, a state of lower stress response and possibly less nociception.
- *Nociceptive flexion reflex threshold (NFR threshold) (NFTS Pain Tracker, Dolosys, Berlin)*: It uses electromyography (EMG) to identify polysynaptic spinal withdrawal reflex that is elicited after the activation of nociceptive A delta afferents.

Two Parameter Monitor

- *Surgical pleth index (SPI) (GE Healthcare, Helsinki, Finland)*: This is based on plethysmographic measures of peripheral sympathetic vasoconstriction and cardiac autonomic tone, generates a proprietary SPI score 0–100 (recommended score is <50).
- *qNOX (qCON 2000 monitor, Fresenius Kabi, Spain)*: Electroencephalographic (EEG) and EMG based monitor, generates a proprietary qNOX score of 0–99.

Multiparameter Monitor

- *Nociception level index (NOL index) (Medasense, Ramat Gan, Israel)*: This is based on 4 parameters (photoplethysmography, galvanic skin response, temperature, and accelerometer), generates a proprietary NOL score 0–100.
- *STeady-state index during general ANesthesia (STAN):*[13] It is a combined measure of bispectral index, blood pressure and heart rate and is still under development and standardization.

Although, larger randomized trials are needed to validate these monitors for OFA, the multiparameter monitors appear promising in future.

OPIOID-FREE ANESTHESIA FOR DIFFERENT SURGERIES

The ultimate goal of surgeons and anesthesiologists in this modern era are fast track recovery after surgery, which is known as ERAS. Nonopioid adjuvants are the cornerstone of these ERAS protocols.[51] These protocolized interventions are required during entire perioperative period, starting from the preoperative timeline and continuing till the postoperative care. The OFA and analgesia approach to various surgeries is discussed here.

Opioid-free Anesthesia for Spine Surgery

Meticulous preanesthetic workup plays a very important part in deciding OFA protocol for spine surgery. Patients should be specifically questioned about pain and its medication preoperatively as the majority of these patients are on chronic pain medication.[53] Preoperative administration of gabapentin

300–650 mg along with 1000 mg of acetaminophen was found to decrease postoperative pain and opioid requirement.[54] A bolus of ketamine 0.5 mg/kg is recommended for chronic pain patients.[53] After attaining unconsciousness, anesthesia is maintained using propofol and sevoflurane. Maintenance of antinociception achieved by intraoperative infusion of ketamine, lidocaine, magnesium and dexmedetomidine. The preoperative use of bilateral erector spinae block may have opioid sparing effect in thoracic and lumbosacral spine surgery.[55] Postoperative pain is controlled by administering acetaminophen and ketorolac.[3] Some surgeons are reluctant to give ketorolac, especially in spine instrumentation surgery, because of fear of delayed fusion but when used for less than 2 days and in the dose of less than 120 mg/day it appears safe.[56] It should be noted that gabapentinoids should be continued if the patient was taking it preoperatively for neuropathic pain.[3]

Opioid-free Anesthesia for Laparoscopic Surgery

Laparoscopic surgeries have now become standard of care in different surgical disciplines. These are now part of ERAS protocol as they hasten patient recovery and decrease hospital stay. However, the perioperative use of opioids during these surgeries can hamper early recovery of this population of patients. Laparoscopy causes great intraoperative hemodynamic perturbation which can be easily prevented by the perioperative amalgam of nonopioid adjuvants.[57] The protocolized approach of OFA for laparoscopic surgeries starts before induction of anesthesia. Dexmedetomidine 1 μg/kg loading dose is given over 10 minutes prior to induction and then an infusion of 0.2–0.5 μg/h continued for the entire intraoperative period.[58] Along with dexmedetomidine infusion of lidocaine and ketamine or magnesium sulfate are used during the intraoperative period. Ketamine appears to be superior to magnesium in terms of postoperative analgesia and recovery. Intraoperative and postoperative administration of acetaminophen and NSAIDs are highly recommended during laparoscopic surgery for adequate pain relief.[59] At the end of surgery, local anesthetics are instilled intraperitoneally to fasten the postoperative recovery and outcome.[60] OFA not only improves postoperative pain but also reduces the PONV and postoperative ileus thereby enhancing the recovery.[7]

Opioid-free Anesthesia for Bariatric Surgery

Patient population requiring bariatric surgery are prone to multitude of medical diseases such as OSA, coronary artery disease, diabetes mellitus, hypertension, etc.[61] Perioperative use of opioids in these patients causes worrisome increase risk of respiratory depression, PONV, postoperative ileus, ICU and hospital stay postoperatively. A protocolized nonopioid anesthesia is the need of hour for this special subset of patients. A Belgian anesthesiologist Jan Paul Mulier created one such protocolized approach publicized as Mulimix, which was modified further. In this modified Mulimix approach, dexmedetomidine is given in the dose of 2 μg/kg over 10 minutes before induction. This is followed by induction of anesthesia using propofol and rocuronium. Intraoperative anesthesia is maintained using desflurane or sevoflurane along with dexmedetomidine infusion which is tapered accordingly.[62] This approach can be further modified using other nonopioid adjuvant such as ketamine, lidocaine as reported in few studies.[63] Postoperative analgesia can be managed by using ketorolac and acetaminophen.

Opioid-free Anesthesia for Orthopedic Surgery

Orthopedic surgeries are one of the most painful procedures. Combination of antinociceptive nonopioid medication perioperatively results in early mobilization and decreases the hospital stay as compared to opioids.[64] The ultimate aim is to provide analgesia and prevent development of chronic surgical pain. Local anesthetic given by different routes such as through regional blocks, neuraxial and intravenously control the somatic pain, whereas the other nonopioid adjuvants not only control the somatic but also the neuropathic pain.[65] Preoperative administration of gabapentin along with NSAIDs and acetaminophen appears to be beneficial. Low dose intraoperative ketamine infusion appears to be beneficial especially, in opioid tolerant and OSA patients.[65] Continuous peripheral nerve blocks or continuous epidural provide superior pain relief and have opioid sparing effects.[43] Postoperative pain management is provided by ketorolac and acetaminophen along with above continuous blocks. Recently liposomal formulations of local anesthetics have become common and appear to provide analgesia for longer duration.[23]

CONTROVERSIES, QUESTIONS, AND THE WAY AHEAD

Like all newer innovations, there are controversies and questions regarding the concept and practice of OFA. This is hardly surprising, given the fact that opium—the original "God's own medicine"—and various opioids have been a part of human history and Pharmacopeia since millennia. Opioids have been a firmly established component of balanced anesthesia ever since the concept was born. Every clinician, especially those dealing with pain, knows the value of opioids for mitigating severe uncontrolled pain whether acute or chronic. Thus, even with the recognition and understanding of the many adverse effects of opioids, it is not easy to displace opioids from its pristine position in providing effective anesthesia and analgesia! This is the reason why there is still ongoing debate about the concept, value and logistics of OFA.[66-68]

The following controversies and questions are raised about OFA:
- Definition of OFA.
- Time-frame of OFA.
- How to choose the effective nonopioid components of OFA?
- How to ensure safety of OFA?
- How to monitor efficacy of OFA?
- How to translate the potential benefits of OFA in postoperative and post-discharge periods?

These are briefly discussed here.

What is the definition of OFA?

OFA stands for opioid-free *anesthesia*, not analgesia. Thus, the term is currently reserved for intraoperative period, or when the patient is under anesthesia. Originally, the term was exclusively used in the context of general anesthesia, with complete loss of consciousness as one of the essential pillars of balanced general anesthesia. However, the use of OFA in local/regional anesthesia/analgesia has diluted the term, because loss of consciousness is not a component of these. Should the term OFA be used in the context of locoregional analgesia then? The scope of OFA is expanding, but the answer is not yet clear. Interestingly, the recently published important systematic review and meta-analysis on the efficacy and adverse effects of OFA by Frauenknecht et al.[69] completely avoided the question of defining OFA! Instead, they exclusively focused on intraoperative use of opioids. The accompanying editorial did propose the following definition for OFA: "a perioperative care strategy that maximizes nonopioid modalities for anesthesia and analgesia and reserves the use of opioids for severe acute pain unrelieved by other methods from admission to discharge from the hospital."[70] As can be seen, this definition is broader, encompassing the perioperative period as well. That brings us to the second related question.

What is the time-frame of OFA?

As can be seen from above, there are different and progressively widening time frames in an anesthesia-providing context when opioids can be used, starting from preoperative period, induction of anesthesia, period of the actual operative procedure, reversal of anesthesia and muscle relaxation, postoperative period, and postdischarge care. Both for clinical and for research purposes, it is important to clarify which of these periods the term "opioid-free" is applied. As mentioned above, the original (and the narrowest) application of OFA is to avoid use of any opioids during the "anesthesia time" (induction to arousal) for general anesthesia.[70] OFA should not mean absolutely no use of opioids in the postoperative period, but where opioid use is kept to a minimum only when unavoidable otherwise.

How to choose the effective nonopioid components of OFA?

As reviewed above, there are many nonopioid components available as alternatives to OFA, from paracetamol to magnesium to pregabalin to nonopioid regional procedures, among others. The question is: which ones of these, and in which combinations, should be used for effective antinociception during operation and quick and safe recovery after operation? In other words, while we all talk of multimodal analgesia (MMA), which specific MMA combination can effectively replace opioids entirely? Various hospitals practicing OFA have their own combinations, or "cocktails", for their patients. It is a matter of complex research to determine which of these cocktails would be the most effective as OFA, for which procedures and/or for which patients? These are difficult questions to answer at present, though work is ongoing, especially for various ERAS protocols.[51,68,71]

How to ensure safety of OFA?

A lot of emphasis is placed on "safety" while noticing the problems with opioid-based anesthesia, from PONV in the immediate postoperative period to opioid abuse in the postdischarge period. In fact, perhaps more than efficacy, safety has been the prime driver of the OFA agenda. Hence, understandably for the sake of fairness, a lot of caution has to be exercised for the components of PFA as well. Although, generally safe, none of the OFA components reviewed above are completely free of adverse effects including high-dose paracetamol. In calling out opioids' adverse effects the onus justifiably comes on the clinician practicing OFA to be mindful of the potential harms of OFA as well.[68,71]

How to monitor efficacy of OFA?

This has already been discussed above. Since, during the intraoperative period, it is not the conscious perception of pain that is relevant, but the unconscious process of nociception (with its secondary effect on other components of balanced anesthesia), hence, the monitoring cannot be done by the usual pain instruments but instead one has to rely on several "proxy" measures, from skin conductance and pupillometry to complex neuromuscular and plethysmographic monitoring, with their own usefulness but also limitations.[52]

How to translate the potential benefits of OFA in postoperative and postdischarge periods?

This is the last, and probably most important, question in the entire area of OFA. Again, one of the most vocal critiques of opioid-based anesthesia is the fact that casual and mindless opioid use during the perioperative period leads to many problems later in the postdischarge period, ranging from the chronic adverse effects of opioids to opioid addiction. To be successful on the ground, patients provided with OFA must be able to document a good quality of recovery and a good quality of life later, without the adverse legacy of chronic opioids but also with a persistent pain-free state.[5,70,71]

CONCLUSION

Opioids still remain the most powerful weapons against pain even when we talk of a new paradigm of analgesia management. Although, OFA techniques have shown some promising results, the anesthesiologists still have to learn how to use these techniques in a protocolized manner for day-to-day clinical practice.[72] The world has moved from opioid-based balanced anesthesia to opioid sparing anesthesia. It awaits to move one step further to OFA if future studies like postoperative and opioid-free anesthesia (POFA) trial shows some promising results.[73]

It may be noted in the end that although this chapter is titled as "opioid-free anesthesia and analgesia", we have dealt only with opioid-free anesthesia. Opioid-free analgesia may be the futuristic progression from opioid based anesthesia to opioid-sparing anesthesia, to OFA and beyond.[67,74] A completely opioid-free analgesia in the postoperative period and in all kinds of severe pain, although possible, will need much more careful consideration. After all, untreated severe pain has its own adverse consequences which are well known.

Hence, a balanced approach, with OFA followed by judicious and minimal use of opioids may be the best option for now.

> **KEY POINTS**
>
> - Opioids have several adverse effects, both in the short-term and in the long-term.
> - Opioid-free anesthesia (OFA) represents a paradigm shift where no opioid is used during the entire intraoperative period, and is followed by opioid use in the postoperative period only if other measures fail to relieve pain.
> - The ultimate goal of OFA is to avoid opioid without compromising intraoperative hemodynamic stability, nociception and postsurgical pain.
> - OFA utilizes various combinations of several nonopioid analgesic and analgesic adjuvant options (paracetamol, nonsteroidal anti-inflammatory drugs, alpha-2 adrenergic receptor antagonists, gabapentinoids, magnesium, ketamine, lidocaine, etc.) with or without local or regional analgesia and chronic pain interventions.
> - OFA is currently favored more in those patients or operations where adverse effects of opioid may be hazardous, e.g., Enhancing Recovery after Surgery (ERAS) protocols, elderly patients with obesity, obstructive sleep apnea, addiction problems, etc.
> - OFA has been used in some orthopedic and neurosurgery, laparoscopic surgery, bariatric surgery, some oncosurgery, etc. Its scope and use are expanding.
> - Although very promising, there are currently a number of issues and controversies with OFA, including its definition, time period, effective and safe combinations of various nonopioid components for different procedures and patients, monitoring antinociception, and translation of the putative benefits of OFA in enhancing recovery and quality of life.

REFERENCES

1. Tonner PH. Balanced anaesthesia today. Best Pract Res Clin Anaesthesiol. 2005;19(3):475-84.
2. Fletcher D, Martinez V. Opioid-induced hyperalgesia in patients after surgery: a systematic review and a meta-analysis. Br J Anaesth. 2014;112(6):991-1004.
3. Brown EN, Pavone KJ, Naranjo M. Multimodal general anesthesia: theory and practice. Anesth Analg. 2018;127(5):1246-58.
4. Forget P. Opioid-free anaesthesia. Why and how? A contextual analysis. Anaesth Crit Care Pain Med. 2019;38(2):169-72.
5. Thota RS, Ramkiran S, Garg R, Goswami J, Baxi V, Thomas M. Opioid free onco-anesthesia: is it time to convict opioids? A systematic review of literature. J Anaesthesiol Clin Pharmacol. 2019;35(4):441-52.
6. Ramaswamy S, Wilson JA, Colvin L. Non-opioid-based adjuvant analgesia in perioperative care. Contin Educ Anaesth Crit Care Pain Oxford Academic. 2013;13:152-7.
7. Hakim KYK, Wahba WZB. Opioid-free total intravenous anesthesia improves postoperative quality of recovery after ambulatory gynecologic laparoscopy. Anesth Essays Res. 2019;13(2):199-203.
8. Kharasch ED, Brunt LM. Perioperative opioids and public health. Anesthesiology. 2016;124(4):960-5.
9. Brummett CM, Waljee JF, Goesling J, Moser S, Lin P, Englesbe MJ, et al. New persistent opioid use after minor and major surgery in US. Adults. JAMA Surg. 2017;152(6):e170504.

10. Weinbroum AA. Role of anesthetics and opioids in perioperative hyperalgesia: one step towards familiarisation. Eur J Anaesthesiol. 2015;32(4):230-1.
11. Mitra S. Opioid-induced hyperalgesia: pathophysiology and clinical implications. J Opioid Manag. 2008;4(3):123-30.
12. Rivat C, Ballantyne J. The dark side of opioids in pain management: basic science explains clinical observation. Pain Rep. 2016;1(2):e570.
13. Lavand'homme P, Estebe JP. Opioid-free anesthesia: a different regard to anesthesia practice. Curr Opin Anaesthesiol. 2018;31:556-61.
14. Ramaswamy S, Langford RM. Antinociceptive and immunosuppressive effect of opioids in an acute postoperative setting: an evidence-based review. BJA Educ. 2017;17(3):105-10.
15. Lee JS, Hu HM, Edelman AL, Brummett CM, Englesbe MJ, Waljee JF, et al. New persistent opioid use among patients with cancer after curative-intent surgery. J Clin Oncol. 2017;35(36):4042-9.
16. Bohringer C, Astorga C, Liu H. The benefits of opioid free anesthesia and the precautions necessary when employing it. Transl Perioper Pain Med. 2020;7(1): 152-7.
17. Kosciuczuk U, Knapp P, Lotowska-Cwiklewska AM. Opioid-induced immunosuppression and carcinogenesis promotion theories create the newest trend in acute and chronic pain pharmacotherapy. Clinics (Sao Paulo). 2020;75:e1554.
18. Buggy DJ, Borgeat A, Cata J, Doherty DG, Doornebal CW, Forget P, et al. Consensus statement from the BJA Workshop on Cancer and Anaesthesia. Br J Anaesth. 2015;114(1):2-3.
19. Kumar K, Kirksey MA, Duong S, Wu CL. A review of opioid-sparing modalities in perioperative pain management: methods to decrease opioid use postoperatively. Anesth Analg. 2017;125(5):1749-60.
20. Soffin EM, Wetmore DS, Beckman JD, Sheha ED, Vaishnav AS, Albert TJ, et al. Opioid-free anesthesia within an enhanced recovery after surgery pathway for minimally invasive lumbar spine surgery: a retrospective matched cohort study. Neurosurg Focus. 2019;46(4):E8.
21. Sultana A, Torres D, Schumann R. Special indications for opioid free anaesthesia and analgesia, patient and procedure related: including obesity, sleep apnoea, chronic obstructive pulmonary disease, complex regional pain syndromes, opioid addiction and cancer surgery. Best Pract Res Clin Anaesthesiol. 2017;31(4):547-60.
22. Cividjian A, Petitjeans F, Liu N, Ghignone M, de Kock M, Quintin L. Do we feel pain during anesthesia? A critical review on surgery-evoked circulatory changes and pain perception. Best Pract Res Clin Anaesthesiol. 2017;31(4):445-67.
23. Mitra S, Carlyle D, Kodumudi G, Kodumudi V, Vadivelu N. New advances in acute postoperative pain management. Curr Pain Headache Rep. 2018;22(5):35.
24. Scott-Warren VL, Sebastian J. Dexmedetomidine: its use in intensive care medicine and anaesthesia. BJA Educ. 2016;16(7):242-6.
25. Kaye AD, Cornett EM, Helander E, Menard B, Hsu E, Hart B, et al. An update on nonopioids: intravenous or oral analgesics for perioperative pain management. Anesthesiol Clin. 2017;35(2):e55-71.
26. Jessen Lundorf L, Korvenius Nedergaard H, Møller AM. Perioperative dexmedetomidine for acute pain after abdominal surgery in adults. Cochrane Database Syst Rev. 2016;2:CD010358.
27. Tonner PH. Additives used to reduce perioperative opioid consumption 1: alpha-2-agonists. Best Pract Res Clin Anaesthesiol. 2017;31(4):505-12.
28. Kaye AD, Granier AL, Garcia AJ, Carlson SF, Fuller MC, Haroldson AR, et al. Non-opioid perioperative pain strategies for the clinician: a narrative review. Pain Ther. 2020;9(1):25-39.

29. Vadivelu N, Schermer E, Kodumudi V, Belani K, Urman RD, Kaye AD. Role of ketamine for analgesia in adults and children. J Anaesthesiol Clin Pharmacol. 2016;32(3):298-306.
30. Assouline B, Tramèr MR, Kreienbühl L, Elia N. Benefit and harm of adding ketamine to an opioid in a patient-controlled analgesia device for the control of postoperative pain: systematic review and meta-analyses of randomized controlled trials with trial sequential analyses. Pain. 2016;157(12):2854-64.
31. Abdallah NM, Salama AK, Ellithy AM. Effects of preincisional analgesia with surgical site infiltration of ketamine or levobupivacaine in patients undergoing abdominal hysterectomy under general anesthesia; A randomized double blind study. Saudi J Anaesth. 2017;11(3):267-72.
32. Buvanendran A, Kroin JS, Rajagopal A, Robison SJ, Moric M, Tuman KJ. Oral ketamine for acute pain management after amputation surgery. Pain Med. 2018;19(6):1265-70.
33. Kurdi MS, Theerth KA, Deva RS. Ketamine: current applications in anesthesia, pain, and critical care. Anesth Essays Res. 2014;8(3):283-90.
34. Beaussier M, Delbos A, Maurice-Szamburski A, Ecoffey C, Mercadal L. Perioperative use of intravenous lidocaine. Drugs. 2018;78(12):1229-46.
35. Weibel S, Jelting Y, Pace NL, Helf A, Eberhart LH, Hahnenkamp K, et al. Continuous intravenous perioperative lidocaine infusion for postoperative pain and recovery in adults. Cochrane Database Syst Rev. 2018;6(6):CD009642.
36. Khan JS, Yousuf M, Victor JC, Sharma A, Siddiqui N. An estimation for an appropriate end time for an intraoperative intravenous lidocaine infusion in bowel surgery: a comparative meta-analysis. J Clin Anesth. 2016;28:95-104.
37. Dunn LK, Durieux ME. Perioperative use of intravenous lidocaine. Anesthesiology. 2017;126(4):729-37.
38. Rodríguez-Rubio L, Nava E, Del Pozo JSG, Jordán J. Influence of the perioperative administration of magnesium sulfate on the total dose of anesthetics during general anesthesia. A systematic review and meta-analysis. J Clin Anesth. 2017;39:129-38.
39. Srebro D, Vuckovic S, Milovanovic A, Kosutic J, Vujovic KS, Prostran M. Magnesium in pain research: state of the art. Curr Med Chem. 2017;24(4):424-34.
40. Ghezel-Ahmadi V, Ghezel-Ahmadi D, Schirren J, Tsapopiorgas C, Beck G, Bölükbas S. Perioperative systemic magnesium sulphate to minimize acute and chronic post-thoracotomy pain: a prospective observational study. J Thorac Dis. 2019;11(2):418-26.
41. Do SH. Magnesium: a versatile drug for anesthesiologists. Korean J Anesthesiol. 2013;65(1):4-8.
42. Schmidt PC, Ruchelli G, Mackey SC, Carroll IR. Perioperative gabapentinoids: choice of agent, dose, timing, and effects on chronic postsurgical pain. Anesthesiology. 2013;119(5):1215-21.
43. Chou R, Gordon DB, de Leon-Casasola OA, Rosenberg JM, Bickler S, Brennan T, et al. Management of Postoperative Pain: A Clinical Practice Guideline From the American Pain Society, the American Society of Regional Anesthesia and Pain Medicine, and the American Society of Anesthesiologists' Committee on Regional Anesthesia, Executive Committee, and Administrative Council. J Pain. 2016;17(2):131-57.
44. Weinbroum AA. Non-opioid IV adjuvants in the perioperative period: pharmacological and clinical aspects of ketamine and gabapentinoids. Pharmacol Res. 2012;65(4):411-29.
45. Fabritius ML, Geisler A, Petersen PL, Nikolajsen L, Kontinen V, Hamunen K, et al. Gabapentin for post-operative pain management: a systematic review with

meta-analyses and trial sequential analyses. Acta Anaesthesiol Scand. 2016;60(9): 1188-208.
46. Fabritius ML, Strøm C, Koyuncu S, Jæger P, Petersen PL, Geisler A, et al. Benefit and harm of pregabalin in acute pain treatment: a systematic review with meta-analyses and trial sequential analyses. Br J Anaesth. 2017;119(4):775-91.
47. Cavalcante AN, Sprung J, Schroeder DR, Weingarten TN. Multimodal analgesic therapy with gabapentin and its association with postoperative respiratory depression. Anesth Analg. 2017;125(1):141-6.
48. Kumar AH, Habib AS. The role of gabapentinoids in acute and chronic pain after surgery. Curr Opin Anaesthesiol. 2019;32(5):629-34.
49. Hah J, Mackey SC, Schmidt P, McCue R, Humphreys K, Trafton J, et al. Effect of perioperative gabapentin on postoperative pain resolution and opioid cessation in a mixed surgical cohort: a randomized clinical trial. JAMA Surg. 2018;153(4): 303-11.
50. Fiore JF Jr, Olleik G, El-Kefraoui C, Verdolin B, Kouyoumdjian A, Alldrit A, et al. Preventing opioid prescription after major surgery: a scoping review of opioid-free analgesia. Br J Anaesth. 2019;123(5):627-36.
51. Echeverria-Villalobos M, Stoicea N, Todeschini AB, Fiorda-Diaz J, Uribe AA, Weaver T, et al. Enhanced Recovery After Surgery (ERAS): A perspective review of postoperative pain management under ERAS pathways and its role on opioid crisis in the United States. Clin J Pain. 2020;36(3):219-26.
52. Ledowski T. Objective monitoring of nociception: a review of current commercial solutions. Br J Anaesth. 2019;123(2):e312-21.
53. Smith J, Probst S, Calandra C, Davis R, Sugimoto K, Nie L, et al. Enhanced recovery after surgery (ERAS) program for lumbar spine fusion. Perioper Med (Lond). 2019;8:4.
54. Chakravarthy VB, Yokoi H, Coughlin DJ, Manlapaz MR, Krishnaney AA. Development and implementation of a comprehensive spine surgery enhanced recovery after surgery protocol: the Cleveland Clinic experience. Neurosurg Focus. 2019;46(4):E11.
55. Chin KJ, Lewis S. Opioid-free analgesia for posterior spinal fusion surgery using erector spinae plane (ESP) blocks in a multimodal anesthetic regimen. Spine. 2019;44(6):E379-83.
56. Li J, Ajiboye RM, Orden MH, Sharma A, Drysch A, Pourtaheri S. The effect of ketorolac on thoracolumbar posterolateral fusion: a systematic review and meta-analysis. Clin Spine Surg. 2018;31(2):65-72.
57. Bhardwaj S, Garg K, Devgan S. Comparison of opioid-based and opioid-free TIVA for laparoscopic urological procedures in obese patients. J Anaesthesiol Clin Pharmacol. 2019;35(4):481-6.
58. Kaye AD, Chernobylsky DJ, Thakur P, Siddaiah H, Kaye RJ, Eng LK, et al. Dexmedetomidine in enhanced recovery after surgery (ERAS) protocols for postoperative pain. Curr Pain Headache Rep. 2020;24(5):21.
59. Barazanchi AWH, MacFater WS, Rahiri JL, Tutone S, Hill AG, Joshi GP, et al. Evidence-based management of pain after laparoscopic cholecystectomy: a PROSPECT review update. Br J Anaesth. 2018;121(4):787-803.
60. Das NT, Deshpande C. Effects of intraperitoneal local anesthetics bupivacaine and ropivacaine versus placebo on postoperative pain after laparoscopic cholecystectomy: a randomised double blind study. J Clin Diagn Res. 2017;11(7):UC08-12.
61. Soleimanpour H, Safari S, Sanaie S, Nazari M, Alavian SM. Anesthetic considerations in patients undergoing bariatric surgery: a review article. Anesth Pain Med. 2017;7(4):e57568.

62. Basha I. A systematic analysis on opioid-free general anesthesia versus opioid-based general anesthesia for bariatric surgery. Nurse Anesth Capstones. 2017; 9:1-22.
63. Aronsohn J, Orner G, Palleschi G, Gerasimov M. Opioid-free total intravenous anesthesia with ketamine as part of an enhanced recovery protocol for bariatric surgery patients with sleep disordered breathing. J Clin Anesth. 2019;52:65-6.
64. Kohring JM, Orgain NG. Multimodal analgesia in foot and ankle surgery. Orthop Clin North Am. 2017;48(4):495-505.
65. Pitchon DN, Dayan AC, Schwenk ES, Baratta JL, Viscusi ER. Updates on multimodal analgesia for orthopedic surgery. Anesthesiol Clin. 2018;36(3):361-73.
66. Veyckemans F. Opioid-free anaesthesia: Still a debate? Eur J Anaesthesiol. 2019;36(4):245-6.
67. Lavand'homme P. Opioid-free anaesthesia: Pro: damned if you don't use opioids during surgery. Eur J Anaesthesiol. 2019;36(4):247-9.
68. Lirk P, Rathmell JP. Opioid-free anaesthesia: Con: it is too early to adopt opioid-free anaesthesia today. Eur J Anaesthesiol. 2019;36(4):250-4.
69. Frauenknecht J, Kirkham KR, Jacot-Guillarmod A, Albrecht E. Analgesic impact of intra-operative opioids vs. opioid-free anaesthesia: a systematic review and meta-analysis. Anaesthesia. 2019;74(5):651-62.
70. Elkassabany NM, Mariano ER. Opioid-free anaesthesia - what would Inigo Montoya say?. Anaesthesia. 2019;74(5):560-3.
71. Albrecht E, Chin KJ. Advances in regional anaesthesia and acute pain management: a narrative review. Anaesthesia. 2020;75(Suppl 1):e101-10.
72. Thiruvenkatarajan V, Wood R, Watts R, Currie J, Wahba M, Van Wijk RM. The intraoperative use of non-opioid adjuvant analgesic agents: a survey of anaesthetists in Australia and New Zealand. BMC Anesthesiol. 2019;19(1):188.
73. Beloeil H, Laviolle B, Menard C, Paugam-Burtz C, Garot M, Asehnoune K, et al. POFA trial study protocol: a multicentre, double-blind, randomised, controlled clinical trial comparing opioid-free versus opioid anaesthesia on postoperative opioid-related adverse events after major or intermediate non-cardiac surgery. BMJ Open. 2018;8(6):e020873.
74. Mulier J. Opioid free general anesthesia: a paradigm shift?. Rev Esp Anestesiol Reanim. 2017;64(8):427-30.

CHAPTER 14

Nonoperating Room Anesthesia: Challenges and Safety

Kamakshi Garg, Neeru Luthra

INTRODUCTION

Nonoperating room anesthesia (NORA) refers to anesthesia for procedures done in places other than operating room (OR) with diverse environment. These procedures offer challenges which are not regularly confronted in the OR. The continued escalation of NORA cases is based on rapid technologic developments and innovations. Most of the patients undergoing NORA procedures are likely to be classified as American Society of Anesthesiologists (ASA) class III–V physical status[1] and are usually considered high risk candidates for surgery. Hence, a support by anesthesiologist is very important in these procedures. An analysis of ASA Closed Claims database found that remote location claims demonstrated a higher proportion of claims for death compared with OR claims (54% vs. 29%) and involved older and sicker patients.[2] 50% of the patients in remote location claims required monitored anesthesia care—a reflection of the importance of close monitoring and management of patients by a skilled anesthesia provider. Respiratory events and inadequate oxygenation and ventilation were more common in these remote location claims than in OR claims.[3]

The purpose of this chapter is twofold: (1) to highlight the inherent, common, as well as unique characteristics of NORA cases that impose unusual challenges for anesthesiologists providing care outside the OR; and (2) to describe the goals, methodologies and pitfalls of interventions in these environment that might be unfamiliar to the anesthesiologist.

NOVEL CHARACTERISTICS OF NORA CASES AND CHALLENGES TO THE ANESTHESIA PROVIDER

The three most important characteristics of NORA are its location, the medical personnel performing and its relative novelty. These are also the major challenges face by the anesthesiologist as the procedure does not occur in the routine operation theater, secondly the procedure is done mainly by a medical personnel who are not aware about the anesthetic techniques and, finally, the procedures and technologies used are usually new or different to the anesthesiologist in one way or another. For many patients undergoing NORA procedures, the scheduling is either urgent, emergent or unknown to the anesthesia provider thereby preventing adequate periprocedural evaluation.

Challenges to Anesthesia Provider

The two most common challenges to the anesthesiologist are: (1) poor communication between providers exacerbated by medicine-anesthesiology culture gap and (2) inadequate physical space to accommodate the needs of the patient requiring anesthesia services. Procedural suites are usually remotely located. This increases the time lag between the request for assistance and the arrival of help, both with technological and medical problems. Hence, anesthesiologist should be ready with a backup plan and at the same time make sure that there is proper supply of working equipment prior to giving anesthesia in remote locations. Moreover, NORA suites are frequently organized from the perspective of the proceduralist, and unfortunately the needs of the anesthesiologist are overlooked. For example, in certain procedures the anesthesiologist may have limited access to the head of the patient or hemodynamic monitors may be difficult to visualize or may not function properly. At certain places intravenous lines may become inaccessible or oxygen and suction outlets may be sub optimally placed. For these reasons' anesthesiologists should be mindful of how best to orient both the patient and providers spatially within the procedure room.

Challenges in Relation to Patient Conditions

Patient conditions precluding the need of sedation or anesthesia for nonoperating room procedures are:
- Children, especially those below 10 years.[4]
- Cerebral palsy, developmental delay, and learning difficulties.
- Movement disorders, seizure disorders, and muscular contractures.
- Pain, both related to procedure and other causes.
- Acute trauma with unstable cardiovascular, respiratory, or neurologic function.
- Increased intracranial pressure (ICP).
- Significant comorbidity and patient frailty (ASA physical status III, IV).
- Children having fear of closed spaces, anxiety, and panic disorders.

SAFETY DURING ANESTHESIA PRACTICE

Safety during anesthesia services outside the OR requires the anesthesiologist to—(1) implement ASA standards for all procedures,[2] (2) improve interpersonal communication skills, and (3) re-evaluate and reaffirm the importance of preoperative assessment.

American Society of Anesthesiologists has issued a statement dealing with minimum standards and the essential monitoring which is must in NORA locations.[2] These include:

- Oxygen presence of reliable source and continuous supply. For a backup supply full E-cylinder should be ready.
- Suction supply must be functional and complete.
- Proper scavenging of inhalational agents should be there.
- Anesthesia apparatus should have:
  - Availability of Ambu bag or a manual resuscitator capable of delivering at least 90% oxygen by positive-pressure ventilation.
  - Complete supply of anesthetic drugs in adherence to ASA standards.
  - Basic monitoring equipment as per ASA standards should be there.
  - Availability of functional anesthesia machine or anesthesia work station equivalent to those in the operation theaters and maintained to the same standards.
- Electric receptacle.
  - The number of wall sockets should be enough for anesthesia machine and monitors.
  - There should be independent power plugs or ground interrupters if the area gets wet.
- Sufficient light for the patient, anesthesia machine, and monitoring equipment along with good battery-operated backup light source.
- Enough area for:
  - Personnel and equipment.
  - Easy and expeditious access to patient, anesthesia machine, and monitoring equipment.
- Immediate availability of cardiopulmonary resuscitation equipment such as cardiac defibrillator, and emergency medicine.
- Ensure competent staff to support the anesthesiologist and a reliable means of two-way communication.
- Safety standards for the building and facilities present must be carefully observed.
- Recovery room facilities:
  - Competent staff to provide postprocedure care.
  - Suitable measures should be taken to allow safe transport of patient to main anesthesia recovery room.

Communication with the medical proceduralist is key to providing an optimal anesthesia, taking time to discuss the procedure. This allows the physician to know about the anesthetist considerations and also various anesthetic options with regards to the procedure and the patient. Medical interventionalists lack experience with relatively rare but serious complications that might arise during the procedure, such as loss of airway. Hence, proper planning and discussion with the medical personnel is mandatory.

PREPROCEDURAL ASSESSMENT FOR OUTPATIENT ANESTHESIA PROCEDURES

Preoperative anesthesia assessment plays an important role in outpatients as a minor case can change into a catastrophe in a compromised individual. All patients should be evaluated preoperatively as per standard guidelines for preanesthetic assessment[5] of 2012, which indicate that a preanesthetic check-up must have:
- A detailed history, physical examination of the patient.
- Check for the various laboratory investigations, and also for radiological information, if any.
- ASA grading of the patient.
- A proper and clear anesthetic plan which should be discussed with the patient.
- Fasting instruction for the patient which should be, at least 8 hours for solids, 6 hours for semi-solids and 2 hours for clear fluids.

MONITORING IN NONOPERATING ROOM ANESTHESIA LOCATIONS

Anesthesia machines may or may not be provided in nonoperating room locations. However, a compatible anesthesia machine along with monitors should be made available, if the arena does not offer a permanent anesthesia work station. Infrequent use may result in degradation of equipment and the use of preprocedural checks, preferably with a standardized checklist, cannot be overemphasized before embarking on NORA. All patients should be monitored by as per ASA standards for basic monitoring, but some difficult cases may require more advanced monitoring.[6,7] Pulse oximeter was the primary monitor used by the anesthesiologist earlier to know about the oxygen status of the patient and it still remains an important monitor for us.[8] Over the past 20 years, the standard of monitoring also includes capnometer. End-tidal carbon dioxide monitoring is a gold standard to look for the quality of ventilation and circulation.[9-12] In case an anesthesiologist is dealing with a more complicated case then the facility for invasive monitoring like arterial line or central venous cannulation should be available. A pre-prepared cart containing essential equipment should be checked and restocked after each case.

SPECIFIC PROCEDURES-RELATED ISSUES

Gastrointestinal Procedures

A number of procedures are done in the endoscopy suite which include routine screening, colonoscopies or complex submucosal dissections. The need for type of anesthesia depends upon the complexities and invasiveness of the procedure. The most common procedures are as follows:

Esophagogastroduodenoscopy: In esophagogastroduodenoscopy (EGD) a fiberoptic endoscope is used for examination of the upper gastrointestinal (GI) tract (esophagus, pylorus, and stomach). Due to the presence of sphincters negotiating the scope into the esophagus and subsequently into the pylorus is the most difficult. Although topicalization, opioid or benzodiazepine sedation is adequate as most patients tolerate this, general anesthesia may be required for those at risk of aspiration, in anxious patients and children.[13] The patients who fall in this high-risk category are those with gastroesophageal reflux disease (GERD), morbid obesity, obstructive sleep apnea, and asthma. General anesthesia can be administered through endotracheal tube or laryngeal mask airways (LMAs), preferably Pro Seal, as it has a gastric drainage port. Terblanche et al. used a refined laryngeal mask in advanced airway management for upper gastrointestinal endoscopy (i.e., the LMA® Gastro™ Airway).[14] It allowed passing of instruments like a gastroscope through its accessory tube into the esophagus. Another new device is an endoscopy mask which has an additional port with a soft silicone membrane to accommodate endotracheal tubes or different endoscopic devices.

Sigmoidoscopy and colonoscopy: This procedure is used for examination of the lower intestinal tract involving the colon and distal ileum. The diagnostic procedures can be performed with combination of benzodiazepines and opioids. However, interventions like biopsies or polyp removal may require intravenous agents such as propofol or inhalational agents such as nitrous oxide, and sevoflurane for anesthesia.[15]

A special concern for upper endoscopy and colonoscopy in today's time is the potential risk for transmission of coronavirus disease 2019 (COVID-19) to health care workers as these procedures are considered aerosol generating. Elective endoscopic procedures should be postponed or should be performed in negative pressure procedure rooms using personal protection equipment. Preference should be for general anesthesia rather than sedation, and rapid sequence induction and intubation should be the norm as far as possible.[16]

Endoscopic retrograde cholangiopancreatography (ERCP): In this procedure endoscopically-guided injection of contrast is given through the duodenal papilla and biliary or pancreatic ducts are examined fluoroscopically. Patients are usually in the prone position. Many patients are compromised with significant comorbidities and require precise intervention during the procedure. Certain procedures such as hemostasis, stent placement, stone extraction, pancreaticobiliary visualization, laser lithotripsy, and sphincterotomy may require general anesthesia.[17] Drugs like antispasmodics (glucagon and intravenous hyoscyamine) which are used to reduce duodenal motility and improve operating conditions during endoscopy by gastroenterologists can cause sinus tachycardia.[18]

Peroral endoscopic myotomy (POEM): This minimally invasive procedure involves endoscopic insufflation of carbon dioxide into the esophagus for the correction of achalasia. General anesthesia is best suited as the procedure is of long duration and an endotracheal tube prevents aspiration of gastric contents. It is important to monitor the end-tidal carbon dioxide to diagnose any subcutaneous emphysema to pneumothorax, pneumomediastinum, and pneumoperitoneum during insufflation. During all these procedures attention should be paid to pressure areas, particularly the eyes, lips, and teeth, and extreme rotation of the neck should be avoided.

Interventional Pulmonary Procedures

Bronchoscopy: Bronchoscopic interventions are complicated as the patients are at high risk and usually have multiple comorbidities including obstructive and restrictive lung diseases. Hence, preoperative planning and assessment is very important.[19] As airway is shared in these procedures, intravenous anesthesia is preferred using propofol with opioids and muscle relaxants.

Common bronchoscopy procedures include:
- *Endobronchial stenting*: Placement of self-expanding metallic stents to treat tracheal stenosis.
- Endobronchial biopsy, laser treatment, and cauterization.
- Balloon dilation and cryotherapy.

ANESTHESIA FOR IMAGE-GUIDED INTERVENTIONS: EVOLUTION OF A NEW INTERFACE

The number of procedures performed in interventional radiology settings is expanding with the advancement in technology. The radiological procedures take place in specialty areas such as catheterization laboratories, neuroradiology suites, computed tomography (CT) scanners, and magnetic resonance imaging (MRI) suites.

Procedures in the CT suite predispose to certain environmental considerations for the anesthesiologist like:
- Unfavorable equipment layout.
- Radiation exposure.
- Occult bleeding risk.
- Contrast allergies.
- Inaccessibility around the patient's head due to X-ray tubes, and moving C-arm.
- Placement of the anesthesia machine.

Staff exposure to radiation can be minimized by a number of precautions:[20] limiting the time of exposure to radiation, increasing the distance from the source of radiation, using protective shields such as lead aprons, thyroid shields, and leaded eyeglasses, and measuring occupational exposure to radiation.

Adverse reactions due to contrast material administration are seen in 5–8% patients and are dependent on the dose and concentration of the media used. Severe reactions such as laryngeal edema, bronchospasm, pulmonary edema, hypotension, and respiratory arrest or seizures are also known to occur. The mainstay of the treatment involves oxygen, epinephrine, and bronchodilators. Contrast-induced nephropathy is more likely to occur in patients with renal insufficiency.

Computed Tomography-guided Interventions

The CT-guided interventional procedures include catheter drainage, ablation of tumors and injections for pain management. As with other anesthetic administrations, patient comorbidities and the techniques of the interventionalists should be discussed. Local anesthesia may suffice for superficial procedures like CT-guided abscess drainage but deep-seated collections may be painful and require general anesthesia. Similar is the case with injections for pain management procedures which includes injection of phenol and alcohol into ganglion, nerve or plexus to achieve neurolysis. Steroid injections are done into joints for local pain management and to minimalize the inflammatory process. There is a risk of injury to the surrounding structures during these interventions.

Vascular Intervention Procedures

Angiography is the imaging of blood vessels and includes both arteriography and venography. Angiography causes minimal discomfort and may be performed under local anesthesia with or without light sedation. Certain procedures like spinal angiography are lengthy and require patients to remain completely motionless, thus warranting the need for general anesthesia. Neurologic disorders such as recent subarachnoid hemorrhage, stroke, and depressed level of consciousness or raised ICP may necessitate anesthesia with intubation for airway protection. It is important to have extensions on all anesthesia breathing circuits, infusion lines, and monitors to prevent these implements from being accidentally dislodged. Using arteriography, we can evaluate atherosclerotic and ischemic disease, define traumatic injury and define the arterial blood supply of tumors.

Similarly, venous system can be imaged by venography. It can be used for placement of stents, inferior vena cava filter placement, pulmonary arteriography and embolization of arteriovenous malformations (AVMs). These procedures require little or no sedation.

Gastrointestinal and Genitourinary Interventions

The most important and commonly performed procedure is transjugular intrahepatic portosystemic shunt (TIPS). TIPS is an interrelation between the hepatic portal and systemic circulations created via a percutaneous catheter inserted in the internal jugular vein and directed into the liver. The TIPS functions to decompress the portal circulation in patients with portal hypertension. It is indicated for patients who have intractable ascites and repeated esophageal variceal bleeding which is refractory to medical treatment. The procedure takes around 2 and 3 hours and can be performed under sedation or general anesthesia.[21] These patients usually have significant hepatic dysfunction, and require careful preoperative assessment. The anesthetic considerations for TIPS are enumerated in **Table 1**.

Other common GI procedures performed are percutaneous gastrostomy (G-tube), cecostomy and jejunostomy tubes placement.[22] Complications such as bleeding, trauma to the adjoining organs, and peritonitis can occur during these procedures.

TABLE 1: Anesthetic consideration for transjugular intrahepatic portosystemic shunt (TIPS) procedure

Airway–risk of aspiration	• Raised intragastric pressure due to ascites • Recent gastrointestinal bleeding • Decreased level of consciousness due to hepatic encephalopathy
CNS	• Hepatic encephalopathy • Altered mental status • Variable response to anesthetic agents
Respiratory system	• Decreased functional residual capacity due to ascites • Pneumonia • Intrapulmonary shunts • Pleural effusion
Cardiovascular system	• Intraperitoneal hemorrhage • Altered volume status • Associated alcoholic cardiomyopathy • Acute hemorrhage from esophageal varices
Hematologic system	• Thrombocytopenia • Coagulopathy
Fluid balance	• Ascites • Risk of hepatorenal syndrome
Endocrine system	• Tendency to hypoglycemia
Pharmacokinetics	• Increased volume of distribution • Decreased protein binding, drug metabolism, and elimination

(CNS: central nervous system)

Genitourinary procedures commonly performed in radiology suites include dilation, stenting, and suprapubic cystostomy. These interventions may require prone positioning of the patient which generates anesthesia concerns regarding airway, pain management, and access to the patient.

Positron Emission Tomography

Positron emission tomography (PET) imaging technique is used to diagnose, stage, and follow-up malignancies. PET is used to distinguish malignant from benign lesions, identify metabolically active portions of necrotic tumors, and monitor responses to treatment. The challenges in the imaging suites are: limited access to the patient and need for long monitoring equipment to provide enough space for motion of the equipment. The procedures take longer to complete which may affect choice of technique/agent. Availability of wall-mounted pipelines, suction, and equipment for monitoring should be strategically planned in these suites.

Magnetic Resonance Imaging

Magnetic resonance imaging (MRI) uses magnetic fields and radio waves to create images. This technique has an advantage of being radiation-free but has certain physical constraints as only MRI compatible equipment can be used in the MRI suite. The magnetic field of the MRI machine tends to pull objects containing iron or stainless steel and damages can occur because of these mobile projectiles. The equipment used in an MRI suite should not be affected by magnetic attractive forces, heating, or current induction. Patient should be assessed for MRI compatible devices such as cochlear implants, implantable cardioverter-defibrillators pacemakers, pumps, nerve stimulators, or other metal objects such as metal fragments, bullets and aneurysm clips. In recent times nonferromagnetic vascular clips, staples, orthopedic implants, heart valves, and other prostheses are available which make it possible to scan such patients. Patients and staff should wear ear protection and staff should minimize time spent in the scanner.

Monitoring

Monitoring in the MRI suite is challenging. Cables and wires wound in loops may cause induction-heating effects and thermal injury may also occur in skin with large tattoos, especially those with ferromagnetic inks. Patient monitors, ventilator equipment, and electrical infusion pumps may all malfunction when they come too close to the magnetic field. The electrocardiogram is sensitive to the changing magnetic signals. The electrodes should be placed close together and toward the center of the magnetic field. MRI-compatible devices have been developed; however, in the absence of MRI-compatible monitors, tube extensions can be used to keep standard infusion pumps and monitors at a distance.[23] Plans for emergencies must be in place as the locations may be isolated and conventional emergency equipment (standard laryngoscope, oxygen cylinders and cardiac defibrillators) may not be MRI compatible.

Anesthesia

Claustrophobia is a concern for up to 15% of all adult patients undergoing MRI necessitating sedation or even general anesthesia for them to complete the imaging studies.[24] Sedation may be provided by the oral route with benzodiazepines, as intravenous sedation or minimum alveolar concentration (MAC). In children, a combination of incomprehension, separation anxiety, and fear can result in noncooperation and intolerance of relatively brief periods of immobility. The choice of sedation or general anesthesia for a particular child is multifactorial.[25] As with all NORA, the standards of care for pediatric patients undergoing sedation and/or general anesthesia for MRI and CT imaging are the same as those in the OR; a useful acronym "SOAPME" (Suction, Oxygen, Airway equipment, appropriate Pharmaceuticals, Monitoring, and special Equipment) has been coined before embarking upon any pediatric sedation or anesthetic.[26]

Magnetic Resonance Imaging-guided Interventions

Biopsies of tumors which are not well visualized, prostate and breast biopsies can be performed under MRI guidance using sedation and local anesthesia. Cryoablation for treatment of liver, kidney, breast, and prostate tumors and uterine fibroid scan be performed in the MRI suite.[27] General anesthesia may be required to manage pain during freezing and heating of tissues. The procedures are lengthy and repeated breath-holds.

Image-guided Procedures in the Neuroradiology Suite

Although a new technology, image-guided neuroradiological have grown due to availability of improved devices (stents, catheters, and coils), better imaging techniques, and safer contrast media. Diagnostic cerebral angiography used for imaging the cerebral vasculature can be performed with mild sedation. Deeper planes of anesthesia are required for complex and lengthy interventions and whenever there is a need for a still patient. Hemodynamic deviations are sometimes associated with these procedures. Neurologic assessment may be required during the procedures (i.e., carotid stenting) so the need to keep the patient awake. Patient comorbidities and status must be taken into consideration. Monitoring includes arterial blood pressure, neuromonitoring technologies as an indirect measure of cerebral perfusion; electroencephalography and somatosensory, motor, and brainstem evoked potentials. Use of inhalational agents is better avoided because of their confounding effects on these parameters being monitoring.

Endovascular Treatment of Cerebral Aneurysms and Arteriovenous Malformations

Arteriovenous malformations allow for percutaneous isolation of aneurysms from the circulation by positioning of a soft platinum coil within the aneurysm. For wide-necked aneurysms a stent is introduced first, followed by the coil through the stent.[28] There is an increased risk of bleeding as the patients need to be given anticoagulants before stent placement. In patients with subarachnoid hemorrhage endovascular treatment with coils has shown better outcomes than surgical clipping. However, clipping shows better resolution of cranial neuropathies.[29] In 2009, a large multicenter study, the International Subarachnoid Aneurysm Trial (ISAT) reported better outcomes in patients with ruptured anterior and posterior circulation aneurysms undergoing interventional neuroradiology compared to surgical clipping.[30] However, complications such as aneurysm rupture or thromboembolism can occur. The procedure should be completed as quickly as possible. The various modalities of treatment for cerebral AVM includes stereotactic radiosurgery, embolization, microsurgical resection, or combination of different treatment methods. The anesthesiologist may facilitate the procedure by manipulating systemic blood pressure and controlling end-tidal carbon dioxide tension. Certain procedures require patients to be awake for part of the procedure, so the titration of anesthetic drugs.

Interventional Neuroradiology Acute Stroke Treatment

Intravenous recombinant-tissue plasminogen activator treatment has been used for thrombolysis. However, intra-arterial thrombolysis is more promising as it gives more time in the treatment time window (3-6 hours). Also, a higher drug concentration of lytic drug can be given in the target vessel thus, yielding higher recanalization rates. These are challenging procedures as there is little time for preoperative assessment. General anesthesia is advocated as most patients are significantly compromised.

ANESTHESIOLOGISTS IN THE CATHETERIZATION LABORATORY

These procedures require fluoroscopy and at times even more sophisticated interventional technologies. Anesthesiologists involved in these procedures are required to provide monitored anesthesia care which in some cases can turn into complete cardiac anesthesia.

Percutaneous Cardiac Procedures

Various percutaneous cardiac procedures, where anesthesiologist is frequently called are angiography and angioplasty. Percutaneous placement of stents is usually performed under mild sedation, and an anesthesiologist is needed, when the patient presents with hemodynamic or respiratory compromise.[31,32]

Placement of intra-aortic balloon pump is usually done with minimal sedation under a monitored care of anesthesiologist, as these patients may have compromised cardiac and respiratory function.[33,34] Percutaneous closure of septal defects includes closure of patent foramen ovale (PFO) and secundum atrial septal defects (ASDs), percutaneous mitral valve repair and percutaneous aortic valve replacement.

Transesophageal echocardiography is performed by the cardiac anesthesiologists inside the operation theaters and is now being done as outpatient procedure routinely to know about the hemodynamic and the functional status of heart.[35] As technology evolves, percutaneous procedures will become more sophisticated involving patients with congenital, acquired and surgically created defects which can be managed by interventional cardiology procedures.

CONCLUSION

With an advancement in the technology, a higher number and complex procedures are being performed in nonoperating room locations. Anesthesiologists need to provide services in areas that are remote and unfamiliar from the OR. During preparation to give anesthesia or sedation in remote locations, an anesthesiologist should follow a three-step approach. These steps involve vigilant evaluation of the patient, being aware of the peculiar challenges posed by the particular procedure and at the same time have a thorough knowledge about the logistics and limitations of the environment. In all cases, we must remember that an anesthesiologist can never compromise on the standards of anesthesia care and monitoring. These remote locations may require no less care and vigilance than our conventional operating theaters.

> **KEY POINTS**
> - Nonoperating room anesthesia (NORA) refers to procedures done in places other than operating room (OR) with diverse environment.
> - These procedures offer challenges which are not regularly confronted in the OR.
> - With the advancement in technology nonoperating room arena is more onerous and exhausting as there are limited resource, but better patient safety is required.
> - Significant differences in practice due to remote locations and procedures being performed by medical proceduralists create additional management challenges.
> - The unfamiliar environment, presence of procedural equipment which restrict access to the patient and fear of radiation hazards are important issues to be considered.
> - The aim of this chapter is to guide the anesthesiologist regarding procedures performed outside the OR, and highlights the measures to be adopted to provide a safe and optimal anesthesia.

REFERENCES

1. Nagrebetsky A, Gabriel RA, Dutton RP, Urman RD. Growth of nonoperating room anesthesia care in the United States: a contemporary trends analysis. Anesth Analg. 2017;124(4):1261-7.
2. ASA. Statement on nonoperating room anesthetizing locations. Committee of Origin: Standards and Practice Parameters. Approved by the ASA House of Delegates on October 19, 1994 and last amended on October 16. 2013 and reaffirmed on Oct 17 2018. Washington, D.C.: ASA; 2018.
3. Metzner J, Posner KL, Domino KB. The risk and safety of anesthesia at remote locations: the US closed claims analysis. Curr Opin Anaesthesiol. 2009;22(4):502-8.
4. Tobias JD. Sedation of infants and children outside of the operating room. Curr Opin Anaesthesiol. 2015;28(4):478-85.
5. Committee on Standards and Practice Parameters, Apfelbaum JL, Connis RT, Nickinovich DG; American Society of Anesthesiologists Task Force on Preanesthesia Evaluation, Pasternak LR, et al. Practice advisory for preanesthesia evaluation: an updated report by the American Society of Anesthesiologists Task Force on preanesthesia evaluation. Anesthesiology. 2012;116(3):522-38.
6. Practice guidelines for preoperative fasting and the use of pharmacologic agents to reduce the risk of pulmonary aspiration: application to healthy patients undergoing elective procedures: an updated report by the American Society of Anesthesiologists task force on preoperative fasting and the use of pharmacologic agents to reduce the risk of pulmonary aspiration. Anesthesiology. 2017;126(3):376-93.
7. ASA. Standards for basic anesthetic monitoring Committee of Origin: Standards and practice parameters (Approved by the ASA House of Delegates on October 21, 1986, last amended on October 20, 2010, and last affirmed on October 28, 2015). Washington, D.C.: ASA; 2015.
8. Elliott M, Tate R, Page K. Do clinicians know how use pulse oximetry? A literature review and clinical implication. Aust Crit Care. 2006;19(4):139-44.
9. Kodali B. Capnography outside the operating rooms. Anesthesiology. 2013;118(1): 192-201.

10. Bhavani-Shankar K, Moseley H, Kumar AY, Delph Y. Capnometry and anaesthesia. Can J Anaesth. 1992;39(6):617-32.
11. American Heart Association: 2005 AHA guidelines for CPR and emergency cardiovascular care. Part 7.1: Adjuncts for Airway Control and Ventilation. Circulation. 2005;112:IV-51-IV-57.
12. Galvano S, Kodali B. Patient monitoring. In: Urman R, Gross WL, Philip B (Eds): Anesthesia outside the operating room, New York: Oxford University Press; 2011.
13. Gromski M, Matthes K. Gastrointestinal endoscopy procedures. In: Urman R, Gross WL, Philip B (Eds). Anesthesia outside the operating room, New York: Oxford University Press; 2011. pp. 151-66.
14. Terblanche NCS, Middleton C, Choi-Lundberg DL, Skinner M. Efficacy of a new dual channel laryngeal mask airway, the LMA® Gastro™ airway, for upper gastrointestinal endoscopy: a prospective observational study. Br J Anaesth. 2018;120(2):353-60.
15. Theodorou T, Hales P, Gillespie P, Robertson B. Total intravenous versus inhalational anesthesia for colonoscopy: a prospective study of clinical recovery and psychomotor function. Anaesth Intensive Care. 2001;29(2):124-36.
16. Sultan S, Lim JK, Altayar O, Davitkov P, Feuerstein JD, Siddique SM, et al. AGA Institute Rapid Recommendations for Gastrointestinal Procedures During the COVID-19 Pandemic. Gastroenterology. 2020;S0016-5085(20)30458-3.
17. Martindale SJ. Anesthetic considerations during endoscopic retrograde cholangiopancreatography. Anaesth Intensive Care. 2006;34(4):475-80.
18. Lynch CR, Khandekar S, Lynch SM, Disario JA. Sublingual L-hyoscyamine for duodenal antimotility during ERCP: a prospective randomized double-blinded study. Gastrointest Endosc. 2007;66(4):748-52.
19. Abdelmalak B. Anesthesia for interventional pulmonology. In: Urman R, Gross WL, Philip B (Eds). Anesthesia outside the operating room, New York: Oxford University Press; 2011. pp. 167-74.
20. Mitchell EL, Furey P. Prevention of radiation injury from medical imaging. J Vasc Surg. 2011;53(1 Suppl):22S-7S.
21. Scher C. Anesthesia for transjugular intrahepatic portosystemic shunt. Int Anesthesiol Clin. 2009;47(2):21-8.
22. Galaski A, Peng W, Ellis M, Darling P, Common A, Tucker E. Gastrostomy tube placement by radiological versus endoscopic methods in an acute care setting: a retrospective review of frequency, indications, complications and outcomes. Can J Gastroenterol. 2009;23(2):109-14.
23. Raiten J, Elkassabany N, Gao W, Mandel JE. Medical intelligence article: novel uses of high frequency ventilation outside the operating room. Anesth Analg. 2011;112(5):1110-3.
24. Dewey M, Schink T, Dewey CF. Claustrophobia during magnetic resonance imaging: cohort study in over 55,000 patients. J Magn Reson Imaging. 2007;26(5):1322-7.
25. Coté CJ, Wilson S, American Academy of Pediatrics, American Academy of Pediatric Dentistry, Work Group on Sedation. Guidelines for monitoring and management of pediatric patients during and after sedation for diagnostic and therapeutic procedures: an update. Paediatr Anaesth. 2008;18(1):9-10.
26. Coté CJ, Wilson S, American Academy of Pediatrics, American Academy of Pediatric Dentistry, Work Group on Sedation. Guidelines for monitoring and management of pediatric patients during and after sedation for diagnostic and therapeutic procedures: an update. Pediatrics. 2006;118(6):2587-602.
27. Tatli S, Morrison PR, Tuncali K, Silverman SG. Interventional MRI for oncologic applications. Tech Vasc Interv Radiol. 2007;10(2):159-70.

28. Thiex R, Frerichs K. Interventional neuroradiology. In: Urman R, Gross WL, Philip B (Eds). Anesthesia outside the operating room, New York: Oxford University Press; 2011. pp. 92-105.
29. Molyneux A, Kerr R, Stratton I, Sandercock P, Clarke M, Shrimpton J, et al. International Subarachnoid Aneurysm Trial (ISAT) of neurosurgical clipping venous endovascular coiling in 2143 patients with ruptured intracranial aneurysms: a randomized trial. Lancet. 2002;360(9342):1267-74.
30. Apfel CC, Kortilla K, Abdallah M, Kerger H, Turan A, Vedder I, et al. A factorial trial of six interventions for the prevention of postoperative nausea and vomiting. New Engl J Med. 2004;350(24):2441-551.
31. Smith Jr SC, Feldman TE, Hirshfeld Jr JW, Jacobs AK, Kern MJ, King SB, et al. ACC/AHA/SCAI 2005 guideline update for percutaneous coronary intervention: a report of the American College of Cardiology/American Heart Association Task Force on Practice Guidelines (ACC/AHA/SCAI Writing Committee to Update the 2001 Guidelines for Percutaneous Coronary Intervention). J Am Coll Cardiol. 2006;47(1):e1-121.
32. Boden WE, O'Rourke RA, Teo KK, Hartigan PM, Maron DJ, Kostuk WJ, et al. Optimal medical therapy with or without PCI for stable coronary disease. N Engl J Med. 2007;356(15):1503-16.
33. Kar B, Adkins LE, Civitello AB, Loyalka P, Palanichamy N, Gemmato CJ, et al. Clinical experience with the TandemHeart percutaneous ventricular assist device. Tex Heart Inst J. 2006;33(2):111-5.
34. Cannon CP, Weintraub WS, Demopoulos LA, Vicari R, Frey MJ, Lakkis N, et al. Comparison of early invasive and conservative strategies in patients with unstable coronary syndromes treated with glycoprotein IIb/IIa inhibitor tirofiban. N Engl J Med. 2001;344(25):1879-87.
35. Gross WL, Shook DC. TEE and interventional cardiology. J Am Soc Echocardiogr. 2011;24(7):A22.

CHAPTER 15

Anesthetic Management in Pediatric Patients with a Congenital Heart Disease Undergoing Noncardiac Surgery

Manjula Sarkar, Anju Gupta

INTRODUCTION

Congenital heart diseases (CHDs) are the most common congenital abnormality found among children, accounting for approximately one-third of all congenital anomalies with a global prevalence of 8–12/1000 live births.[1] The prevalence in India was found to be much higher at 19.4/1000 live births in a survey conducted from 2011 to 2014.[2] Ventricular septal defect (VSD) was the most common CHD (33%) followed by atrial septal defect (ASD) and tetralogy of Fallot (TOF) with prevalence of 19% and 16% in the children aged 0–5 years. Children with CHD have similar childhood illnesses as healthy children requiring elective and emergency surgery. Such children have high morbidity and mortality. Due to the complexity of cardiac anomalies and a range of noncardiac surgeries which may need to be done, management of such patients is difficult to generalize.

CLASSIFICATION OF CONGENITAL HEART DISEASE

Congenital heart disease patients have a structural and functional cardiac malformation present at birth affecting the heart valves, atrial or ventricular walls or large central vessels. There are two types of CHD: (1) cyanotic and (2) acyanotic **(Table 1)**.[2,3] The cyanotic CHDs are typified by a defect leading to right → left shunt resulting in deoxygenated blood from pulmonary circulation entering the systemic circulation. This results in hypoxia manifesting clinically as cyanosis, which may occur as sudden episodes of severe life-threatening hypoxemia. Acyanotic CHDs are cardiac malformations that present at birth which do not usually interfere with the tissue oxygenation or perfusion.

PATHOPHYSIOLOGY

Circulation has two components: (1) systemic and (2) pulmonary. In normal circulation, systemic and pulmonary blood flows (PBFs) in series. Most types of repaired CHD such as American Society of Anesthesiologists (ASA), VSD, etc., have this type of circulation. In parallel or balanced circulation, there is usually

TABLE 1: Different types of congenital heart disease (CHD)

Types of CHD	Examples
Cyanotic CHD	• Tetralogy of Fallot (TOF): Most common CHD has four components: 　1. Right ventricular wall hypertrophy (RVH) 　2. Ventricular septal defect 　3. Right ventricular outflow obstruction 　4. Overriding arch of aorta that overrides both right and left ventricle
	• Common ventricle • Tricuspid valve atresia • Transposition of great vessels • Total anomalous pulmonary venous return (TAPVR) • Ebstein's anomaly
Acyanotic CHD with left to right shunt	• Patent ductus arteriosus (PDA) 　– Most commonly distal to left subclavian artery, connecting descending aorta to left pulmonary artery • Atrial septal defect (ASD) 　– Ostium primum 　– Ostium secundum 　– Sinus venosus type • Ventricular septal defect (VSD) 　– Membranous 　– Muscular 　– Just below aortic valve 　– Atrioventricular canal defect
Without left to right shunt	• Coarctation of aorta • Aortic stenosis • Subaortic membrane

an abnormality leading to some kind of communication [e.g., septal defect, patent ductus arteriosus (PDA), etc.] between the systemic and pulmonary circulations and physiologically work in parallel. In these patients, the amount of blood flow to the pulmonary and systemic circulation is balanced with the relative proportion of systemic and pulmonary vascular resistances (PVRs).[3] Increased PBF may lead to desaturation due to pulmonary congestion, edema or pneumonia with reduced systemic perfusion. Lower PBF also leads to desaturation and acidosis. Right to left (R to L) shunt leads to hypoxemia due to venous and systemic blood mixing. To maintain oxygenation, following compensatory mechanisms take place in the form of polycythemia, increased blood volume, alveolar hyperventilation, and development of aortopulmonary collaterals. Left to right shunt leads to enhanced PBF causing elevated PVR with consequent pulmonary arterial hypertension, right ventricular hypertrophy (RVH), and eventually heart failure. The pathophysiological changes evolve later to manifest as various coagulation defects in the form of thrombocytopenia, factor deficiency, fibrinolysis, and disseminated intravascular coagulation. These systemic changes increase the incidence of various complications during perioperative period which include infective endocarditis, cardiac arrhythmias, heart blocks, pulmonary and systemic hypertension, thromboembolism, coagulopathy, brain abscess and sudden death.

SIGNS AND SYMPTOMS

Children rarely present with the symptoms typically associated with cardiac disease in adults (e.g., chest pain, dyspnea on exertion, pedal edema). The signs and symptoms vary with the anomaly and as the child grows in age. In infants, the various signs and symptoms include tachycardia, cyanosis, frequent respiratory tract infections, failure to thrive, heart murmur, and failure. In older children, the signs and symptoms would include dyspnea, cyanosis (in cyanotic CHDs), clubbing (with uncorrected cyanotic CHD), history of squatting episodes (in patients with R to L shunting), hypertension, slow physical and mental development, reduced exercise tolerance, heart murmur, and congestive cardiac failure.

RISK CATEGORIZATION

Children with CHDs are at higher risk of perioperative morbidity and perioperative cardiac arrest.[4] Complex lesions carry the highest perioperative risk of complications and include aortic stenosis, parallel circulation physiology [e.g., truncus arteriosus (TA), large unrepaired atrioventricular (AV) septal defect or VSD, hypoplastic left heart syndrome (HLHS), etc.], single ventricle circulation, cardiomyopathy.[5] Single ventricle physiology poses a very high risk with up to 30% mortality from arrhythmias.[6] CHD children with documented pulmonary hypertension (PHT) are 8 times the risk of major perioperative complication.[7,8] Children with severe cardiac failure stand a very high risk and must be optimized preoperatively and surgery done in a specialized center.[4] CHD patients with a well-compensated physiology can undertake elective surgeries at a low perioperative risk, while patients with poorly compensated physiology posted for emergency or major surgeries are at high risk. It is important to stratify these children based on their perioperative risk into three categories: (1) high, (2) intermediate, and (3) low-risk **(Table 2)** for formulating anesthesia plan, perioperative decision making and optimizing perioperative care.[9]

ANESTHETIC MANAGEMENT

Preoperative Evaluation and Preparation

Failure to thrive is an important history pertaining to poorly compensated cardiac lesions due to poor peripheral oxygenation and organ perfusion with or without PHT. Previous records related to the cardiac condition and any ongoing drug therapy should be checked. Physical examination should seek to ascertain any signs/symptoms of congestive heart failure, such as easy fatiguability, diaphoresis, irritability, tachycardia, crepitations, jugular

TABLE 2: Risk categorization of pediatric patients with congenital heart disease undergoing noncardiac procedures/surgery

Category	High risk	Intermediate risk	Low risk
Physiologic compensation	Physiological compromise and/or complicated physiology • Cyanosis • Pulmonary hypertension • Arrhythmias • Cardiac failure	Well compensated	Well compensated
Type of lesion	Complex	Simple	Simple
Type of surgery	Supra-major prolonged invasive surgeries (intrathoracic, intraperitoneal, expected massive blood loss)	Major (intraperitoneal, intrathoracic, blood loss needing transfusion)	Minor
Age	<2 years	<2 years	>2 years
ASA status	IV or V	III and emergency surgery	I–III
Emergency/elective procedure	Emergency	Emergency	Elective
Preoperative hospital stay	>10 days	Up to 10 days	<10 days

(ASA: American Society of Anesthesiologists)

venous distention, and congestive hepatomegaly. Clinical examination should focus on assessment of clubbing, cyanosis, pedal edema, pulse volume and character, and blood pressure. Jugular venous pressure may be difficult to assess in children <5 years who have chubby necks and who move around a lot. Hepatomegaly may be better indicator of increased venous pressures. Other co-existing extracardiac congenital anomalies should be sought which may be present in up to 20% of children.[10] Cardiac auscultation would reveal murmurs depending on the type of lesion. Child's age and weight should be noted. Parents should be counseled and a written informed high-risk consent for administration of anesthesia should be taken. Other important aspects of preoperative anesthesia evaluation are mentioned in **Box 1**.[5,9,11-13]

Investigations

Investigations which should be routinely undertaken include blood grouping and cross matching, hemoglobin/hematocrit, complete and differential blood counts, coagulation profile (platelet count, prothrombin and partial thromboplastin times), serum electrolytes, blood urea nitrogen and serum creatinine and baseline arterial oxygen saturation on room air, chest X-ray (CXR) and electrocardiogram (ECG). C-reactive protein (CRP)

BOX 1: Points to ponder in preoperative assessment and optimization.

- The type of lesion and circulation should be evaluated along with its repercussions on SVR and PVR
- Evidence of long-term complications should be looked for (e.g., arrhythmias, cardiomyopathy, cardiac failure, pulmonary hypertension, cerebral thromboembolism, etc.)
- Phlebotomy may be considered in cyanotic CHD especially with hemoglobin >20 g/dL
- The main anesthetic concern in cyanotic patients are polycythemia and coagulopathy and subsequent hyperviscosity resulting in cerebral vein and sinus thrombosis especially in children <5 years of age
- Anemia and URTI should be treated. Current infections of the respiratory tract or a recent history can increase airway reactivity and lead to poorly tolerated PVR perturbations
- Children on diuretic therapy especially those receiving digoxin are at risk for hypokalemia
- Possibility of difficult venous access should be established as it may alter the choice of anesthesia in favor of inhalational technique
- Routine cardiac medications should be continued before operation. Though adult literature advocates omitting ACE inhibitors, current evidence in children is lacking. Electrolyte imbalances should be anticipated. Aspirin has to be continued, and patients on warfarin need INR monitoring and intravenous heparin bridging therapy
- Premedication with sedatives avoids stress and anxiety, reduces oxygen demands and may lessen the requirement of induction agent (thereby reducing subsequent declines in SVR)
- Availability of blood and blood products should be ensured
- Antibiotic prophylaxis for infective endocarditis is advocated for all CHD patients according to national and local guidelines
- Perioperative hydration should be maintained
- Blood pressure should be recorded in all four-limbs in children with prior surgery to the aorta
- Ventricular ectopics on ECG is ominous sign, particularly children with a single ventricle physiology should be reviewed with a specialist and surgery should preferably be undertaken in a specialized center[6]
- Syndromic association of other co-existing congenital disorders and their systemic repercussions (e.g., difficult airway) should be carefully ruled out[14]

(PVR: pulmonary vascular resistance; SVR: systemic vascular resistance; URTI: upper respiratory tract infection; CHD: congenital heart disease; ACE: angiotensin-converting enzyme; INR: international normalized ratio; ECG: electrocardiogram)

and complete leukocyte count provide indication of any existing infection. Cyanotic CHD cases may have polycythemia with remarkably high hemoglobin and hematocrit which may need intervention. Serum electrolytes may be deranged in patients on diuretics. CXR may reveal cardiomegaly with right atrial and/or RVH/dilatation, dilatation of main pulmonary artery segment and prominent pulmonary vasculature markings in volume overload due to left to right shunts.[14,15] ECG should be done in all children with CHD.[5] It may reveal arrhythmias, signs of right ventricular volume overload can be seen as right bundle branch block (RBBB), RVH, and right atrial enlargement. PR prolongation and complete AV block may be seen in patients with AV septal defects. Latest two-dimensional (2D) echocardiography report should be reviewed. It is the key tool not only for the diagnosis of CHD, but also for establishing its location and exact nature, assessment of pulmonary artery pressure and pulmonary venous drainage, left or right heart dilation and for evaluating for the suitability for device closure of the defects. Transesophageal echocardiography (TEE) may be required if transthoracic windows are suboptimal.

Investigations which are selectively done on case to case basis depending upon the cardiac lesion and patient conditions include diagnostic cardiac catheterization, cardioangiography, magnetic resonance imaging (MRI) or computed tomography (CT), serum digoxin levels, and arterial blood gases. Diagnostic cardiac catheterization provides valuable information about cardiac chamber pressures, shunt fraction and coronary anatomy. It may be helpful in patients with suspected pulmonary vascular disease.[16] Cardioangiography is one of the main cardiac imaging techniques but has limitations including the overlying of neighboring vascular structures, catheter-related problems (especially in younger children), difficulty in simultaneous demonstration of systemic and pulmonary vascular systems, and exposure to high dosages of ionizing radiation and contrast. Multisection spiral CT scan or MRI can be used to accurately outline the normal and pathologic morphologic features of the cardiovascular system in CHD patients especially in complex cardiac pathologies. Patients on digoxin therapy may manifest its toxicity perioperatively since it has a narrow therapeutic index. Serum digoxin levels may be done in cases where its toxic symptoms are suspected. Arterial blood gases may be needed in hypoxic patients, patients with pulmonary congestion or severely decompensated disease preoperatively and perioperatively to guide management.

Premedication

Premedication decreases the likelihood of sympathetic stimulation that may predispose the child to cardiovascular compromise which may eventually result in cyanotic spell or congestive heart failure. However, excessive sedation can lead to loss of protective airway reflexes or hemodynamic compromise and reduced or titrated dose should be given particularly in children with pre-existing cardiac compromise. Midazolam and fentanyl are relatively cardiostable and can be used safely.[17]

Intraoperative Monitoring

Monitoring modalities to be employed for intraoperative management of CHD cases have been mentioned in **Table 3**.[18] Appropriate essential monitors should be in place prior to induction of anesthesia if the child is co-operative. Baseline room air saturation should be obtained. At a minimum, ECG and noninvasive blood pressure (NIBP) should be attached which is generally possible even in a child who is moving. Depending on surgical invasiveness and preoperative patient condition addition monitors are used as indicated. Pulmonary artery pressure monitoring is generally not favored nowadays. TEE

TABLE 3: Intraoperative monitoring modalities for CHD children undergoing noncardiac surgery

Essential	Case specific
• Electrocardiogram • Pulse oximetry (SpO$_2$) • End tidal CO$_2$ (EtCO$_2$) • Arterial blood gas (ABG) • Noninvasive blood pressure (NIBP) • *Temperature monitoring*: Rectal and nasopharyngeal • Precordial or esophageal stethoscope	• Invasive BP monitoring • Central venous pressure • Urine output • Pulmonary artery pressure monitoring • Transesophageal echocardiography

(BP: blood pressure; CHD: congenital heart disease)

is usually indicated during cardiac surgery in children and for interventional procedures in the cardiac catheterization lab.[19] In children with CHD, TEE assessment should concentrate on imaging particular cardiac structures rather than any specific views.[20]

RECOMMENDATION FOR MANAGEMENT OF CONGENITAL HEART DISEASE CHILDREN POSTED FOR ELECTIVE PROCEDURES[5]

High-risk patients should be referred to specialized center with advanced monitoring and intensive care back-up. Regarding management of intermediate risk children, concerned specialist should be consulted and patient transferred if advised. Low-risk patients can be managed in local hospital with basic facilities.

RECOMMENDATION FOR MANAGEMENT OF CONGENITAL HEART DISEASE CHILDREN POSTED FOR EMERGENCY SURGERIES[5]

Patients standing at high or intermediate risk should take advice from the pediatric intensivist about feasibility of transfer to higher center with onsite access to pediatric cardiologist and intensive care therapy unit. If transfer is difficult, advice should be sought from cardiologist and a pediatric cardiac anesthetist from higher center for planning the perioperative management. The child should be transferred only when stable. Low-risk patients can be managed locally. If required, expert advice can be taken.

Drugs to be Kept Ready in Emergency/Crash Trolley for Surgery

All the emergency drugs should be stocked in the operation room where a CHD patient is to be operated and their doses should be precalculated according to the child's weight and displayed for use in case of emergency.

- *Adrenaline* for refractory hypotension (refractory to dopamine) and in cardiac arrest (dose of 1:10,000 adrenaline solution: 0.005–0.01 mg/kg).
- *Noradrenaline* for the treatment of profound hypotension and cardiac arrest.
- *Dopamine* for correction of hypotension due to reduced systemic vascular resistance (SVR).
- *Phenylephrine* causes increased SVR; used in hypotension, shock, and supraventricular tachycardia.
- *Milrinone* is usually started perioperatively in patients with pulmonary arterial hypertension. It reduces PVR and improves surgical outcomes. It is given in an intravenous (IV) loading dose of 50 µg/kg by an infusion at the rate of 0.25–0.75 µg/kg/min.
- *Nitroglycerin* for induced hypotension; given intraoperatively as continuous IV infusion in the dose of 1–3 µg/kg/min.
- *Isoprenaline* is used in bradycardia and heart block.
- *Antiarrhythmic drugs,* viz., amiodarone, beta-blockers.

GENERAL PRINCIPLES OF ANESTHETIC MANAGEMENT

The possibility of difficult airway due to narrow subglottis should be considered. IV access may be difficult to establish in patients who had previous surgery and history of pediatric critical care unit admissions. Due to the dynamic nature of physiological and pathological shunts during anesthesia and surgery, systemic air emboli are a constant hazard in patients with CHD, regardless of the shunt.[21] Therefore, air trap is prudent for all IV lines, but should not be substituted for careful attention and constant attentiveness and purging of any air bubbles in the IV lines. Cyanotic children frequently have simultaneous heart failure, arrhythmias, and PHT making them a very high-risk group.[13] The risk of thrombotic complications is increased in these children with fever, dehydration, and anemia and these should be corrected preoperatively. Infective endocarditis prophylaxis should be ensured in children with CHD. Avoiding fluid overload and maintaining proper temperature to avoid hypothermia are important precautions while managing these cases. Identification of high-risk factors is important during preoperative evaluation. The predominant direction of shunt and the impact of alterations in PVR and SVR on the magnitude of shunt flow across the lesions is important to identify as the appropriate manipulation of SVR and PVR intraoperatively is vital to ensure favorable hemodynamics.

Patients with left to right (L to R) shunt: Common L to R shunts encountered are PDA, VSD and ASD. It is characterized by increased PBF. Therefore, any factor that decreases SVR or increases PVR decreases the pressure gradient across the defect, thereby leading to decreased shunting across them.[22] Inspired oxygen concentration of 100% and hyperventilation should be avoided in these patients as it will lead to pulmonary vasodilation, which can increase shunt fraction and further aggravate pulmonary congestion.

Patients with right to left (R to L) shunt: This includes TOF, Eisenmenger's, Ebstein's anomaly and tricuspid atresia. These lesions are characterized by

TABLE 4: Factors affecting pulmonary and systemic vascular resistance

Increased pulmonary vascular resistance	• Acidosis • Hypoxia • Hypercarbia • Hypoxemia • Light plane of anesthesia • Sepsis • High airway pressures • Atelectasis • Pain
Decreased pulmonary vascular resistance	• High FiO_2 • Hypocarbia • Alkalosis • Vasodilation
Increased systemic vascular resistance	• Alpha agonist • Beta blocker • Increase in intra-abdominal pressure • Compression of aorta
Decreased systemic vascular resistance	• Inhaled anesthetic agents • Vasodilator • Alpha antagonist • Beta agonists • Calcium channel blockers

decreased PBF and hypoxemia. Therefore, any event that leads to increased PVR or decreased SVR increases the degree of shunting thereby precipitating severe hypoxemia.[23]

Factors affecting the PVR and SVR are mentioned in **Table 4**.[18,24,25]

Choice of Anesthetic Agents

The choice of anesthetic agents in these children is mainly directed by presence and type of cardiac shunt, ventricular function (presence or absence of cardiac failure) and the plan to extubate or mechanically ventilate the child following surgery. Many different anesthetic techniques have been described for management of CHD patients, but there is limited literature in support or against any particular technique.[21]

Induction of Anesthesia

Intravenous Induction

Onset of IV induction agent may be faster in patients with R to L shunt.[26] Therefore, drug bolus should be administered slowly in these patients to avoid high plasma levels. On the other hand, onset of IV induction agent may be delayed in L to R shunt patients due to recirculation of the drug. Propofol should be avoided as it may cause a fall in cardiac output.[27,28] Ketamine (2 mg/kg) is the IV induction agent of choice in cyanotic heart disease as it increases SVR.[29] A combination of potent opioid (fentanyl) with an amnesic agent (midazolam) or etomidate (0.3 mg/kg) due to its cardiostability are other possible alternatives.

Inhalational Induction

Securing IV access may not be feasible prior to induction in all children. Inhalational induction using sevoflurane has minimal effect on cardiac contractility is safe for children with CHD.[26] However, use of high inspired sevoflurane concentrations for prolonged time can lead to sudden precipitous fall in SVR, hence use of lower inspired concentrations and graded increase in sevoflurane concentrations is recommended. Inhalation induction with sevoflurane has a slow onset of action in patients with R to L shunt with limited PBF.[30] In case of pure L to R shunt there is no significant effect on uptake of inhaled anesthetic agent.

REGIONAL ANESTHESIA

Regional anesthesia (RA) is relatively safe in patients with CHD. Establishment of any regional block before the surgery reduces anesthetic drug requirements, decreases stress response, provides exceptional analgesia, rapid pain-free emergence, avoids harmful effects of opioids, improved postoperative pulmonary, and gastrointestinal function.[31] The various regional techniques are wound infiltration, peripheral nerve blocks (e.g., penile block, ilioinguinal block, etc.) and central neuraxial analgesia. They are either used independently or along with general anesthesia. Central neuraxial block (spinal, epidural, etc.) can be safely administered provided sudden precipitous fall in SVR and hypotension are avoided.[32] Caudal block using lower dilution of local anesthetic and an adjuvant like clonidine can be safely given. Ultrasound use allows visualization of various anatomic structures and spread of local anesthetic drug and, reduce volume of drugs.[33] Various adjuvants to local anesthetics have been found to significantly prolong the duration of analgesia, e.g., morphine (mean 15 hours), clonidine (mean 10 hours), fentanyl (mean 6 hours), and dexmedetomidine (mean 10 hours).[34]

Intravenous Fluid Administration

Intravenous fluid of choice is a combination of crystalloids and colloids.[35] Plasmalyte is a balanced salt solution having electrolyte constitution similar to that of plasma and hence is preferred to Ringer lactate.[36] Fluid overload and hypovolemia should both be avoided.

Maintenance of Anesthesia

Muscle relaxation can be maintained using intermittent bolus doses of neuromuscular blockers such as rocuronium, cisatracurium, vecuronium, and pancuronium at regular intervals along with an inhalational agent. Sevoflurane and isoflurane have insignificant cardiac depressant effect or on the shunt fraction and they are widely used in these patients. Desflurane use has been described but its effects in these children are not established. Alternatively, a mixture of a sedative (midazolam), an analgesic (fentanyl) and a muscle relaxant drug (vecuronium) can be administered as continuous infusion throughout the surgery to maintain homogeneous plasma drug levels and ensure a deep plane of anesthesia. Total IV anesthesia with propofol infusions is not advised in cases where a fall in SVR would be deleterious. Nitrous oxide is generally not preferred in patients with cardiac shunts as it aggravates cerebral air embolism and alter PVR. Pulmonary hypertensive crisis episodes should be treated with 100% oxygen, prostacyclin analogs, inhaled nitric oxide, phosphodiesterase inhibitors, inotropic agents and other methods to maintain PBF and cardiac output.[25]

Emergence from Anesthesia

Tachycardia and hypertension during emergence can be detrimental in lesions like TOF. Removal of supraglottic airway device should preferably be done in a deeper plane of anesthesia. Desflurane and sevoflurane are preferred agents due to rapid recovery profile. Endotracheal tube should be taken out when all protective reflexes have returned.

Postoperative Care and Pain Management

These patients should be observed in a high-dependency bed or intensive care unit. Postoperative complications include cardiac ischemia, arrhythmia, pain, dehydration, and ventilatory issues. Postoperative care includes prevention of tachycardia, hypothermia, shivering, hypoxia, pain and any factor producing a sympathetic response.[37] Hypoventilation leading to hypoxia and hypercarbia should be avoided due to risk of increase in PVR in patients with R to L shunts and PHT.[8] Elective postoperative mechanical ventilation or nasal continuous positive airway pressure may be required in some cases with compromised physiology. Acute postoperative pain following a surgery due to nociceptor stimulation can lead to release of inflammatory mediators and catecholamines which affect major organ systems, thereby increasing postoperative morbidity. Aggressive control of postoperative pain prevents adverse hemodynamic, immunologic, hemostatic and metabolic effects. Adequate analgesia attenuates increased levels of stress hormones released intraoperatively. A balance is maintained between coronary blood flow and myocardial oxygen demand that prevents perioperative myocardial ischemia.

Modalities of postoperative analgesia include the following:
- *Opioids* as IV bolus or infusion.
- *Nonsteroidal anti-inflammatory drugs (NSAIDs)* which act by inhibiting cyclo-oxygenase (COX) enzyme, thus helping to reduce opioid dose, e.g., nonselective NSAIDs such as diclofenac, ibuprofen, ketorolac, indomethacin and selective COX2 inhibitors such as celecoxib, parecoxib, etc.

- *Alpha-adrenergic agents* provide cardiovascular stability but associated with sedation, bradycardia and hypotension; reduce sedative and analgesic requirements, e.g., dexmedetomidine, clonidine.
- *Local anesthetic infiltration* at the surgical incision site; commonly used are lidocaine, bupivacaine, levobupivacaine, and ropivacaine.
- *Peripheral nerve blocks* using local anesthetics.
- *Multimodal analgesia* literatures support the combination of two analgesics which have different mechanism of action as they provide better analgesia with lesser side effects.

ANESTHETIC CONSIDERATIONS OF MANAGEMENT OF SPECIFIC CARDIAC LESIONS

Patent Ductus Arteriosus

Increasing survival of premature low birth weight neonates has ensured increasing number of them presenting for PDA ligation. Conservative management includes administration of indomethacin, a prostaglandin synthetase inhibitor, which leads to smooth muscle constriction of the ductus and thus, may lead to its closure. Nonetheless, these tiny premature neonates lack the smooth muscle in ductal tissue, whereby indomethacin may not be effective. Many of these children may be in respiratory and cardiac failure and would be at very high risk in addition to their increased risk because of prematurity. They have small circulatory volume and delicate transitional circulation. The neonates who are in congestive cardiac failure need meticulous preoperative optimization with restriction of IV fluids, diuretic and inotropic agents. Availability of blood should be ensured as sudden, catastrophic bleeding during ligation of PDA is a real danger if the ductus arteriosus ruptures. Therefore, warmed crystalloid, albumin, and blood should be immediately available. The other common cause of hypotension is compression of the lungs, heart, and kinking of great vessels by the surgeon while gaining surgical exposure. The procedure may be performed at bed side or in the operating room. Special care should be taken to ensure normothermia, ventilation, and oxygenation. It is imperative to secure two good peripheral venous accesses. Arterial line should be secured on the opposite side of arch of aorta. Some practitioners prefer an inhalation induction as it decreases SVR and therefore shunting. An opioid-based technique with muscle relaxant is a safe and commonly used technique for anesthesia. Surgery in right lateral position ensures proper positioning. Systolic blood pressure should be brought down to 70–90 mm Hg at the time of dissection and ligation of ductus arteriosus depending on the age of the patient. These patients usually remain intubated after procedure. Video-assisted thoracoscopic surgery (VATS) using endoscopes inserted through a series of small thoracotomy ports is gaining popularity.[38] Complications can arise during intraoperative period such as bleeding, bradycardia, increased blood pressure (especially diastolic) after ligation of ductus arteriosus and recurrent laryngeal nerve palsy.

Tetralogy of Fallot

Tetralogy of Fallot accounts for 10% of patients with CHD.[39] The child presents with cyanosis from birth and may develop hypercyanotic or Tet "spells" in infancy, due to spasm of infundibular muscle in the right ventricular outflow in response to sympathetic stimulation, e.g., when the child is disturbed or crying or may become limp and unresponsive. An older child with uncorrected pathology may "squat" in an attempt to improve PBF (by increasing SVR) and will manifest clubbing.

These patients commonly present for palliative shunt surgeries before corrective surgery can be performed. Three types of shunts can be done:
1. Blalock-Taussig shunt. Classic and modified.
2. Waterston shunt.
3. Potts shunt.

Objectives of anesthesia in these patients include:[39]
- *Maintaining SVR.*
- *Decreasing PVR* (avoid hypoxia, hypercapnia, and metabolic/respiratory acidosis).
- *Maintaining mild myocardial depression.*
- *Slower heart rate.*

Ketamine induction is preferred as it maintains SVR.[37] Inhalational induction is not preferred as it decreases SVR and can precipitate cyanotic attack. Right lateral position is given for surgery. Take care of oxygen saturation and bradycardia—intraoperative compression of lung tissue and clamping of pulmonary artery during anastomosis can decrease saturation and can cause severe bradycardia.[40] Frequent arterial blood gas analysis and correction of acidosis should be done. Watch out for hypercyanotic spell manifested by intraoperative sudden desaturation, hypotension and bradycardia.[13]

Treatment includes:
- *Hyperventilation* with 100% warm humidified oxygen.
- *Beta-blocker*, e.g., propranolol at a dose of 0.1 mg/kg IV takes care of infundibular spasm.
- *Phenylephrine* 5–10 µg/kg IV increases SVR.
- *Morphine* at a dose of 0.1–0.2 mg/kg IV.
- *Fluid administration* to maintain right ventricular filling.
- *Increase in depth of anesthesia.*
- *Treatment of metabolic acidosis.*
- *Direct aortic compression* to increase SVR.

Complications of shunt surgery include bleeding, hypoxemia, pneumothorax, thrombosis and kinking of shunt and pulmonary edema due to overcorrection of shunt.

Examples of assessment and management of two cases of CHD are given in **Table 5** to understand the physiology, identify risk factors, and plan perioperative management.

TABLE 5: Example of perioperative management plan for two cases of CHD posted for noncardiac surgeries

Case 1: A 25-day-old baby with unrepaired tetralogy of Fallot for emergency laparotomy

Physiology	Compromised (moderate cardiac failure, failure to thrive, cyanosis, feeding poor)
Risk category	High risk (Heart failure, cyanosis, emergency major surgery, <2 years old)
Lesion	Simple
Management	Refer to higher specialized center
Anesthetic considerations	• Child should be kept calm by using sedative premedication • Slow inhalational or titrated IV induction with ketamine • Balanced anesthesia with good perioperative analgesia • Avoid dehydration and sympathetic stimulation to avoid hypercyanotic spells • Diligently avoid air bubbles into IV lines • Give high-inspired oxygen and avoid factors which increase PVR or decrease SVR • Be prepared to deal with hypercyanotic spells during surgery

Case 2: A 5-year-old child with repaired VSD for toe abscess drainage

Physiology	Well compensated (No failure to thrive, good exercise tolerance, no cyanosis/clubbing, no signs of congestive heart failure, ECG normal)
Lesion	Simple
Risk category	Low
Management	Locally managed
Anesthesia considerations	• Inhalational or IV induction • Support ventilation intraoperatively and use balanced anesthetic technique • Caudal block or ankle block • Endocarditis prophylaxis not required

(PVR: pulmonary vascular resistance; SVR: systemic vascular resistance; IV: intravenous; VSD: ventricular septal defect; ECG: electrocardiogram)

LIMITATIONS IN MANAGING CONGENITAL HEART DISEASE PATIENTS

There is limited evidence in literature for definitively categorizing CHD children as high, intermediate or low risk. Furthermore, there is no consensus on perioperative management which may be due to the lack of advancement in the treatment approaches and the diversity and intricacy of CHD making it difficult to have a single approach to management. Lack of skilled staff in the operating theater and nonavailability of advanced monitors in a noncardiac operating theater can pose a challenge to the anesthetist in managing such cases. Additionally, absence of a well-equipped coronary care unit (CCU) can hamper proper postoperative care in such children. Primary care hospitals lack the infrastructure required for the management of such high-risk CHD children undertaking noncardiac elective or emergency surgeries and referral to appropriately equipped set-up would be prudent for successful outcome.

CONCLUSION

Dealing with pediatric CHD needs constant vigilance, accurate monitoring, experienced anesthesiologist, good infrastructure, and proper communication between surgeon, anesthesiologist, nursing staff and patient relatives. For a successful patient outcome, it is imperative to have a sound foundation in understanding of the pathophysiologic and hemodynamic perturbations of the particular cardiac lesion and the pharmacological principles.

ACKNOWLEDGMENT

The authors wish to acknowledge the unconditional hard work done by Dr Ananki Chakravarty during writing of this chapter.

KEY POINTS

- Children with congenital heart disease (CHD) being taken-up for noncardiac surgeries are at higher risk.
- Main factors posing the highest risk in these patients include compromised physiology, complex disease, and existence of long-term complications.
- Intermediate risk factors are considered as patients posted for major and/or emergency operations, age <2 years, American Society of Anesthesiologists (ASA) physical status of ill patients for emergency procedure and prolonged preoperative hospital stay.
- High-risk patients should be referred to a higher center for definitive management.
- Induction using sevoflurane/ketamine, maintenance with sevoflurane/isoflurane, and opioid analgesia are appropriate anesthesia techniques.
- Proper diagnosis, optimization, preoperative preparation, no air bubble, no arrhythmias, optimal perioperative hemodynamics, good analgesia, good monitoring and postoperative care should be the mainstay for a good outcome.

REFERENCES

1. Hoffman JI, Kaplan S. The incidence of congenital heart disease. J Am Coll Cardiol. 2002;39(12):1890-900.
2. Dixit R, Rai SK, Yadav AK, Lakhotia S, Agrawal D, Kumar A, et al. Epidemiology of congenital heart disease in India. Congenit Heart Dis. 2015;10(5):437-46.
3. Junghare SW, Desurkar V. Congenital heart diseases and anaesthesia. Indian J Anaesth. 2017;61(9):744-52.
4. Ramamoorthy C, Haberkern CM, Bhananker SM, Domino KB, Posner KL, Campos JS, et al. Anesthesia-related cardiac arrest in children with heart disease: data from the Pediatric Perioperative Cardiac Arrest (POCA) registry. Anesth Analg. 2010;110(5):1376-82.

5. Hennein HA, Mendeloff EN, Cilley RE, Bove EL, Coran AG. Predictors of postoperative outcome after general surgical procedures in patients with congenital heart disease. J Pediatr Surg. 1994;29(7):866-70.
6. Garson A Jr, Randall DC, Gillette PC, Smith RT, Moak JP, McVey P, et al. Prevention of sudden death after repair of tetralogy of Fallot: treatment of ventricular arrhythmias. J Am Coll Cardiol. 1985;6(1):221-7.
7. Taylor CJ, Derrick G, McEwan A, Haworth SG, Sury MR. Risk of cardiac catheterization under anaesthesia in children with pulmonary hypertension. Br J Anaesth. 2007;98(5):657-61.
8. Carmosino MJ, Friesen RH, Doran A, Ivy DD. Perioperative complications in children with pulmonary hypertension undergoing noncardiac surgery or cardiac catheterization. Anesth Analg. 2007;104(3):521-7.
9. White MC, Peyton JM. Anesthetic management of children with congenital heart disease for non-cardiac surgery. Contin Educ Anaesth Crit Care Pain. 2012;12(1):17-22.
10. Greenwood RD, Rosenthal LA, Parisi L, Fyler DC, Nadas AS. Extracardiac abnormalities in infants with congenital heart disease. Pediatrics. 1975;55(4):485-92.
11. Murphy TW, Smith JH, Ranger MR, Haynes SR. General anesthesia for children with severe heart failure. Pediatr Cardiol. 2011;32(2):139-44.
12. White MC. Anesthetic implications of congenital heart disease for children undergoing non-cardiac surgery. Anaesth Int Care Med. 2012;13(9):432-7.
13. Malviya S, Voepel-Lewis T, Siewert M, Pandit UA, Riegger LQ, Tait AR. Risk factors for adverse postoperative outcomes in children presenting for cardiac surgery with upper respiratory tract infections. Anesthesiology. 2003;98(3):628-32.
14. Litman RS. The difficult pediatric airway. In: Litman RS (Ed). Pediatric anesthesia: The requisites. St. Louis: Mosby; 2004.
15. DeFilippis AP, Law K, Curtin S, Eckman JR. Blood is thicker than water: the management of hyperviscosity in adults with cyanotic heart disease. Cardiol Rev. 2007;15(1):31-4.
16. Diaz LK, Andropoulos DB. New developments in pediatric cardiac anesthesia. Anesthesiol Clin North Am. 2005;23(4):655-76.
17. Newstead B. Premedication drugs useful in children. Update in Anaesthesia. 2005;19(4):6.
18. Frankville D. Anesthesia for children and adults with congenital heart disease. In: Lake CL, Booker PD (Eds). Pediatric Cardiac Anesthesia. Philadelphia: Lippincott Williams and Wilkins; 2005. pp. 601-32.
19. Weintraub R, Shiota T, Elkadi T, Golebiovski P, Zhang J, Rothman A, et al. Transesophageal echocardiography in infants and children with congenital heart disease. Circulation. 1992;86(3):711-22.
20. Puchalski MD, Lui GK, Miller-Hance WC, Brook MM, Young LT, Bhat A, et al. Guidelines for performing a comprehensive transesophageal echocardiographic examination in children and all patients with congenital heart disease: recommendations from the American Society of Echocardiography. J Am Soc Echocardiogr. 2019;32(2):173-215.
21. Menghraj SJ. Anesthetic considerations in children with congenital heart disease undergoing non-cardiac surgery. Indian J Anaesth. 2012;56(5):491-5.
22. Laird TH, Stayer SA, Rivenes SM, Lewin MB, McKenzie ED, Fraser CD, et al. Pulmonary-to-systemic blood flow ratio effects of sevoflurane, isoflurane, halothane, and fentanyl/midazolam with 100% oxygen in children with congenital heart disease. Anesth Analg. 2002;95(5):1200-6.

23. Cannesson M, Piriou V, Neidecker J, Lehot JJ. Anaesthesia for non-cardiac surgery in patients with grown-up congenital heart disease. Ann Fr Anesth Reanim. 2007;26(11):931-42.
24. Widrich J, Shetty M. Physiology, Pulmonary Vascular Resistance. [Updated 2020 May 29]. In: StatPearls [Internet]. Treasure Island (FL): StatPearls Publishing; 2020 Jan. [online] Available from https://www.ncbi.nlm.nih.gov/books/NBK554380/. [Last accessed November, 2020].
25. Friesen RH, Williams GD. Anesthetic management of children with pulmonary arterial hypertension. Paediatr Anaesth. 2008;18(3):208-16.
26. Mellor J. Induction of anaesthesia in paediatric patients. Update Anaesth. 2004;18.
27. Flick RP, Sprung J, Harrison TE, Gleich SJ, Schroeder DR, Hanson AC, et al. Perioperative cardiac arrests in children between 1988 and 2005 at a tertiary referral center: a study of 92,881 patients. Anesthesiology. 2007;106(2):226-37.
28. Williams GD, Jones TK, Hanson KA, Morray JP. The hemodynamic effects of propofol in children with congenital heart disease. Anesth Analg. 1999;89(6):1411-6.
29. Oklu E, Bulutcu FS, Yalcin Y, Ozbek U, Cakali E, Bayindir O. Which anesthetic agent alters the hemodynamic status during pediatric catheterization? Comparison of propofol versus ketamine. J Cardiothorac Vasc Anesth. 2003;17(6):686-90.
30. Steward DJ. Manual of Pediatric Anesthesia, 5th edition. New York: Churchill Livingston; 2001.
31. Lofland GK. The enhancement of hemodynamic performance in Fontan circulation using pain free spontaneous ventilation. Eur J Cardiothorac Surg. 2001;20(1):114-8.
32. Kachko L, Birk E, Simhi E, Tzeitlin E, Freud E, Katz J. Spinal anesthesia for noncardiac surgery in infants with congenital heart diseases. Paediatr Anaesth. 2012;22(7):647-53.
33. Shah RD, Suresh S. Applications of regional anaesthesia in paediatrics. Br J Anaesth. 2013;111(Suppl 1):114-24.
34. Ansermino M, Basu R, Vandebeek C, Montgomery C. Nonopioid additives to local anesthetics for caudal blockade in children: a systematic review. Paediatr Anaesth. 2003;13(7):561-73.
35. Bhardwaj N. Perioperative fluid therapy and intraoperative blood loss in children. Indian J Anaesth. 2019;63(9):729-36.
36. NICE. (2015). NICE guidelines [NG29]: Intravenous fluid therapy in children and young people in hospital. [online] Available from https://www.nice.org.uk/guidance/ng29. [Last accessed November, 2020].
37. Walker A, Stokes M, Moriarty A. Anesthesia for major general surgery in neonates with complex cardiac defects. Paediatr Anaesth. 2009;19(2):119-25.
38. Jacobs JP, Giroud JM, Quintessenza JA, Morell VO, Botero LM, van Gelder HM, et al. The modern approach to patent ductus arteriosus treatment: complementary roles of video-assisted thoracoscopic surgery and interventional cardiology coil occlusion. Ann Thorac Surg. 2003;76(5):1421-27.
39. Hamid M. Anesthetic considerations for congenital heart disease patient. In: Narin C, (Ed). Perioperative Considerations in Cardiac Surgery. InTech; 2012. [online] Available from http://www.intechopen.com/books/perioperative-considerations-in-cardiac-surgery/anaesthesia-forcongenital-heart-surgery. [Last accessed November, 2020].
40. Tandale SR, Kelkar KV, Ghude AA, Kambale PV. Anesthesia considerations in neonate with tetralogy of Fallot posted for laparotomy. Ann Card Anaesth. 2018;21(4):465-6.

CHAPTER 16

Panorama of Postdural Puncture Headache: Current Evidence

Pratibha Jain Shah

INTRODUCTION

Postdural puncture headache (PDPH) or meningeal puncture headache or spinal headaches are postural headaches following any interference that violates the integrity of the meninges. This can follow deliberate puncture with a spinal needle or an accidental dent with an epidural or other needle.[1] PDPH is an important iatrogenic cause of patient morbidity following modern anesthesia, pain management procedures, after attempted epidural blocks, and after spinal taps. The risk of accidental dural puncture (ADP) with large bore epidural needle is around 1.5% in obstetric patients compared to less than 0.5% in nonobstetric, even in experienced hands and more than half of these patients develop PDPH.[2,3] A number of studies have reported a PDPH rate in the range 75–85%.[1] The risk of PDPH with a spinal needle is almost similar in obstetric and nonobstetric patients, i.e., 1.5–11.2% depending on size and type of needle.[3] Postlumbar puncture incidence of headache is around 10–30%.[4]

Postdural puncture headache accounts for 12% of lawsuits pertaining to obstetric anesthesia in the American Society of Anesthesiologists (ASA) Closed-Claims Project Database for dereliction involving anesthesia, regional anesthesia and chronic pain management.[1] This necessitates its consideration in informed consent involving any anesthetic procedures with risk of PDPH and proper attention to procedure-related factors to reduce incidence.[1] Occasionally, inadvertent dural puncture and PDPH could be an unavoidable complications. Therefore, anesthesiologists need to be familiar with the preventive and treatment modalities. Prophylaxis and treatment of PDPH have been studied and discussed for more than a century, but for the most part, a clear consensus is still lacking.

HISTORY

A German surgeon Karl August Bier wrote about PDPH in 1898 after he injected 10–15 mg of spinal cocaine into himself, his assistant, and seven of his patients. Four of the nine people, including him, developed PDPH. He reported his experience "I had a feeling of very strong pressure on my skull and became rather dizzy when I stood up rapidly from my chair. All these symptoms vanished at once when I lay down flat, but returned when I stood up. I was forced to take to bed and remained there for 9 days because all the manifestations recurred as soon as I got up. The symptoms finally resolved nine days after the lumbar puncture".[1] Before the beginning of the 20th century, serious and sustained headache following spinal anesthesia was very frequent and this questioned the effectiveness of this modality. "The most notable successful attempts to reduce the loss of cerebrospinal fluid (CSF) were by Vandam and Dripps and Hart and Whitacre, using narrower-gauge and "noncutting" needles in the 1950s".[1,3] Epidural blood patch (EBP), a remarkably innovative technique, has proven to be the greatest advance in PDPH management. In the late 1960 Dr James Gormley, a general surgeon, introduced the idea of using autologous blood to "patch" a hole in the meninges. This procedure was later popularized in anesthesiology circles, by Dr Anthony DiGiovanni and Burdett Dunbar. Unfortunately, there were no preventive steps prior to the implementation of the EBP that could be defined as major changes over the mere passage of time. Rates of PDPH following spinal anesthesia have been steadily declining from an incidence exceeding 50% in Bier's time to around 10% in the 1950s, largely due to changes in practice following the identification of risk factors, until now a rate of 1% or less can be reasonably expected. Still worse, 1.7% of obstetric patients tend to experience PDPH following spinal anesthesia.

PATHOPHYSIOLOGY

Despite much research, controversy on the exact etiology of PDPH symptoms continues. The original theory of leakage of CSF hypothesized that PDPH is the result of a disturbance of normal CSF homeostasis. CSF is produced mainly in the choroid plexus at an approximate rate of 0.35 mL/min. The total CSF volume of around 150 mL (1.5–2 mL/kg) in adults is maintained by reabsorption of excess CSF through the arachnoid villi. This exerts 5–15 cmH$_2$O lumbar opening pressures in horizontal posture and 40–50 cmH$_2$O pressure in upright position.[1] Whenever the rate of CSF leakage (0.084–4.5 mL/sec) through a meningeal puncture site exceeds the rate of CSF production, CSF volume and pressure decrease.[1,3-7] The symptoms of PDPH occur when 10% of CSF is lost and resolve quickly with this deficit rejuvenation. The resultant low CSF pressure leads to **(Flowchart 1)**:
- Sagging of brain (shift downward) due to the deprivation of the cushioning effect of intracranial fluid. This causes friction and pressure on the surrounding pain-sensitive structures such as cranial nerves, dura, upper cervical nerves, venous sinuses and bridging veins, within the cranium, specifically in the upright position. Traction on the 5th cranial nerve causes a frontal headache, 9th and 10th cranial nerves cause occipital pain, the upper cervical nerves including C1, C2, and C3 cause pain in the neck and shoulders. Due to its long and arduous intracranial path, the 6th cranial nerve (abducens) is most vulnerable to traction and is responsible for visual symptoms. Nausea is attributed to vagal stimulation. Sagging of the brain in upright position contributes to orthostatic symptoms.[1,3,7]

Flowchart 1: Pathophysiology of postdural puncture headache (PDPH).

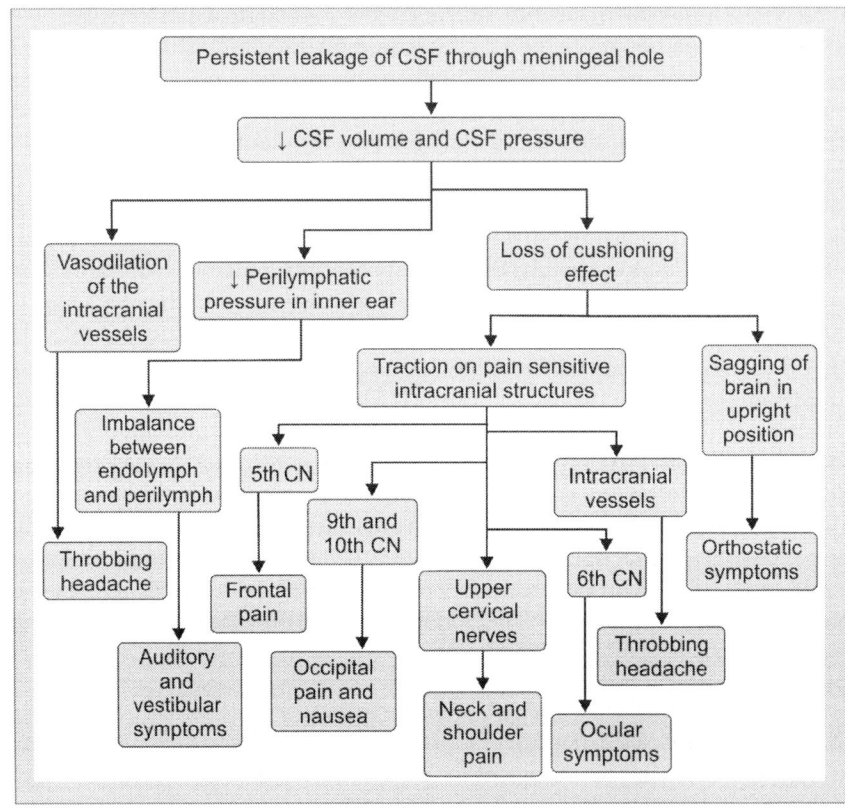

(CSF: cerebrospinal fluid; CN: cranial nerve)

- Adenosine-mediated reflex vasodilation of the intracranial vessels (especially cerebral veins) to maintain a constant intracranial volume (Monro-Kellie hypothesis),[1] and reflex cerebral venodilation due to traction on intracranial vessels contribute to throbbing headache.
- Diminishing perilymphatic pressure in the inner ear due to direct communication between the CSF and the perilymph via the cochlear aqueduct.[1] This disturbs the balance between the endolymph and perilymph and alters of hair cell position which is manifested as auditory and vestibular symptoms.[1,3]

Second theory (high CSF pressure headache) which is not well accepted, postulated that headache is caused by meningeal irritation, secondary to chemical or bacterial invasion. CSF pressure is normal or high.

Clinical Presentation

Postdural puncture headache presents as a bilaterally symmetrical, dull aching or throbbing or pressure type pain with a frontal-occipital distribution. Usually, the headache has a postural dimension, aggravated in upright posture

> **BOX 1:** Diagnostic criteria for PDPH: The International Headache Society's ICHD-3.
> - Headache has developed in temporal relation to the low CSF pressure or CSF leakage or led to its discovery
> - Dural puncture has been performed
> - Headache develops within 5 days after dural puncture
> - Not better accounted for by another ICHD-3 diagnosis
>
> (ICHD-3: the International Classification of Headache Disorders; CSF: cerebrospinal fluid; PDPH: postdural puncture headache)

and relieved or at least improved with lying down.[1,3,5] The onset of headache is usually within 3 days in >90% (6-72 hours) and within 48 hours in 60% individuals but is rarely seen after 5 days following a meningeal puncture. PDPH usually remits spontaneously within 3-15 days in 72% patients after dural puncture with spinal needle[7] and 87% recover by 6 months. PDPH with an epidural needle has not been well studied, but is likely to last longer than that after a spinal needle.

Associated Symptoms

Other nonspecific symptoms present in severe PDPH may be nausea, vomiting, neck stiffness, ocular complaints such as difficulty in accommodation, photophobia and diplopia, and auditory complaints such as tinnitus, hearing loss (in the low-frequency range), vertigo and hyperacusis.[1] Headache is the only complain in 29% of patients with PDPH.[1,7]

Other rare symptoms associated with PDPH are seizures, vertigo, bilateral forearm pain, abdominal pain, and diarrhea.

The revised diagnostic criteria for PDPH is published in international classification of headache disorders (ICHD) by the International Headache Society (IHS) in 2017-18 (**Box 1**).[8]

The severity of headache varies considerably among patients. Lybecker et al. classified headache severity by physical activity limitation, degree of bed confinement, and related symptoms and found mild, moderate, and severe PDPH in 11%, 23%, and 67% cases after spinal anesthesia, respectively (**Table 1**).[9] Another severity grading system described by Corbey et al. combines visual analog scores (VAS) and the patient's functional ability (**Table 2**).[10] The reliability of the various measures of severity of PDPH has not yet been determined.

RISK FACTORS

Patient-related Risk Factors

Age

Peak incidence of PDPH is in teens and the early 20s, and is less frequent after 50 years of age. It may be due to: (1) inelastic dura that is less likely to tear after punctures, (2) impedance of CSF leakage due to adhesions and calcification,

TABLE 1: Modified Lybecker classification of severity of PDPH

Mild PDPH	Moderate PDPH	Severe PDPH
• Light restriction of daily activities • Not bedridden • No associated symptoms • Responds well to nonopiate analgesics	• Significant restriction of daily activities • Bedridden most of the day • Associated symptoms may or may not be present • Requires the addition of opiates	• Complete restriction of daily activities • Bedridden all day • Associated symptoms present • Not responsive to conservative management

(PDPH: postdural puncture headache)

TABLE 2: Corbey classification of severity of PDPH

Grade I	Headache does not interfere with normal daily activity VAS pain score 1–3 out of 10
Grade II	Headache relieved by periodical bed rest VAS pain score 4–7 out of 10
Grade III	Headache prevents the patient from sitting up to eat VAS pain score 8–10 out of 10

(VAS: visual analog scores; PDPH: postdural puncture headache)

(3) less reactive cerebrovascular system, (4) less active physically, and (5) less likely to complain (11.0% in 31–50 years of age vs. 4.2% others).[7,11]

Gender

The risk of PDPH is twofold higher in female compared to male (11.1% vs. 3.6%), because of enhanced vascular reactivity due to hormonal changes.[5,7,11,12]

Pregnancy

High incidence of PDPH in pregnancy may be attributed to increased estrogen levels, which increases the cerebral vascular distension in response to CSF hypotension.[3,11]

Vaginal Delivery

Vaginal delivery is linked with a higher rate of PDPH than C-section delivery (74% vs. 53%). Following UDP during epidural catheter placement for labor analgesia, there is increased CSF leakage secondary to the mechanical consequences of expulsive efforts during the 2nd stage of labor.[11,13]

Morbid Obesity

Obesity is associated with a lower rate of PDPH [39% vs. 56% at a body mass index (BMI) of 31.5 kg/m^2 above and below, respectively], though pain intensity is the same. This is apparently due to the beneficial effect of increased abdominal pressure on the magnitude of CSF leakage and reduce physical activity and a higher cesarean delivery rate in these patients.[11]

Dural Thickness

Dura has varying thickness. Some people do not develop a PDPH if the dural puncture occurs in a thicker area.[6,14]

Cigarette Smoking

Smokers have lower risk of PDPH compared to nonsmokers (13.7% vs. 34.1%). This could be because smoking promotes blood clotting and may facilitate closure of the dural hole by a clot.[15]

History of Headache

Patients with history of headache within a week prior to lumbar puncture and chronic bilateral tension-type headache are at increased risk of PDPH.[1]

Previous Postdural Puncture Headache

Patients who have experienced PDPH previously are 4.3 times increase risk of subsequent PDPH because of the predisposition of certain individuals to the development of PDPH.[7,11]

Procedural-related Risk Factors

The occurrence of PDPH is affected by numerous technical factors linked to neuraxial technique which is described here.

Needle Size and Tip Design

Needle size is directly linked to the incidence, severity, associated symptoms, period and need for concrete steps of intervention. The bigger the needle, the greater the incidence of PDPH. Cutting needle has the highest impact of needle size. Cutting needles (Quincke and Atraucan) have a higher risk for PDPH comparing with noncutting, pencil-point needle (Whitacre and Sprotte) (6.6% vs. 1.7%).[6] Electron microscopy has shown that pencil point needles are more traumatic to the dura than the cutting needles. It is postulated that a pencil point needle produces an irregular tear in the dura and the subsequent inflammatory reaction reduces CSF leakage more effectively than the clean U-shaped puncture seen with a cutting needle.[14] The incidence of PDPH is also high when UDP occurs with a 16 G compared with an 18 G epidural needle (88% vs. 64%) **(Fig. 1)**.

Orientation of Bevel

Clinically, a longitudinal orientation of the needle bevel reduces the risk of PDPH by 70% compared to perpendicular orientation (5.7% with parallel vs. 16.1% with perpendicular bevel orientation).[7] Dural fibers were once believed to run longitudinally; therefore inserting the needle bevel in parallel with long axis of the spine caused less trauma to the dura by separating dural fibers

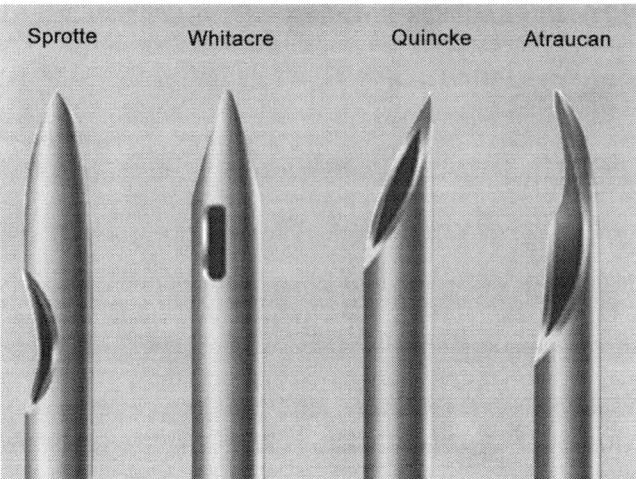

Fig. 1: Tip design of spinal needles.

rather than cutting. Nevertheless, microscopic dissection of the dura mater from corpses showed that the dura consists of multidirectional interlacing collagen fibers with transverse and longitudinal elastic fibers.[14,16] Some authors proposed that the parallel-oriented insertion of the bevel would more likely result in less stress on the dural hole and therefore a smaller opening with less CSF leak.[11] Despite confusing anatomic evidence, clinical experience is in favor of the insertion of the parallel oriented Quincke's needle. A matter of controversy still exists for insertion of epidural needles bevel orientation, despite a substantially high incidence of post ADP intermediate to extreme PDPH with perpendicular placement than parallel (70% vs. 24 %). A variety of worries about parallel needle insertion such as lateral needle deviation, catheter insertion problems, and dural needle rotation trauma, etc., tend to be of concern to practitioners.[1]

Midline or Paramedian Approach

Currently, neither paramedian nor median approach is recommended due to insufficient data. Paramedian approach to the subarachnoid space has been suggested as a means of reducing PDPH, particularly when using cutting needles because it creates dural puncture with a "flap valve" that seals the hole and check CSF leakage which is not formed with midline puncture.[11]

Air versus Saline for Locating the Epidural Space

Both saline/air medium which is used in the loss-of-resistance technique to define the epidural space, was not clearly shown to affect the incidence of PDPH.[11]

Multiple Dural Punctures

Incidence of PDPH is significantly high after second spinal injection compared to single dural puncture (4.2% vs. 1.6%).[3,11]

TABLE 3: Various factors affecting the incidence of PDPH		
Factors that may increase		**Factors that do not increase**
• Age	Younger > old	• Continuous spinal
• Gender	Females > males	• Timing of ambulation
• Needle size	Larger > smaller	• Concentration of local anesthetic
• Type of needle	Cutting > noncutting	
• Bevel orientation	Perpendicular > parallel	• Presence or absence of opioids and
• Number of punctures	Multiple > Single	
• Pregnancy	More in pregnant	• The type of opioid
• Previous H/o PDPH	More	

Intrathecal Injectate

A higher incidence of PDPH is reported with hyperbaric lidocaine-bupivacaine than tetracaine-procaine for spinal anesthesia.[11] It is unclear whether the difference was caused by the type of local anesthetic (LA) (ester vs. amide) or because of the absence or presence of glucose in the drug.

Continuous Spinal Anesthesia and Combined Spinal-epidural Anesthesia

Both techniques, continuous spinal anesthesia or the combined spinal-epidural anesthesia, do not influence the risk for PDPH.[1,3]

Various factors influencing the incidence of PDPH are listed in **Table 3**.

ASSOCIATED PROBLEMS

The immediate problems associated with PDPH are the helplessness to perform daily routine tasks, such as providing care for the newborn; an extended duration of hospitalization and a higher number of hospital visits in emergency.[1,3]

Rare but serious complications of PDPH include subdural hematoma, cerebral venous sinus thrombosis, chronic headache, backache, neck ache, diplopia, and hearing loss.

PREVENTION

In an effort to minimize the occurrence of PDPH after spinal or after UDP, many techniques and procedures were employed, although with minimal success. Nevertheless, they are helpful in reducing the likelihood of serious PDPH, symptom span, or need for EDP.

General Measures

Appropriate patient selection is crucial in reducing the incidence of PDPH. One has to weigh the risk of PDPH with benefits of regional anesthesia in every case considering patient-related risk factors.

Bed rest and aggressive hydration (oral and intravenous) is suggested as prophylactic steps against PDPH by a significant majority, but there is no evidence to support this widespread practice. Early mobilization may actually decrease the risk of PDPH. Furthermore, since pregnant women are hypercoagulable and are at higher risk of thrombosis of the deep veins and pulmonary embolism. So, immobility should not be used as a preventive measure.[1] Normal hydration should be maintained orally. Intravenous fluids are required to prevent dehydration only if oral intake is not feasible.[17]

Precautions during Neuraxial Technique

The smallest size, noncutting spinal (24-27 G needles are ideal) should be used for spinal anesthesia, and for epidural anesthesia a 18 G epidural needle should be used. The stylet should be replaced prior to needle withdrawal. This effectively lowers the incidence of PDPH with 21 G Sprotte needle from 16.3 to 5.0% due to decrease chances of wicking strand of arachnoid mater from extending across the dura but this difference is not significant with 25 G Quincke needle on replacement of stylet. The needle should be inserted with parallel orientation of bevel and the number of punctures should be minimized. The use of ultrasound to evaluate the location, depth and angle of the spinal processes has promising role to reduce ADP and PDPH risk. Other measures such as use of paramedian approach, use of saline for loss of resistance testing, maternal pushing for vaginal delivery do not have strong convincing clinical evidence.

Preventive Measures to Reduce Postaccidental Dural Puncture Risk of Postdural Puncture Headache

Not all patients with ADP will develop PDPH and only a portion of them will require definitive treatment. The effectiveness of various PDPH prophylactic interventions is debatable.[18] Therefore, it is important to weigh risk-benefit ratio of particular preventive measure, inform patient about high risk of PDPH and regular follow-up until discharge in event of confirm ADP.[1]

Stylet replacement could be helpful prior to epidural needle removal ones ADP occur as replacing the stylet is found to be a simple and effective means to lower the incidence of PDPH after lumbar puncture.[5,11,12] Though supportive evidence is lacking.

The duration of the 2nd stage of labor should be confined (up to 30-60 minutes), and pushing effort should be avoided by the use of forceps in the event of ADP during epidural for labor analgesia. This may reduce the risk of PDPH.[1]

Prophylactic *caffeine* is not advocated because of no benefit on incidence of headaches. Intravenous *cosyntropin* (1 mg), an adrenocorticotropic hormone (ACTH) analog, considerably lowers PDPH incidence and need of EBP because of unknown mechanism.[19] This beneficial effect may be related to volume expansion by aldosterone-stimulating effect, modulation of pain perception via central endorphin-like action, or enhance CSF production through stimulation of sodium ion transport.[3] These limited encouraging data will require further studies to validate.

Intrathecal saline was first described by Jacobaeus et al. in 1923. Intrathecal injection of 10 mL preservative-free saline immediately after ADP through epidural needle or through an intrathecal catheter prior to removal may reduce the incidence of PDPH (32% vs. 62%) and need of EBP.[3,20] This should be injected only when residual LA effects have cleared up.

Intrathecal catheters (ITC): Even though ITC placement is becoming frequent, reattempting epidural at an adjacent interspace still remains the common choice following ADP. The benefit of ITC to reduce the risk of PDPH after ADP especially, if left in situ for 24 hours may be due to inflammation or edema secondary to reaction to catheter which prevent further CSF loss after removal; though the supportive evidence is extremely limited.[1,3,21] ITC placement immediately after ADP has added advantages of providing rapid spinal analgesia and reducing the danger of another ADP.

Epidural saline to treat PDPH was first reported by Rice and Dabbs in 1950. A bolus or continuous infusion of saline in epidural space restores CSF volume and increases intracranial pressure. Besides reduction in severity and delay in onset of symptoms, there is no convincing evidence regarding prophylactic epidural saline on the incidence of PDPH or the subsequent need for EBP.[1]

Epidural opiates: Epidural morphine 3 mg in 10 mL saline has long been utilized for the treatment of PDPH. It was recently revisited as prophylaxis after ADP, and found beneficial. But it would require prolonged monitoring for respiratory depression.[22]

Prophylactic epidural blood patch (PEBP): Epidural blood patch has majestic efficacy as a treatment, but has fueled interest as prophylaxis for PDPH. Research regarding PEBP has yielded mixed results. It reduces total duration of symptoms (from a median of approximately 5 to 2 days) and overall pain burden. It should be performed only after the LA effect has resolved, as premature administration may cause excessive cephalad displacement of LA. Residual LA may interfere with coagulation and further decrease the efficacy of the EBP.[1,3,23] PEBP is not currently recommended as a routine measure due to inconclusive evidence.

Prophylactic epidural dextran-40 patch (20 mL) is effective for preventing PDPH following ADP. Though its safety and efficacy remain unclear.[3,18]

DIAGNOSTIC EVALUATION

Postdural puncture headache remains a clinical diagnosis of exclusion. While headache after meningeal puncture is suspected to be PDPH,[8] the exclusion of other benign and severe etiologies is important **(Table 4)**. A comprehensive history and physical examination, particularly blood pressure, temperature and basic neurological examination must be carried out before making the diagnosis of PDPH. Headache associated with meningeal puncture worsens with firm bilateral jugular venous pressure for 10–15 seconds and improve for

TABLE 4: Differential diagnosis of postdural puncture headache (PDPH)

Benign causes	Serious causes
Nonspecific headache	Meningitis (septic or aseptic)
Exacerbation of chronic headache	Subdural hematoma
Hypertensive headache	Subarachnoid hemorrhage
Pneumocephalus (symptoms within 1 hour)	Pre-eclampsia/eclampsia
Sinusitis	Intracranial venous thrombosis
Intrathecal steroids induced arachnoiditis	Intracranial mass lesion
Caffeine withdrawal	Cerebral aneurysm
Spontaneous intracranial hypotension	Spinal abscess
Myofascial syndrome	Anterior spinal artery syndrome

15–30 seconds with sitting epigastric pressure test.[1] Laboratory studies are not usually required for PDPH diagnosis but complete blood count (CBC), blood culture, magnetic resonance imaging (MRI), cerebral computed tomography (CT) scan or cerebral Doppler could be performed to exclude the possibility of developing serious complications. CSF leak and pressure can be detected by radionuclide cisternography, radionuclide myelography, and manometric studies.

Gadolinium enhanced MRI in PDPH suggests low intracranial pressure characterized by diffuse non-nodular pachymeningeal enhancement due to dilation of thin walled vessels, descent of the cerebellar tonsils and/or medulla, obliteration of basilar cisterns, decreased ventricular size, enlargement of the pituitary gland, and subdural fluid collections.[3]

TREATMENT

Early detection and treatment of PDPH avoids not only the perpetual cycle of immobility, fatigue and depression, but also severe complications.

Supportive Measures

Psychological Support

As PDPH is an iatrogenic complication, many patients are furious, resentful, frustrated and tearful. Hence, good communication and reassurance is very important. Reassure them that it resolves spontaneously with a quick passage of time.

Posture

The horizontal position provides remarkable relief. However, evidence regarding beneficial effect of prolong supine position is lacking. The prone position relieves PDPH in some patients, but unfortunately not comfortable for many patients.[11,18]

Abdominal Binders

Abdominal binders are uncomfortable and available evidence is insufficient to recommend its use in the treatment of PDPH.[3]

Pharmacologic Treatment

Many pharmacological agents have been advocated for the treatment of PDPH, but are not usually recommended in view of insufficient evidences.[1,3,11,24] One should have guarded expectations, especially when dealing with severe PDPH because many of the treatment have initial optimistic role but eventually disproven in the literature **(Table 5)**.

Simple oral analgesics such as paracetamol, nonsteroidal anti-inflammatory drugs, and weak opioids for 24–48 hours are helpful in mild to moderate PDPH.

Opioid analgesics such as morphine, oxycodone may be offered if simple oral analgesia is ineffective, but long-term therapy is not recommended.

Methylxanthine derivatives such as aminophylline, theophylline and caffeine, are commonly used to treat PDPH due to their cerebral vasoconstrictor

TABLE 5: Various medications used for prophylaxis and treatment of PDPH

Agent	Mechanism of action	Route	Effect on PDPH	Adverse effect
Opioids	Interact with receptors	Oral/IV	Pain relief	Nausea/vomiting
Caffeine	CNS stimulant, blocks cerebral adenosine receptors	Oral 300 mg IV 500 mg	Temporary relief	Headache return within 48 hours after IV Seizures
Sumatriptan	Serotonin type 1d agonist	6 mg SC	Variable results	Pain at injection site, chest tightness
Gabapentin	Increase concentration of GABA in the brain	300–800 mg 8 hourly for 4 days	Decrease severity	Sedation
Hydrocortisone	Agonist	100–200 mg TDS for 48 hours	Decrease VAS 50% by 6 hours 75% by 24 hours	Hyperglycemia, weight gain, hypokalemia, fluid accumulation
Cosyntropin	Increase CSF production, fluid and electrolyte retension	60 U IM 1.5 U/kg IV	Pain relief for 3–7 days	Caution in HTN, diabetes

(CSF: cerebrospinal fluid; CNS: central nervous system; HTN: hypertension; PDPH: postdural puncture headache; VAS: visual analog scores; GABA: gamma-aminobutyric acid)

effect and increased CSF production by Na-K pumps stimulation. *Caffeine* can be used orally (300 mg) or intravenously (500 mg caffeine sodium benzoate which contains 250 mg caffeine) in PDPH. Dose should not exceed 300 mg BD with a maximum 900 mg in 24 hours as more than 1 g caffeine can cause seizures. Lactating women should not receive more than 200 mg in 24 hours. It provides a significant improvement in mild to moderate PDPH for 1–4 hours in 70% cases after 2 hours of administration. Repeat dosages are required due to short half-life (<6 hours). Long-term (>24 hours) caffeine therapy cannot be recommended. Caffeine is contraindicated in seizure disorders, pregnancy induced hypertension and supraventricular tachyarrhythmias.[1] *Theophylline* is not commonly used despite prolonged action due to narrow safety profile.

Adrenocorticotropic hormone and its synthetic analogs (tetracosactrin and cosyntropin) increase circulating volume by elevating endogenous aldosterone levels, increase CSF production, and stimulate β-endorphin release and thus, improve symptoms of PDPH.

Miscellaneous medications: Many drugs such as steroids (hydrocortisone, dexamethasone, and methylprednisolone), gabapentinoids (gabapentin, pregabalin), antidiuretic hormone analog (desmopressin), sumatriptan (6 mg subcutaneous), methylergonovine, ondansetron, mannitol, neostigmine, and atropine are effective in improving the severity of PDPH.[24] But the evidences are inconclusive to use these drugs for the treatment of PDPH **(Table 4)**.

Invasive Procedures

Few invasive procedures which have been used to treat PDPH include the following:

Acupuncture may promote release of endorphins and relieve muscle spasm.[3]

Sphenopalatine ganglion block inhibits parasympathetic outflow to cerebral vasculature and prevents vasodilation. A simple technique, the operator places a cotton pledget soaked with LA in the nose and allows diffusion across the nasal mucosa. Currently, insufficient evidence to validate its role in PDPH.[25]

Greater occipital nerve block inhibits pain transmission to the trigeminal nucleus caudalis reducing central sensitization, which switches off the headache. More evidence is required on the role of greater occipital nerve block (GONB) in PDPH.[26]

Epidural Therapies

These are recommended only when access to epidural space is considered logical, or an epidural catheter is in situ.

Epidural morphine (3.5–4.5 mg) successfully relieves headache. It should be used with caution in case of large size puncture due to the risk of respiratory depression.[1,3,22]

Epidural saline as 20–30 mL bolus or infusion offers quick and nearly complete relief, but the procedure is riddled by an exceptionally high rate of recurrence of headache.[1,3]

Epidural blood patch (**Table 6**) is regarded as the most successful therapeutic modality for PDPH in which freshly drawn autologous blood is injected into epidural space.[3,11,27,28]

TABLE 6: Epidural blood patch (EBP)	
Indication	*Severe PDPH affecting daily activities*
Mechanisms of action	The actual mechanism is unknown, but proposed theories are: • Tamponade effect of the blood in the epidural space compressing the thecal sac, and displacing CSF cephalad toward the brain • Fibrin clot around the dural puncture seals the hole and stops CSF leakage until the dura heals • A quick rise in intrathecal pressure deactivates adenosine receptors and reverses vasodilatation
Blood volume injected	• 20 mL (adequate to form a well-organized clot over the rent and create some degree of epidural tamponade)[1] • Stop injection earlier, if not tolerated by the patient
Timing of injection	The ideal timing is still a matter of debate and research. For greater efficacy, it is recommended 48 hours after dural puncture, however, may be considered earlier in severe PDPH for symptomatic relief. If performed within 48 hours, there is reduced efficacy and increased need of repeat EBP, due to the detrimental effect of lidocaine and CSF on coagulation
Contraindication	Same as for epidural needle placement: infection at the site, coagulopathy, systemic sepsis, fever, 'red-flag' symptoms suggesting an alternative diagnosis and patient refusal
Prerequisite	Confirmation of diagnosis; informed consent that includes procedural details, success rate, anticipated side effects and risk involved; establish intravenous access
Preprocedure blood culture and antibiotic	No sufficient evidence to recommend
Level for EBP	Same level or one space below the original site of dural puncture as blood in epidural space predominately spreads cephalad due to high negative pressure gradient within the epidural space at higher spinal levels. Average spread is 3.5 levels above and 1 level below the site of injection[1]
Recommended monitoring	Noninvasive blood pressure, heart rate and SpO_2
Postprocedure instructions	Supine position for 1–2 hours; avoid lifting, straining and air travel for 24 hours; regular pulse, blood pressure and temperature monitoring; over-the-counter analgesics even for mild residual discomfort; stool softeners and cough suppressants; review by anesthesiologist till 4 hours of the procedure and then daily until discharge or symptoms resolve; report for inadequate relief, recurrence of symptoms and any complications after discharge
Success rate	70 to 98% if performed at least 24 hours after the dural puncture

Contd...

Contd...

Indication	*Severe PDPH affecting daily activities*
Complications	Backache (50%), neck pain, leg pain, paresthesia, paraparesis, cauda equine syndrome, radicular pain, meningeal irritation, elevated intracranial pressures, seizures infection, subdural hematoma, and temporary cranial nerve palsy
Indications for repeat EBP	Partial relief or recurrence after complete relief with 1st EBP. Though evidence is limited, it is reasonable to wait for 24 hours before repeating EBP
Indication for consulting other specialties	Failure of EBP, change in the nature of headache, and atypical presentation

Alternatives to epidural blood patching: Although evidence is limited, various colloid solutions such as dextran 40, gelatin, hydroxyethyl starch can be used to provide prolong epidural tamponade to seal meningeal rent in patients who refuse an EBP or when an EBP is ineffective.[1,3] *Fibrin sealant patch* composed of fibrinogen and thrombin and prepared from human pooled plasma. It forms a firm, nonretractable fibrin clot and found to be effective in preventing dural leakage after spinal surgery, treatment of persistent PDPH, spontaneous intracranial hypotension, and CSF leakage after long-term intracellular catheterization.[29]

Surgery

There are limited evidence regarding curative surgical closure of dural rent for intractable PDPH.[3]

Postdural Puncture Headache in Children

Though PDPH is considered to be rare complication in children but the actual occurrence is 10–50% in aged between 10 and 18 years.[30] It is uncommon in children under 10 years because of high CSF volume, (approximately 4 mL/kg) and low intracranial pressure, (30–40 mm H_2O lower than an adult). Preventive measures and treatment of PDPH in children remain on the same line as adults.[31] If conservative measures are ineffective after 48 hours, it is reasonable to consider EBP with 0.2–0.3 mL/kg of autologous blood in epidural space until child feels discomfort or pressure in the back.[32]

CONCLUSION

Postdural puncture headache, an iatrogenic complication can be miserable for both the recipient and the anesthesiologist. There is a large variation on prophylactic and conservative therapeutic treatments because of the lack of enough large randomized controlled clinical trials to provide satisfactory evidence-based recommendations. EBP is still the most effective gold standard treatment for severe PDPH. Several other treatment modalities for PDPH are available, but high-level evidence supporting their efficacy is still needed.

> **KEY POINTS**
> - Postdural puncture headache (PDPH) is an iatrogenic complication following dural puncture intentionally with spinal needle or unintentionally with an epidural needle.
> - It is a low-pressure headache caused by persistent cerebrospinal fluid (CSF) leakage through meningeal rent.
> - It is characterized by a bilaterally symmetrical, dull aching or throbbing, or pressure type postural fronto-occipital pain that is exacerbated in an upright position, and relieved with recumbency.
> - It develops within 3–5 days of dural puncture and resolves spontaneously.
> - Associated risk factors include female gender, younger age, pregnancy, cutting large diameter needles, multiple punctures and previous history of PDPH and chronic headache. The approach of the needle (median or paramedian), the bevel orientation, and the intrathecal injectate do modify the risk of PDPH to little extent.
> - No therapies reliably prevent the development of PDPH after unintentional dural puncture (UDP) with an epidural needle.
> - The best way to treat PDPH is to prevent it from developing.
> - No evidence supports prolong bed rest and vigorous hydration for prophylaxis or therapy for PDPH.
> - Epidural blood patching (EBP) is a gold standard therapy for severe or refractory PDPH.
> - High-level evidence supporting efficacy of several available treatment modalities for PDPH is still awaited.
> - An informed consent related to PDPH should be endorsed for procedures with a risk of PDPH because of associated medicolegal liability.

REFERENCES

1. NYSORA. Harrington and Miguel Angel Reina. Postdural puncture headache. Brian E, Reina MA. [online] Available from https://www.nysora.com/foundations-of-regional-anesthesia/complications/postdural-puncture-headache/. [Last accessed November, 2020].
2. Choi PT, Galinski SE, Takeuchi L, Lucas S, Tamayo C, Jadad AR. PDPH is a common complication of neuraxial blockade in parturients: a meta-analysis of obstetrical studies. Can J Anaesth. 2003;50(5):460-9.
3. Peralta F, MacArthur A. Postpartum headache. In: David H, Chestnut HD, Cynthia A, Tsen LC, Kee WD, Beilin Y (Eds). Chestnut's Obstetric Anesthesia: Principles and Practice, 6th edition. Philadelphia: Elsevier; 2020. pp. 730-45.
4. Bezov D, Lipton RB, Ashina S. Post-dural puncture headache: part I diagnosis, epidemiology, etiology, and pathophysiology. Headache. 2010;50(7):1144-52.
5. Kwak KH. Postdural puncture headache. Korean J Anesthesiol. 2017;70(2):136-43.
6. Turnbull DK, Shepherd DB. Post-dural puncture headache: pathogenesis, prevention and treatment. Br J Anaesth. 2003;91(5):718-29.
7. Amorim JA, Gomes de Barros MV, Valença MM. Post-dural (post-lumbar) puncture headache: risk factors and clinical features. Cephalalgia. 2012;32(12):916-23.
8. Headache Classification Committee of the International Headache Society (IHS). The international classification of headache disorders, 3rd edition. Cephalalgia. 2018;38(1):1-211.

9. Lybecker H, Djernes M, Schmidt JF. Postdural puncture headache (PDPH): onset, duration, severity, and associated symptoms. An analysis of 75 consecutive patients with PDPH. Acta Anaesthesiol Scand. 1995;39(5):605-12.
10. Corbey MP, Bach AB, Lech K, Frorup AM. Grading of severity of postdural puncture headache after 27-gauge Quincke and Whitacre needles. Acta Anaesthesiol Scand. 1997;41(6):779-84.
11. Alice L, Oswald. Postdural puncture headache. In: Suresh M (Ed). Shnider and Levinson's anesthesia for obstetrics, 5th edition. Philadelphia: Lippincott Williams and Wilkins, a Wolters Kluwer Business; 2013.
12. Ghaleb A, Khorasani A, Mangar D. Postdural puncture headache. Int J Gen Med. 2012;5:45-51.
13. Nath G, Subrahmanyam M. Headache in the parturient: Pathophysiology and management of post-dural puncture headache. J Obstet Anaesth Crit Care. 2011;1(2):57-66.
14. Reina MA, de Leon-Casasola OA, Lopez A, De Andres J, Martin S, Mora M. An in vitro study of dural lesions produced by 25-gauge Quincke and Whitacre needles evaluated by scanning electron microscopy. Reg Anesth Pain Med. 2000;25(4):393-402.
15. Dodge HS, Ekhator NN, Jefferson-Wilson L, Fischer M, Jansen I, Horn PS, et al. Cigarette smokers have reduced risk for post-dural puncture headache. Pain Physician. 2013;16(1):E25-30.
16. Richman JM, Joe EM, Cohen SR, Rowlingson AJ, Michaels RK, Jeffries MA, et al. Bevel direction and postdural puncture headache: a meta-analysis. Neurologist. 2006;12(4):224-8.
17. Arevalo-Rodriguez I, Ciapponi A, Roque I Figuls M, Munoz L, Bonfill Cosp X. Posture and fluids for preventing post-dural puncture headache. Cochrane Database Syst Rev. 2016;3(3):CD009199.
18. Apfel CC, Saxena A, Cakmakkaya OS, Gaiser R, George E, Radke O. Prevention of postdural puncture headache after accidental dural puncture: a quantitative systematic review. Br J Anaesth. 2010;105(3):255-63.
19. Hakim SM. Cosyntropin for prophylaxis against postdural puncture headache after accidental dural puncture. Anesthesiology. 2010;113(2):413-20.
20. Charsley MM, Abram SE. The injection of intrathecal normal saline reduces the severity of postdural puncture headache. Reg Anesth Pain Med. 2001;26(4):301-5.
21. Heesen M, Klöhr S, Rossaint R, Walters M, Straube S, van de Velde M. Insertion of an intrathecal catheter following accidental dural puncture: a meta-analysis. Int J Obstet Anesth. 2013;22(1):26-30.
22. Al-metwalli RR. Epidural morphine injections for prevention of post dural puncture headache. Anaesthesia. 2008;63(8):847-50.
23. Scavone BM, Wong CA, Sullivan JT, Yaghmour E, Sherwani SS, McCarthy RJ. Efficacy of a prophylactic epidural blood patch in preventing post dural puncture headache in parturients after inadvertent dural puncture. Anesthesiology. 2004;101(6):1422-7.
24. Basurto Ona X, Martínez García L, Solà I, Bonfill Cosp X. Drug therapy for treating post-dural puncture headache. Cochrane Database Syst Rev. 2011;(8):CD007887.
25. Cohen S, Ramos D, Grubb W, Mellender S, Mohiuddin A, Chiricolo A. Sphenopalatine ganglion block: a safer alternative to epidural blood patch for postdural puncture headache. Reg Anesth Pain Med. 2014;39(6):563.
26. Hasoon J, Berger A, Urits I, Orhurhu V. Greater occipital nerve blocks for the treatment of postdural puncture headache after labor epidural. Saudi J Anaesth. 2020;14(2):262-3.

27. Russell R, Laxton C, Lucas DN, Niewiarowski J, Scrutton M, Stocks G. Treatment of obstetric post-dural puncture headache. Part 2: epidural blood patch. Int J Obstet Anesth. 2019;38:104-18.
28. Boonmak P, Boonmak S. WITHDRAWN: Epidural blood patching for preventing and treating post-dural puncture headache. Cochrane Database Syst Rev. 2013;(11):CD001791.
29. Crul BJ, Gerritse BM, van Dongen RT, Schoonderwaldt HC. Epidural fibrin glue injection stops persistent postdural puncture headache. Anesthesiology. 1999;91(2):576-7.
30. Wee LH, Lam F, Cranston AJ. The incidence of post dural puncture headache in children. Anaesthesia. 1996;51(12):1164-6.
31. Janssens E, Aerssens P, Alliet P, Gillis P, Raes M. Postdural puncture headaches in children. A literature review. Eur J Pediatr. 2003;162(3):117-21.
32. Ylonen P, Kokki H. Management of postdural puncture headache with epidural blood patch in children. Paediatr Anaesth. 2002;12(6):526-9.

CHAPTER 17

Perioperative Venous Thromboembolism: A Review

Nitin Sethi, Jayashree Sood

INTRODUCTION

The disease spectrum of venous thromboembolism (VTE) comprises of superficial vein thrombosis (SVT), deep vein thrombosis (DVT) and pulmonary embolism (PE). VTE incidence in United States is 1-2 per 1000 population,[1] whereas in Asian patients the incidence varies from 14 to 57 per 100,000 person years.[2] Up to 10% of all inpatient deaths can be attributed to VTE. A significant cause of VTE in inpatients is surgical intervention, up to 25% of surgical patients are affected by it.[3] The highest reported incidence of VTE in surgical patients is after arthroplasty and cancer surgeries.[4] A major challenge in treatment of VTE is the diagnosis of the condition. Nearly half of the patients with a diagnosis of PE, have asymptomatic DVT on presentation.[5] In the recent past, several recommendations and guidelines for perioperative VTE prophylaxis have been developed but largely they have not been able to make any significant impact on the incidence of patient morbidity.[2,6,7] Therefore, it is essential that active surveillance protocols be developed at the institutional level to detect DVT at the earliest in at risk surgical patients prior to onset of any fatal complication.

PATHOPHYSIOLOGY

The onset of venous thrombosis can be explained by the Virchow's triad: hypercoagulability venous stasis and endothelial injury. The normal peripheral venous flow comprises of two components—first is a continuous or laminar flow and second is the pulsatile flow. The laminar flow occurs secondary to pressure generated during left ventricular contraction and elastic recoil of the arterial vasculature. Any increase in microvascular resistance due to excessive sympathetic outflow results in increased venous pressure resulting in blood stasis. Pulsatile flow occurs due to the compression of muscles around the deep veins which pushes the blood toward the heart and is facilitated by antireflex venous valves. Prolonged bed rest and general anesthesia largely abolishes this flow resulting in stasis of blood around the venous valve pockets.[8,9] Furthermore, absence of pulsatile flow makes the valve cusps hypoxic, which are entirely dependent on oxygen diffusion from the deoxygenated venous blood for their nutrition.[10] Hypoxia of the venous valve cusps in addition to surgical stress triggers release of inflammatory mediators, that activate the endothelial cells resulting in an imbalance between procoagulant and anticoagulant factors with preponderance of procoagulant factors such as tissue factor (TF) and Ul-Von Willebrand factors (UI-VWF), and decreased levels of anticoagulant factors such as thrombomodulin and endothelial cell protein C receptor thus promoting thrombosis.[11,12]

The activated endothelial cells cause accumulation of monocytes, neutrophils, and TF-releasing circulating microvesicles (MVs) due to the expression of selectins, in particular P-selectin. UI-VWF in the venous blood causes further accumulation of platelets and neutrophils resulting in formation of platelet adhesions and neutrophil extracellular traps (NETs). TF further causes formation of thrombin and promotes fibrinogen conversion to fibrin. Amalgamation of fibrin, platelets, NETs, red blood cells, and neutrophils results in formation of the initial thrombotic nidus.[13,14]

The flow of venous blood into and out of the venous valve pocket causes enlargement of the venous thrombus which becomes striated and subsequently extends from the valve pocket to occupy the main venous conduit. These thrombi, if left untreated, can extend proximally and eventually embolize toward the pulmonary circulation causing obstruction to pulmonary artery blood flow. Approximately 30–50% obstruction of pulmonary artery cross-sectional area is required to elevate the pulmonary artery pressure and increase the pulmonary vascular resistance.[15] Pulmonary artery obstruction results in ventilation-perfusion mismatch secondary, to dead space ventilation resulting in hypoxemia. The patient initially compensates for hypoxemia by increasing the minute ventilation which results in respiratory alkalosis, but as the compensating mechanisms fail hypercapnia will set in, resulting in respiratory failure.[16] The right ventricular afterload increases due to elevation of pulmonary vascular resistance resulting in an elevated right ventricular pressure. Prolonged elevation of right ventricular pressure can cause deviation of the interventricular septum to the left, compromising left ventricular filling during diastole, and fall in cardiac output resulting in systemic hypoperfusion. Prolonged elevation of right ventricular pressure can also result in increased ventricular oxygen demand leading to right ventricular ischemia which further compromises left ventricular preload and cardiac output. If timely intervention is not done biventricular failure may occur.[17,18]

DIAGNOSIS OF VENOUS THROMBOEMBOLISM

Deep Vein Thrombosis

Clinical Features

The Wells' model[19] for predicting DVT is the commonly used scoring system for risk stratification of DVT (**Table 1**). The classical clinical features of DVT include limb pain, swelling and erythema. On examination the patient may have dilated veins, calf swelling, pitting edema and tenderness. Differential diagnosis of DVT includes hematoma, osteoarthritis, cellulitis and superficial thrombophlebitis.[20]

TABLE 1: Wells' criteria for prediction of deep vein thrombosis[19]

Clinical presentation	Score*
Active cancer (patient either receiving treatment for cancer within the previous 6 months or currently receiving palliative treatment)	1
Paralysis, paresis, or recent cast immobilization of the lower extremities	1
Recently bedridden for ≥3 days, or major surgery within the previous 12 weeks requiring general or regional anesthesia	1
Localized tenderness along the distribution of the deep venous system	1
Entire leg swelling	1
Calf swelling at least 3 cm larger than that on the asymptomatic side (measured 10 cm below tibial tuberosity)	1
Pitting edema confined to the symptomatic leg	1
Collateral superficial veins (nonvaricose)	1
Previously documented deep vein thrombosis	1
Alternative diagnosis at least as likely as deep vein thrombosis	-2

*Wells scoring system for DVT: -2 to 0: low probability, 1 to 2 points: Moderate probability, 3 to 8 points: high probability.

Source: Modi S, Deisler R, Gozel K, Reicks P, Irwin E, Brunsvold M, et al. Wells criteria for DVT is a reliable clinical tool to assess the risk of deep venous thrombosis in trauma patients. World J Emerg Surg. 2016;11:24.

Permission: Open access article distributed under the terms of creative common CC by license. (http://creativecommons.org/licenses/by/4.0/).

Investigations

D-dimer test: D-dimer, a fibrin degradation product is generated during breakdown of cross-linked thin clot. D-dimer assay has a high sensitivity and low specificity for diagnosis of VTE. However, in patients of high risk or clinical suspicion of VTE, even if only the D-dimer is negative, imaging modalities should be used to further confirm the diagnosis.[21]

Ultrasonography: Venous compression ultrasonography is a widely used noninvasive test for diagnosing DVT. The diagnosis of DVT is confirmed by lack of compressibility in the venous segment affected by thrombosis along with absence of blood flow. The common methods used for compression ultrasonography are either two-point compression in the groin and popliteal fossa to detect proximal DVT or whole leg scanning of both the proximal and dorsal venous system. A negative whole leg scan rules out the presence of DVT.[22]

Pulmonary Embolism

Clinical Features

The probability of PE can be determined using the modified Wells'[23] (**Table 2**) or the revised Geneva scoring system[24] (**Table 3**). Patients with PE commonly present with cough, shortness of breath, chest pain which may be pleuritic or

TABLE 2: Modified Wells' model for prediction of pulmonary embolism[23]

Clinical presentation	Score*
Previous pulmonary embolism or deep vein thrombosis	1.5
Heart rate >100 per minute	1.5
Deep vein thrombosis signs	3
Hemoptysis	1
Diagnosis less likely than pulmonary embolism	3
Ongoing cancer	1
Surgery or immobilization within 4 weeks	1.5

Interpretation of score: 0-1 low probability; 2-6 intermediate probability; >6 high probability.

Source: Chagnon I, Bounameaux H, Aujesky D, Roy PM, Gourdier AL, Cornuz J, et al. Comparison of two clinical prediction rules and implicit assessment among patients with suspected pulmonary embolism. Am J Med. 2002;113(4):269-75.

TABLE 3: Revised Geneva model for prediction of pulmonary embolism[24]

Clinical presentation	Score *
Age >65 years	1
Previous DVT or pulmonary embolism	3
Surgery under GA or lower limb procedure within 1 month	2
Ongoing cancer or cured within 1 years	2
Symptoms	
Lower limb pain (unilateral)	3
Hemoptysis	2
Clinical signs	
Heart rate 75–94 per minute	3
Heart rate >95 per minute	5
Lower limb deep venous palpation resulting in pain or unilateral edema	4

Interpretation of score: 0-3 low probability; 4-10 intermediate probability; >11 high probability.

(DVT: deep vein thrombosis; GA: general anesthesia)

Source: Le Gal G, Righini M, Roy PM, Sanchez O, Aujesky D, Bounameaux H, et al. Prediction of pulmonary embolism in the emergency department: the revised Geneva score. Ann Intern Med. 2006;144(3):165-71.

present as substernal discomfort, and hemoptysis. On examination patient may be hypoxic with tachypnea and tachycardia. If the PE is massive, features of cardiogenic shock may be present.[25]

Investigations

Chest X-ray: The classical radiological sign of PE, the "Hampton's hump" or peripheral wedge-shaped opacity secondary to a large pulmonary infarct may not be always present. Another radiological feature which is specific for PE is the "Westermark sign", i.e., oligemia distal to a large occluded pulmonary vessel is seen in only 2% of the patients.[26]

Electrocardiography: Patients with PE will show right heart strain pattern characterized by T-wave inversion in leads V_1–V_4, II, III and aVF, large S-wave in lead I and Q wave in lead III along with right axis deviation.[27]

Echocardiography: Transthoracic or transesophageal echocardiography may demonstrate right ventricular dilatation or hypokinesia. In about 10% patients it may also be able to visualize thrombus within the right heart.[28]

Ventilation perfusion scan: In ventilation/perfusion (V/Q) scan technetium (Tc)-99m labeled macroaggregated albumin particles are injected intravenously (IV) and inhaled radioisotopes like xenon-153 are used to evaluate pulmonary circulation and ventilation respectively. The results of V/Q scan are classified as, normal or low probability, nondiagnostic and high probability. 70% of V/Q scans result may be nondiagnostic, therefore objective confirmation of DVT with a venous compression ultrasound will add to the diagnosis.[29]

Computed tomography pulmonary angiography: The diagnostic modality of choice for PE is computed tomography pulmonary angiography (CTPA). It allows detailed evaluation of lung parenchyma, as it acquires a high-resolution image and can even detect areas of peripheral pulmonary infarction. It has replaced pulmonary angiography for diagnosis of PE which was earlier considered to be the gold standard. An alternative to CTPA is the contrast-enhanced magnetic resonance angiography (CE-MRA) but requires expertise in interpretation of results.[30]

TREATMENT OF PULMONARY EMBOLISM

The initial treatment goal is to ensure hemodynamic and respiratory stability prior to initiation of anticoagulation therapy. Patients with suspected PE should be started on parenteral anticoagulation till a definitive diagnosis is made.

Unfractionated Heparin

Unfractionated heparin (UFH) is administered IV, with a half-life of 1–2 hours. The anticoagulant effect of UFH is monitored using activated partial thromboplastin time (aPTT) and antifactor Xa activity. UFH is administered as 80 U/kg bolus followed by an infusion of 18 U kg/h. Dose adjustment is done by measuring aPTT values every 6 hours, with a target range of 1.5–2.5 times the baseline control value.[31]

Low-molecular-weight Heparin

Low-molecular-weight heparin (LMWH) is administered subcutaneously (SC) and has a long half-life enabling once or twice daily dosing. Complications associated with heparin therapy such as bleeding and thrombocytopenia are least with LMWH as compared to UFH. The two commonly used LMWH are dalteparin, 200 U SC OD and enoxaparin, 1 mg/kg SC OD. No routine laboratory monitoring for LMWH therapy is recommended.[31] After a minimum of 5 days treatment with UFH or LMWH, long-term oral anticoagulant with oral vitamin K antagonist or a direct oral anticoagulant is initiated.

Factor Xa Inhibitor

Fondaparinux is a synthetic indirect factor Xa inhibitor with an efficacy similar to UFH and LMWH. Its dosing regimen is 5.0 mg SC for weight <50 kg, 4.5 mg SC for weight 50-100 kg and 10 mg SC for weight >100 kg.[32]

Oral Medication

The most commonly used vitamin K antagonist for long term treatment of VTE is warfarin. It is started along with heparin in a dose of 5 mg/day and overlapped with IV heparin for a minimum of 5 days or until warfarin's therapeutic effect is achieved as determined by the international normalized ratio (INR). Target INR for VTE treatment is between 2 and 3. Warfarin is administered in a dose of 2.5-10 mg/day and titrated as per INR values.[33]

Direct acting oral nonvitamin K antagonist or direct oral anticoagulants (DOACs) have emerged as alternatives to heparin-warfarin regimen. These include the direct thrombin inhibitors such as dabigatran[34] and direct factor Xa inhibitors such as rivaroxaban and apixaban.[35,36] Dabigatran is administered in a dose of 150 mg BD after 5-10 days of initial treatment with a parenteral anticoagulant usually LMWH.[34] Rivaroxaban (15 mg BD for first 21 days, then 20 mg OD)[35] and apixaban (10 mg BD first 7 days, then 5 mg BD)[36] can be used for primary treatment of VTE, without the need for starting parenteral anticoagulants.

Thrombolytic Therapy

In patients with acute PE presenting with hemodynamic instability thrombolytic therapy is preferred. It is most beneficial if the therapy is initiated within 48 hours of symptoms onset. Incidence of a major bleeding episode especially intracranial hemorrhage is increased with thrombolytic therapy. These drugs cause rapid clot lysis by converting plasminogen to plasmin. Specific fibrinolytic drugs which activate plasmin in fibrin already bond to the blood clots are now used, these include alteplase (dose: 100 mg IV over 2 hours), reteplase (dose: 10 U IV over 2 minutes, and after 30 minutes 10 U IV over 2 minutes) and tenecteplase (dose: 50 mg IV over 5 seconds).[37]

GUIDELINES FOR PERIOPERATIVE VENOUS THROMBOEMBOLISM PROPHYLAXIS

Thromboprophylaxis should be initiated after application of a risk assessment model for VTE. The most widely used VTE risk assessment tool for surgical patients is the modified Caprini risk assessment scale (**Table 4**).[38] In the past couple of years, two major guidelines on perioperative VTE prophylaxis have

TABLE 4: Modified Caprini risk assessment scale* for venous thromboembolism in surgical patients[38]

1 Point	2 Points	3 Points	4 Points
Age 41–60 years	Age 61–74 years	Age >75 years	Recent onset stroke: <1 month
Nature of surgery: minor	Arthroscopic surgery	History of venous thromboembolism	Elective hip or knee arthroplasty
BMI > 25 kg/m²	Major open surgery >45 minutes duration	Family history of venous thromboembolism	Fracture of pelvis, hip or leg
Lower limb edema	Major laparoscopic surgery >45 minutes duration	Presence of factor V Leiden thrombophilia	Recent spinal cord injury: <1 month
Lower limb varicose veins	Cancer	Mutation in prothrombin 20210A gene	
Ongoing pregnancy or postpartum period	Confinement to bed >72 hours	Presence of lupus anticoagulant	
Unexplained or recurrent miscarriages	Plaster cast with immobilization	Presence of anticardiolipin antibodies	
Use of oral contraceptives or hormone replacement therapy	Indwelling central venous catheter	Increased serum homocysteine levels	
Recent sepsis: <1 month		Additional congenital or acquired thrombophilia disorders	
Recent debilitating pulmonary disease including pneumonia: <1 month		Heparin-induced thrombocytopenia	
Altered pulmonary function tests			
Acute myocardial infarction			
Recent congestive cardiac failure: <1 month			
History of inflammatory bowel disease			
Patient requiring bed rest			

Interpretation of score for surgical risk category: 0 very low risk; 1-2 low risk; 3-4 moderate risk, >5 high risk.

(BMI: body mass index)

Source: Urbanek T, Krainski Z, Kostrubiec M, Sydor W, Wysocki P, Antoniewicz A, et al. Venous thromboembolism prophylaxis in cancer patients - guidelines focus on surgical patients. Acta Angiol. 2016;22(3):71-102.

been published, the European guidelines on preoperative VTE prophylaxis in 2018,[6] and the American Society of Hematology (ASH) guideline in 2019.[7] A summary of both these guidelines is presented below.

European Guidelines for Perioperative Venous Thrombosis Prophylaxis

The European perioperative VTE prophylaxis guidelines have been made in 12 chapters.[6] A brief overview of all these chapters is presented.

Mechanical Prophylaxis

In patients who have contraindication to pharmacological thromboprophylaxis, mechanical prophylaxis with either graduated compression stockings (GCS) or intermittent pneumatic compression (IPC) device should be used. However, IPC should be preferred over GCS. GCS alone can be used in patients not at high VTE risk.[39]

No recommendation for routine use of GCS or IPC is made in patients on pharmacological thromboprophylaxis, not at extremely high risk of VTE.[39]

In very high risk VTE patients combination therapy with mechanical and pharmacological prophylaxis should be used, with IPC preferred over GCS.

Aspirin

In patient undergoing high risk orthopedic procedures such as total knee arthroplasty and hip fracture surgery, aspirin is preferred in patients who are not at high VTE risk or have an increased bleeding risk. Furthermore, aspirin in combination with IPC can be used in high risk orthopedic surgical procedures.[40]

In patients undergoing low risk orthopedic surgical procedures without high risk for VTE, no pharmacological prophylaxis is recommended. However, if such patients have a high VTE risk then aspirin can be used.[40] Aspirin is not recommended for prophylaxis if patients undergoing general surgical procedures.[40]

Inferior Vena Cava Filters

No definite evidence regarding the use of inferior vena cava filter (IVCF) in the surgical setting is available. Temporary IVCF placement can be considered in high VTE risk patients in whom both pharmacological and mechanical prophylaxis is completely contraindicated. Also, in patients with recent history of DVT having contraindication to anticoagulation, IVCF placement should be considered.[41]

Cardiovascular and Thoracic Surgery

Cardiovascular surgery: Venous thromboembolism risk in patients scheduled for coronary artery bypass graft and aortic valve replacement is moderate. However, if the bleeding risk is high then mechanical prophylaxis with IPC should be considered. The presence of one or more of the following risk factors; age >70 years, >4 units blood/blood products transfusion, mechanical ventilation >24 hours duration, any postoperative complication such as acute kidney injury or sepsis makes the cardiac surgical patients at high risk necessitating pharmacological prophylaxis on achieving hemostasis.[42]

Long-term anticoagulation is required in patients with atrial fibrillation requiring valve surgery.[42] Peripheral vascular surgery carries a low VTE risk and medical therapy alone can control bleeding. Abdominal aortic aneurysm repair carries a VTE and bleeding risk necessitating initiation of pharmacological prophylaxis as soon as hemostasis is achieved. Due to high heparin induced thrombocytopenia (HIT) risk with UFH it should be used only for short duration and replaced by LMWH.[42]

Thoracic surgery: Thoracic surgical procedures are low risk for developing VTE and mechanical prophylaxis with IPC should suffice. However, patients undergoing surgery for cancer are at high VTE risk and require pharmacological prophylaxis in addition to IPC.[42]

Neurosurgery

Craniotomy: In all patients undergoing craniotomy the use of IPC should be started from the preoperative period. If patients have a high VTE risk then pharmacological prophylaxis with low dose unfractionated heparin (LDUFH) or LMWH should begin once the bleeding risk is minimized.[43] For patients with nontraumatic intracranial hemorrhage, consider LMWH or LDUFH in addition to IPC once the bleeding risk in minimal.[43]

Spine surgery: No other thromboprophylaxis is recommended in patients undergoing spine surgery, if they lack any additional risk factors such as ongoing cancer, complex surgical procedures, and limited ambulation. For patients with additional risk factors start with mechanical prophylaxis in the preoperative period with addition of LMWH postoperatively after at least 24 hours, once the risk of bleeding is considered to be minimal.[43]

Surgery in Obese Patients

The risk of VTE with laparoscopic bariatric surgery is less as compared to an open procedure. Obese patients at low VTE risk require either mechanical or pharmacological prophylaxis. Obese patients with high VTE risk [age >55 years, body mass index (BMI) >55 kg/m^2, previous VTE history, hypercoagulability, obstructive sleep apnea, pulmonary arterial hypertension] require a combination of anticoagulants and IPC. LMWH is the preferred anticoagulant in obese patients. In low risk VTE obese patients, the recommended dose is 3,000–4,000 IU SC every 12 hours. Whereas in high-risk VTE obese patients, the dose is 4,000–6,000 IU SC every 12 hours.[44]

Obese patients undergoing nonbariatric surgery with BMI > 40 kg/m^2 require LMWH prophylaxis in a dose of 3,000–4,000 IU SC every 12 hours.[44]

Surgery in Pregnant Patient

Pregnant patient undergoing nonobstetric surgery during pregnancy or immediate postpartum period require thromboprophylaxis. Thromboprophylaxis is recommended in all patients undergoing cesarean section apart from low-risk patients. The duration of thromboprophylaxis should be at least 6 weeks for high-risk patients and at least 7 days for rest of the patients.[45]

Surgery in Elderly Patient

The risk of perioperative VTE increases with age greater than 70 years. Any comorbidity that increases VTE risk in elderly should be identified and treated beforehand. The dosing of anticoagulant is same as in nonelderly population, but use of LDUFH in patients with renal dysfunction and weight adjusted dosing of LMWH is recommended.[46] A combination of IPC, LMWH or direct oral vitamin-K antagonist and early postoperative mobilization is warranted in elderly patients, especially after major orthopedic surgery.[46]

Ambulatory Surgery

Low-risk surgical procedures without any additional risk factors in ambulatory patients require only supportive measures such as early ambulation and adequate hydration. In low-risk surgical procedures with additional risk factor or high-risk surgical procedures without any additional risk factors consider pharmacological prophylaxis with LMWH. In high-risk procedures with additional risk factors, pharmacological prophylaxis with LMWH should be considered and if there is high bleeding risk then consider mechanical prophylaxis. Pharmacological prophylaxis should be for a minimum duration of 7-days or could be limited to the duration of hospitalization. For high-risk surgical procedures, a 4-weeks duration of therapy is recommended.[47]

Critical Care

Mechanical thromboprophylaxis with IPC should be used in all critical care patients. Patients who are critically ill should receive pharmacological prophylaxis with LMWH or low-dose unfractionated heparin (LDUH), but LMWH is preferred over LDUH. In renal insufficiency patients either LDUH or reduced doses of LMWH (enoxaparin) should be used. LDUH or LMWH can be used in patients with liver dysfunction but requires regular laboratory monitoring. In patients with high bleeding risk or with platelet count <50,000 cells/mm^3 avoid both mechanical and pharmacological prophylaxis. IVC filter is not recommended for primary prevention of VTE, there use is warranted only if both pharmacological and mechanical prophylaxis is contraindicated. In patients with HIT all forms of heparin anticoagulants should be discontinued, nonheparin anticoagulants such as argatroban (in renal insufficiency), bivalirudin (after cardiac surgery) or fondaparinux can be considered.[48]

Chronic Treatment with Antiplatelet Drugs

Patients on chronic treatment with antiplatelet drugs (APDs) should receive pharmacological prophylaxis if the risk of VTE outweighs bleeding risk. Patient on dual APDs undergoing procedure with high VTE risk the priority should be early resumption of APD over pharmacological prophylaxis. If combination use of APD and anticoagulant increase the bleeding risk over VTE then consider using IPC without stopping APD. Patients on aspirin should receive the first dose postsurgery as soon as adequate hemostasis is achieved whereas, clopidogrel should be started 24–48 hours postsurgery without the loading dose. In patients on APD therapy avoid nonsteroidal anti-inflammatory drugs.[49]

Patients with Pre-existing Coagulation Disorder and After Severe Perioperative Bleeding

In patients with inherited bleeding disorder the risk of VTE occurrence versus perioperative bleeding should be assessed prior to initiation of VTE prophylaxis. Mechanical thromboprophylaxis is recommended in patients with factor VII deficiency. In patients with hemophilia A or B use of pharmacological prophylaxis is not recommended. If the risk of VTE is high, then LMWH should be administered while maintaining factor VIII/IX levels at 0.6–1.0 IU/mL. Patients with hemophilia requiring perioperative factor correction, daily factor levels should be measured for the initial 3–5 days to guide treatment. For major surgery the factor levels should be maintained at 0.8–1 IU/mL. In the postoperative period also, the levels should be measured every 12 hours for the first 24 hours and daily thereafter. The use of factor XI concentrate should be minimal in order to avoid risk of thrombosis. If patient with factor VII deficiency require VTE prophylaxis, then pharmacological prophylaxis should be considered. Monitor fibrinogen levels after major surgery to maintain a level of 1–1.5 g/L till 10–14 days postoperatively. In patients with thrombocytopenia (platelet count <50,000 cells/mm^3) reduced dosages of LMWH should be used and monitor factor Xa levels to adjust LMWH dose. In prosthetic heart valves with high thrombotic risk, warfarin therapy should be resumed at the earliest. Monitor INR to guide warfarin therapy, if patient is having bleeding. If the risk of postoperative bleeding is greater than VTE then consider starting full dose anticoagulation 46–72 hours after surgery.[50]

American Society of Hematology Guidelines for Prevention of Venous Thromboembolism

The ASH guidelines 2019 have given a set of recommendation for VTE prevention during major general surgery, orthopedic surgery, neurosurgery, urological surgery, cardiovascular surgery, trauma and gynecological surgery.[7] Presented below is a brief overview of these recommendations.

Major Surgery in General

In patients undergoing major surgery either mechanical or pharmacological prophylaxis should be used as no difference in VTE-related mortality has been seen. Mechanical prophylaxis is favored in patients at high risk of bleeding and in those who have not received any pharmacologic prophylaxis. IPC device is to be preferred over graduated compression stocking for mechanical prophylaxis. Mechanical and pharmacological prophylaxis combination should be used if patient is at high VTE risk. Standalone pharmacological prophylaxis is not preferred and should always be in combination with mechanical prophylaxis. IVC filter use for VTE prophylaxis in patients undergoing major surgery is not recommended. Antithrombotic prophylaxis administered postoperatively can be either early (within 12 hours postoperatively) or late (after 12 hours postoperatively) and should be extended postoperatively in major surgical procedures for a duration of 19-42 days.

Orthopedic Surgery

In patients undergoing total knee replacement (TKR) or total hip replacement (THR), either aspirin or anticoagulants can be used for prophylaxis. If anticoagulants are used, then DOAC is preferred over LMWH. There is no benefit of using any class of DOAC over other. The use of LMWH is preferred over UFH or warfarin if DOAC is not used. Use of LMWH or UFH is preferred rather than no pharmacological prophylaxis at all in patients undergoing hip fracture surgery.

Major General Surgery

Prophylaxis with either LMWH or UFH is preferred over no pharmacological prophylaxis at all in all patients undergoing major surgical procedures.

Laparoscopic Cholecystectomy

No role of pharmacological prophylaxis laparoscopic cholecystectomy patients apart from patients with risk factor for VTE, who may benefit from pharmacological prophylaxis.

Neurosurgery

Mechanical prophylaxis is recommended in patients undergoing major neurosurgical procedures. It is only in patients who are expected to have prolonged immobility postsurgery or wherein surgery carries a low risk for major blood loss, pharmacological prophylaxis with LMWH should be considered.

Urological Procedures

During transurethral resection of the prostate (TURP) the use of pharmacological prophylaxis is not recommended. Only those patients with risk factors for VTE may benefit from pharmacological prophylaxis using either LMWH or UFH. Also, in patients undergoing radical prostatectomy pharmacological prophylaxis has no role apart from those requiring extensive lymph node dissection or an open radical prostatectomy. Pharmacological prophylaxis can be with either LMWH or UFH.

Cardiovascular Surgery

Either pharmacological prophylaxis or no pharmacological prophylaxis at all has demonstrated any benefit in patients undergoing cardiac or major vascular surgery. If pharmacological prophylaxis is needed like in high-risk VTE patients then either LMWH or UFH can be used.

Major Trauma

Patients having major trauma with low to moderate bleeding risk pharmacological prophylaxis can be used with either LMWH or UFH. However, if the bleeding risk is high then no pharmacological prophylaxis is recommended.

Major Gynecological Surgery

In patient undergoing major gynecological surgery pharmacological prophylaxis with either LMWH or UFH can be used.

PHARMACOLOGICAL PROPHYLAXIS DRUGS

Drugs used for pharmacological prophylaxis should be started within 2–12 hours preoperatively, except for fondaparinux which is administered 6–8 hours after surgery. VTE prophylaxis is continued postoperatively till the patient becomes ambulatory or is fit for hospital discharge, the usual duration is up to 10 days postoperatively. However, high risk surgical patients for VTE such as those with cancer may need postoperative prophylaxis till 10–14 days. This prophylaxis may be extended till 3–4 weeks postdischarge in patients who have undergone major abdominal or pelvic surgery for cancer.[51,52] LMWH is the preferred drug for extended postoperative prophylaxis.[51]

Unfractionated Heparin

It is administered in a dose of 5,000 U SC 2 hours preoperatively, thereafter every 8–12 hours.[52] In obese patients the starting dose for UFH is 5,000–6,500 U. There is no need to modify UFH dose in patients with renal dysfunction. Platelet count should be monitored at regular intervals in patients on UFH, and it should be discontinued if HIT develops.[53]

Low-molecular-weight Heparin

Various LMWH preparations are available such as enoxaparin, dalteparin, tinzaparin and nadroparin.[54,55]

Enoxaparin

It is administered in a dose of 40 mg SC 2 hours before abdominal surgery or 12 hours prior to nonabdominal surgery and 40 mg SC OD 2–72 hours after surgery, once adequate hemostasis is achieved. In cancer patients, enoxaparin 40 mg SC is given 10-12 hours before surgery and thereafter 40 mg SC 6-12 hours after surgery.[53]

Dalteparin

It is administered in a dose of 5,000 U SC 12 hours before surgery and thereafter 5,000 U daily. If the risk of VTE is low, then a dose of 2,500 U SC 1-2 hours preoperatively followed by 2,500 U daily is administered. In patient undergoing major orthopedic surgery thromboprophylaxis should be started at 12 hours or more preoperatively followed by 12 hours or more postoperatively.[53,55]

Fondaparinux

It is started 6-8 hours postoperatively in a dose of 2.5 mg SC OD.[56]

Direct Oral Anticoagulants

Direct oral anticoagulants such as rivaroxaban, dabigatran, and apixaban have been recommended for used in patients undergoing TKR or THR surgery. These drugs are started in the postoperative period and have shown to reduce the incidence of VTE. Rivaroxaban is started in a dose of 10 mg OD 6-10 hours after surgery and continued for a maximum of 2 weeks after TKR and 5 weeks after THR.[57] Dabigatran is started in a dose of 110 mg 1-4 hours postoperatively followed by 220 mg daily and is continued for 28-35 days after THR and for 10 days after TKR.[58] Apixaban is started in a dose of 2.5 mg BD 12-24 hours after surgery for a duration of 32-38 days after THR and 10-14 days after TKR.[59]

Aspirin

Several trials have reported the use of aspirin for extended postoperative prophylaxis after TKR and THR. It is commonly used in a dose of 81 mg OD or occasionally in a dose 160 mg OD.[60]

CONCLUSION

Venous thromboembolism in patients undergoing major surgical procedures is an important cause of postoperative morbidity and mortality. Although, timely diagnosis and treatment is essential but adhering to perioperative thromboprophylaxis guidelines can significantly reduce the burden of VTE. Mechanical and pharmacological prophylaxis combination is necessary in all patients undergoing major surgeries, however, if there is any contraindication to pharmacological prophylaxis then at least mechanical prophylaxis with IPC devices should be initiated.

KEY POINTS

- The disease spectrum of venous thromboembolism (VTE) comprises of superficial vein thrombosis (SVT), deep vein thrombosis (DVT) and pulmonary embolism (PE), with up to 25% patients undergoing surgery being affected by it.
- Prolonged bed rest and general anesthesia results in stasis of blood around the venous valve pockets triggering release of inflammatory mediators which result in an imbalance between procoagulant and anticoagulant factors causing formation of thrombus. These thrombi, if left untreated, can extend proximally and eventually embolize toward the pulmonary circulation.
- The initial treatment goal for PE is to ensure hemodynamic and respiratory stability prior to initiation of anticoagulation therapy.
- After a minimum of 5 days treatment with unfractionated heparin (UFH) or low molecular weight heparin (LMWH), long-term oral anticoagulant treatment with oral vitamin K antagonist or a direct oral anticoagulant (DOAC) is initiated.
- Thrombolytic therapy is reserved for patients with acute PE who have clinical factors of hemodynamic instability.
- Pharmacological prophylaxis with either LMWH or UFH is preferred over no pharmacological prophylaxis at all in patients undergoing major surgical procedures.
- In patients having contraindication to pharmacological thromboprophylaxis, mechanical prophylaxis using either graduated compression stockings (GCS) or intermittent pneumatic compression (IPC) device should be used. However, IPC should be preferred over GCS.
- In patient undergoing total knee replacement (TKR) or total hip replacement (THR), either aspirin or anticoagulants can be used for prophylaxis. If anticoagulants are used them DOAC is preferred over LMWH.
- In all patients undergoing craniotomy, the use of IPC should be started from the preoperative period. For high-risk VTE patients pharmacological prophylaxis with low dose unfractionated heparin (LDUFH) or LMWH should be started once the bleeding risk is minimized.
- Obese patients who are high risk for VTE require a combination of anticoagulants and IPC. LMWH is the preferred anticoagulant in obese patients.
- There is no benefit in favor of either using or not using pharmacological prophylaxis at all in patients undergoing cardiac or major vascular surgery. If needed either LMWH or UFH can be used.
- Drugs used for VTE prophylaxis should be started within 2–12 hours preoperatively and is continued postoperatively till the patient becomes ambulatory or is fit for hospital discharge, the usual duration is up to 10 days postoperatively.

REFERENCES

1. Cardell JA, Amankwah KD. Venous Thromboembolism: Prevention, diagnosis and treatment. In: Cameron JL, Cameron AM (Eds). Current Surgical Therapy, 13th edition. Philadelphia: Elsevier Inc.; 2020. pp. 1072-82.
2. Liew NC, Alemany GV, Angchaisuksiri P, Bang SM, Choi G, DE Silva DA, et al. Asian venous thromboembolism guidelines: updated recommendations for the prevention of venous thromboembolism. Int Angiol. 2017;36(1):1-20.
3. Gordon RJ, Lombard FW. Perioperative venous thromboembolism: A review. Anesth Analg. 2017;125(2):403-12.

4. Sweetland S, Green J, Liu B, Berrington de González A, Canonico M, Reeves G, et al. Duration and magnitude of the postoperative risk of venous thromboembolism in middle aged women: prospective cohort study. BMJ. 2009;339:b4583.
5. Righini M, Le Gal G, Aujesky D, Roy PM, Sanchez O, Verschuren F, et al. Diagnosis of pulmonary embolism by multidetector CT alone or combined with venous ultrasonography of the leg: a randomised non-inferiority trial. Lancet. 2008;371(9621):1343-52.
6. Afshari A, Ageno W, Ahmed A, Duranteau J, Faraoni D, Kozek-Langenecker S, et al. European Guidelines on perioperative venous thromboembolism prophylaxis: executive summary. Eur J Anaesthesiol. 2018;35(2):77-83.
7. Anderson DR, Morgano GP, Bennett C, Dentali F, Francis CW, Garcia DA, et al. American Society of Hematology 2019 guidelines for management of venous thromboembolism: prevention of venous thromboembolism in surgical hospitalized patients. Blood Adv. 2019;3(23):3898-944.
8. López JA, Chen J. Pathophysiology of venous thrombosis. Thromb Res. 2009;123 (Suppl 4):S30-4.
9. Agutter PS, Malone PC, Silver IA. Experimental Validation of Methods for Prophylaxis against Deep Venous Thrombosis: a review and proposal. Thrombosis. 2012;2012:156397.
10. Malone PC, Agutter PS. Deep venous thrombosis: the valve cusp hypoxia thesis and its incompatibility with modern orthodoxy. Med Hypotheses. 2016;86:60-6.
11. Watson SP. Platelet activation by extracellular matrix proteins in haemostasis and thrombosis. Curr Pharm Des 2009;15(12):1358-72.
12. Williams MR, Azcutia V, Newton G, Alcaide P, Luscinskas FW. Emerging mechanisms of neutrophil recruitment across endothelium. Trends Immunol. 2011;32(10):461-9.
13. Martinod K, Wagner DD. Thrombosis: tangled up in NETs. Blood. 2014;123(18):2768-76.
14. Van der Meijden PE, Ozaki Y, Ruf W, de Laat B, Mutch N, Diamond S, et al. Theme 1: pathogenesis of venous thromboembolism (and post-thrombotic syndrome). Thromb Res. 2015;136 (Suppl 1):S3-7.
15. Smulders YM. Pathophysiology and treatment of haemodynamic instability in acute pulmonary embolism: the pivotal role of pulmonary vasoconstriction. Cardiovasc Res. 2000;48(1):23-33.
16. Kostadima E, Zakynthinos E. Pulmonary embolism: pathophysiology, diagnosis, treatment. Hellenic J Cardiol. 2007;48(2):94-107.
17. Marcus JT, Gan CT, Zwanenburg JJ, Boonstra A, Allaart CP, Götte MJ, et al. Interventricular mechanical asynchrony in pulmonary arterial hypertension: left-to-right delay in peak shortening is related to right ventricular overload and left ventricular underfilling. J Am Coll Cardiol. 2008;51(7):750-7.
18. Mauritz GJ, Marcus JT, Westerhof N, Postmus PE, Vonk-Noordegraaf A. Prolonged right ventricular post-systolic isovolumic period in pulmonary arterial hypertension is not a reflection of diastolic dysfunction. Heart. 2011;97(6):473-8.
19. Modi S, Deisler R, Gozel K, Reicks P, Irwin E, Brunsvold M, et al. Wells criteria for DVT is a reliable clinical tool to assess the risk of deep venous thrombosis in trauma patients. World J Emerg Surg. 2016;11:24.
20. Kesieme E, Kesieme C, Jebbin N, Irekpita E, Dongo A. Deep vein thrombosis: a clinical review. J Blood Med. 2011;2:59-69.
21. Gibson NS, Sohne M, Gerdes VE, Nijkeuter M, Buller HR. The importance of clinical probability assessment in interpreting a normal d-dimer in patients with suspected pulmonary embolism. Chest. 2008;134(4):789-93.

22. Gornik HL, Gerhard-Herman MD, Misra S, Mohler ER 3rd, Zierler RE. Peripheral vascular ultrasound and physiological testing part II: testing for venous disease and evaluation of hemodialysis access technical panel; appropriate use criteria task force. ACCF/ACR/AIUM/ASE/IAC/SCAI/SCVS/SIR/SVM/SVS/SVU 2013 appropriate use criteria for peripheral vascular ultrasound and physiological testing part II: testing for venous disease and evaluation of hemodialysis access: a report of the American College of Cardiology foundation appropriate use criteria task force. J Am Coll Cardiol. 2013;62(7):649-65.
23. Chagnon I, Bounameaux H, Aujesky D, Roy PM, Gourdier AL, Cornuz J, et al. Comparison of two clinical prediction rules and implicit assessment among patients with suspected pulmonary embolism. Am J Med. 2002;113(4):269-75.
24. Le Gal G, Righini M, Roy PM, Sanchez O, Aujesky D, Bounameaux H, et al. Prediction of pulmonary embolism in the emergency department: the revised Geneva score. Ann Intern Med. 2006;144(3):165-71.
25. Lavorini F, Di Bello V, De Rimini ML, Lucignani G, Marconi L, Palareti G, et al. Diagnosis and treatment of pulmonary embolism: a multidisciplinary approach. Multidiscip Respir Med. 2013;8(1):75.
26. Lu P, Chin BB. Simultaneous chest radiographic findings of Hampton's hump, Westermark's sign, and vascular redistribution in pulmonary embolism. Clin Nucl Med. 1998;23(10):701-2.
27. Ullman E, Brady WJ, Perron AD, Chan T, Mattu A. Electrocardiographic manifestations of pulmonary embolism. Am J Emerg Med. 2001;19(6):514-9.
28. Dabbouseh NM, Patel JJ, Bergl PA. Role of echocardiography in managing acute pulmonary embolism. Heart. 2019;105(23):1785-92.
29. Qaseem A, Snow V, Barry P, Hornbake ER, Rodnick JE, Tobolic T, et al. Joint American Academy of Family Physicians/American College of Physicians' panel on deep venous thrombosis/pulmonary embolism. Current diagnosis of venous thromboembolism in primary care: a clinical practice guideline from the American Academy of Family Physicians and the American College of Physicians. Ann Fam Med. 2007;5(1):57-62.
30. Albrecht MH, Bickford MW, Nance JW Jr, Zhang L, De Cecco CN, Wichmann JL, et al. State-of-the-art pulmonary CT angiography for acute pulmonary embolism. Am J Roentgenol. 2017;208(3):495-504.
31. Hirsh J, Bauer KA, Donati MB, Gould M, Samama MM, Weitz JI. Parenteral anticoagulants: American College of Chest Physicians' evidence-based clinical practice guidelines (8th edition). Chest. 2008;133(6 Suppl):141-159S.
32. Büller HR, Davidson BL, Decousus H, Gallus A, Gent M, Piovella F, et al. Matisse Investigators. Subcutaneous fondaparinux versus intravenous unfractionated heparin in the initial treatment of pulmonary embolism. N Engl J Med. 2003;349(18):1695-702.
33. Agnelli G, Becattini C. Anticoagulant treatment for acute pulmonary embolism: a pathophysiology-based clinical approach. Eur Respir J. 2015;45(4):1142-9.
34. Büller HR, Décousus H, Grosso MA, Mercuri M, Middeldorp S, Prins MH, et al. Edoxaban versus warfarin for the treatment of symptomatic venous thromboembolism. N Engl J Med. 2013;369(15):1406-15.
35. Büller HR, Prins MH, Lensin AW, Decousus H, Jacobson BF, Minar E, et al. Oral rivaroxaban for the treatment of symptomatic pulmonary embolism. N Engl J Med. 2012;366(14):1287-97.
36. Agnelli G, Buller HR, Cohen A, Curto M, Gallus AS, Johnson M, et al. Oral apixaban for the treatment of acute venous thromboembolism. N Engl J Med. 2013;369(9):799-808.

37. Martin C, Sobolewski K, Bridgeman P, Boutsikaris D. Systemic thrombolysis for pulmonary embolism: a review. P T. 2016;41(12):770-5.
38. Urbanek T, Krainski Z, Kostrubiec M, Sydor W, Wysocki P, Antoniewicz A, et al. Venous thromboembolism prophylaxis in cancer patients—guidelines focus on surgical patients. Acta Angiol. 2016;22(3):71-102.
39. Afshari A, Fenger-Eriksen C, Monreal M, Verhamme P; ESA VTE Guidelines Task Force. European guidelines on perioperative venous thromboembolism prophylaxis: mechanical prophylaxis. Eur J Anaesthesiol. 2018;35(2):112-5.
40. Jenny JY, Pabinger I, Samama CM; ESA VTE Guidelines Task Force. European guidelines on perioperative venous thromboembolism prophylaxis: aspirin. Eur J Anaesthesiol. 2018;35(2):123-9.
41. Comes RF, Mismetti P, Afshari A; ESA VTE Guidelines Task Force. European guidelines on perioperative venous thromboembolism prophylaxis: inferior vena cava filters. Eur J Anaesthesiol. 2018;35(2):108-11.
42. Ahmed AB, Koster A, Lance M, Faraoni D; ESA VTE Guidelines Task Force. European guidelines on perioperative venous thromboembolism prophylaxis: cardiovascular and thoracic surgery. Eur J Anaesthesiol. 2018;35(2):84-9.
43. Faraoni D, Comes RF, Geerts W, Wiles MD; ESA VTE Guidelines Task Force. European guidelines on perioperative venous thromboembolism prophylaxis: neurosurgery. Eur J Anaesthesiol. 2018;35(2):90-5.
44. Venclauskas L, Maleckas A, Arcelus JI; ESA VTE Guidelines Task Force. European guidelines on perioperative venous thromboembolism prophylaxis: surgery in the obese patient. Eur J Anaesthesiol. 2018;35(2):147-53.
45. Ducloy-Bouthors AS, Baldini A, Abdul-Kadir R, Nizard J; ESA VTE Guidelines Task Force. European guidelines on perioperative venous thromboembolism prophylaxis: surgery during pregnancy and the immediate postpartum period. Eur J Anaesthesiol. 2018;35(2):130-3.
46. Kozek-Langenecker S, Fenger-Eriksen C, Thienpont E, Barauskas G; ESA VTE Guidelines Task Force. European guidelines on perioperative venous thromboembolism prophylaxis: surgery in the elderly. Eur J Anaesthesiol. 2018;35(2):116-22.
47. Venclauskas L, Llau JV, Jenny JY, Kjaersgaard-Andersen P, Jans Ø; ESA VTE Guidelines Task Force. European guidelines on perioperative venous thromboembolism prophylaxis: day surgery and fast-track surgery. Eur J Anaesthesiol. 2018;35(2):134-8.
48. Duranteau J, Taccone FS, Verhamme P, Ageno W; ESA VTE Guidelines Task Force. European guidelines on perioperative venous thromboembolism prophylaxis: intensive care. Eur J Anaesthesiol. 2018;35(2):142-6.
49. Llau JV, Kamphuisen P, Albaladejo P; ESA VTE Guidelines Task Force. European guidelines on perioperative venous thromboembolism prophylaxis: Chronic treatments with antiplatelet agents. Eur J Anaesthesiol. 2018;35(2):139-41.
50. Ahmed A, Kozek-Langenecker S, Mullier F, Pavord S, Hermans C; ESA VTE Guidelines Task Force. European guidelines on perioperative venous thromboembolism prophylaxis: Patients with preexisting coagulation disorders and after severe perioperative bleeding. Eur J Anaesthesiol. 2018;35(2):96-107.
51. Rausa E, Kelly ME, Asti E, Aiolfi A, Bonitta G, Winter DC, et al. Extended versus conventional thromboprophylaxis after major abdominal and pelvic surgery: systematic review and meta-analysis of randomized clinical trials. Surgery. 2018;164(6):1234-40.
52. Felder S, Rasmussen MS, King R, Sklow B, Kwaan M, Madoff R, et al. Prolonged thromboprophylaxis with low molecular weight heparin for abdominal or pelvic surgery. Cochrane Database Syst Rev. 2019;8(8):CD004318.

53. Lyman GH, Bholke K, Falanga A, Seattle WA, Alexandria VA; American Society of Clinical Oncology, et al. Venous thromboembolism prophylaxis and treatment in patients with cancer: American Society of Clinical Oncology clinical practice guideline update. J Clin Oncol 2015;11(3):e442-4.
54. Joy M, Tharp E, Hartman H, Schepoff S, Cortes J, Sieg A, et al. Safety and efficacy of high-dose unfractionated heparin for prevention of venous thromboembolism in overweight and obese patients. Pharmacotherapy. 2016;36(7):740-8.
55. Gould MK, Garcia DA, Wren SM, Karanicolas PJ, Arcelus JI, Heit JA, et al. Prevention of VTE in nonorthopedic surgical patients: antithrombotic therapy and prevention of thrombosis, 9th ed: American College of Chest Physicians' evidence-based clinical practice guidelines Chest. 2012;141(2 Suppl):e227S-77S.
56. Kumar A, Talwar A, Farley JF, Muzumdar J, Schommer JC, Balkrishnan R, et al. Fondaparinux sodium compared with low-molecular-weight heparins for perioperative surgical thromboprophylaxis: a systematic review and meta-analysis. J Am Heart Assoc. 2019;8(10):e012184.
57. Kakkar AK, Brenner B, Dahl OE, Eriksson BI, Mouret P, Muntz J, et al. Extended duration rivaroxaban versus short-term enoxaparin for the prevention of venous thromboembolism after total hip arthroplasty: a double-blind, randomised controlled trial. Lancet. 2008;372(9632):31-9.
58. Eriksson BI, Dahl OE, Rosencher N, Kurth AA, van Dijk CN, Frostick SP, et al. Dabigatran etexilate versus enoxaparin for prevention of venous thromboembolism after total hip replacement: a randomised, double-blind, non-inferiority trial. Lancet. 2007;370(9591):949-56.
59. Lassen MR, Gallus A, Raskob GE, Pineo G, Chen D, Ramirez LM. Apixaban versus enoxaparin for thromboprophylaxis after hip replacement. N Engl J Med. 2010;363(26):2487-98.
60. Anderson DR, Dunbar M, Murnaghan J, Kahn SR, Gross P, Forsythe M, et al. Aspirin or rivaroxaban for VTE prophylaxis after hip or knee arthroplasty. N Engl J Med. 2018;378(8):699-707.

CHAPTER 18

Carbon Footprint Analysis in Perioperative Care

Shashi Kiran, Neha Aeron

INTRODUCTION

A carbon footprint is defined as total greenhouse gas (GHG) emissions by an individual, event, organization, or product.[1] Carbon dioxide (CO_2) is the dominant man-made GHG, which is emitted when fossil fuels are burnt in homes, factories or power stations. However, there are many other important GHGs, e.g., methane (CH_4), mainly emitted by agriculture and landfill sites, which is 25 times more potent than CO_2.[2] Similarly, nitrous oxide (N_2O), though emitted in smaller quantities, is about 300 times more potent than CO_2 and is released mainly from industries and farming. Gases released from refrigerators are thousand times more potent than CO_2.[3]

Like other walks of life, healthcare activities are also responsible for significant emission of GHGs. Perioperative medicine worldwide is associated with pollution of air, soil, and water with sulfur, nitrogen, anesthetic gases, toxic materials, particulate matter, and persistent organic materials. In United States, it has been estimated that healthcare contributes to 8% of the nation's greenhouse emissions.[4] In United Kingdom, the National Health Service (NHS) is responsible for 25% of total public sector emissions.[5] In India and China, healthcare accounts for approximately 5% of the national CO_2 footprint.[6] These ongoing climate changes are putting an additional burden on an already stressed healthcare systems across most parts of the world. Globally there is a significant cost impact of health care at local and national level. However, its adverse environmental impact remains largely overlooked especially in a country such as India. Moreover, advances in health care are expected to increase proportionately with increase in life expectancy and population growth which may result in increased CO_2 footprint.

TECHNIQUE OF ESTIMATION OF CARBON FOOTPRINT

The rise in temperature, as caused by GHG is calculated mathematically in terms of Global warming potential and is expressed in terms of carbon dioxide equivalents (CO_2e).[7] Carbon footprint is a quantitative expression of GHG emission. The most common method of its estimation is life cycle assessment (LCA).[8,9] It includes estimation and addition of the entire amount of GHG emitted in the complete life cycle of a particular product right from its manufacturing to its consumption and disposal (Cradle to grave analysis). Common resources available for GHG accounting are GHG protocol of World Resource Institute, International Organization for Standardization (ISO) and Public available specifications 2050 of British standard institution.

Carbon footprint analysis may be done in either a bottom-up (process analysis) method or a top-down (input-output) method. While bottom-up method is more accurate for small entity calculations; top-down process is better for large scale calculations.[8] However, in practice a combination of both the processes is used and is also known as the economic input-output life cycle assessment analysis hybrid (EIO-LCA).[3] It is emerging as a gold standard technique as it is not only robust and accurate but also flexible and reliable. This process is done in three steps:[10-13]

1. *Selection of greenhouse gas*: The selection of GHG emission that needs to be estimated depends on the type of activity for which calculation of carbon footprint is required. For example; while, in a thermal plant the most common GHG emitted is CO_2; cattle farms emit CH_4 and N_2O apart from CO_2. Same gases are also emitted during perioperative period.
2. *Setting the boundary*: It is done to establish the exact fraction of an organization that causes GHG emission.
3. *Collection of data*: This is done using the GHG protocol of World Resource Institute, ISO and Public available specifications 2050 of British standard institution. GHG emissions are then calculated using a complex algebraic conversion factors provided by the above said resources in terms of CO_2e.

ROLE OF PERIOPERATIVE CARE IN CO_2 FOOTPRINT

Carbon footprint starts occurring the moment a particular patient leaves home to reach the hospital till the period he reaches back to his home after discharge from the hospital. Major sources of CO_2 footprint emissions in perioperative care are production and use of disposables including single-use surgical devices, anesthetic gases and energy used for heating, ventilation and air conditioning (HVAC) **(Box 1)**.[14] Further, common practice of many hospitals to classify all operating room (OR) waste as "clinical waste" results in requirement for its disposal of by incineration.

Over 1 year period, a carbon foot printing study of operating theaters was done in three quaternary-care hospitals in Canada [Vancouver General Hospital, (VGH)], USA [University of Minnesota Medical Center, (UMMC)] and UK [John Radcliffe Hospital, (JRH)]. GHG emissions were estimated using primary activity data and applicable emission factors; and reported according to the GHG protocol. It was observed that operating rooms (ORs) under consideration had a carbon footprint of 5,187, 936 kg of CO_2e at JRH, 4,181,864 kg of CO_2e at UMMC, and 3,218,907 kg of CO_2e at VGH annually. However, on a per unit area basis, JRH had the lowest carbon intensity at 1,702 kg CO_2e m^{-2} as compared to 1,951 kg CO_2e m^{-2} at VGH and 2,284 kg CO_2e m^{-2} at UMMC. Based on case volumes at all three sites, VGH had the lowest carbon intensity per operation at 146 kg CO_2e per case compared with 173 kg CO_2e per case at JRH and 232 kg CO_2e per case at UMMC. Major sources of GHG emissions

> **BOX 1:** Various causes of carbon footprint in perioperative period.
>
> - Anesthesia-related
>   - Volatile agents
>   - Intravenous anesthetic agents
>   - Anesthesia-related medical waste
> - HVAC system
>   - Heating, cooling, ventilation, lights
>   - Plug loads
> - Surgical waste
>   - Civic solid waste, hazardous waste, liquid effluents, sharps, black box waste (acutely toxic and infectious), reusable linen
>   - Transport of all wastes to their designated areas
> - Miscellaneous
>   - Plastics, glass and plastic vials/bottles, aluminum wrapping for sutures, gloves, basins, disposable gowns, drapes, cotton towels/swabs, laparotomy pads
> - Anesthesia/surgical material supply chain
>
> (HVAC: heating, ventilation and air conditioning)

in this study were anesthetic gases and energy consumption with ORs being three to six times more energy-intense than the hospital as a whole, primarily due to HVAC requirements which amounted to 90–99% of overall energy use. This shows that OR is associated with more aggressive energy use as compared to inpatient department. As a whole HVAC system was reportedly responsible for 52% of energy needs of inpatient areas. Overall, the carbon footprint of surgery in the three countries studied was estimated to be 9.7 million tons of CO_2e per year.[10]

Pichler et al. carried out the first comparable estimates of CO_2 emissions of health care across all Organization of Economic Cooperation and Development (OECD) countries (except Chile), China and India for the years 2000–2014. The OECD countries were selected due to the availability of their harmonized and disaggregated healthcare expenditure data, while China and India were included due to their size and global significance, using aggregated health care expenditure data provided by the World Health Organization (WHO)/World Bank. The countries in their sample covered around 54% of the world's population and 78% of world gross domestic product (GDP) in 2014. The novelty of their study was the methodologically consistent cross-country comparison of the health carbon footprint of these countries in time-series spanning 15 years with health care, on average, accounting for 5% of the national CO_2 footprint making it comparable in importance to the food sector. The largest amount of carbon footprint was seen to be generated by China (601 metric tons CO_2) followed by US, Japan, India and Germany (480, 115, 74 and 55 metric tons CO_2 respectively). Latvia had the lowest carbon footprint (0.5 metric tons CO_2). They reported that the carbon intensity of the domestic energy system, the energy intensity of the domestic economy and healthcare expenditure together explained half of the variance in per capita health carbon footprints. Their results indicated that important leverage points existed inside and outside the health sector.[6]

The environmental impact of hysterectomy in the United States by LCA was studied by Thiel et al. Hysterectomy was chosen as it was considered 2nd most commonly performed surgery in US and all four commonly used surgical approaches, i.e., (1) vaginal, (2) abdominal, (3) laparoscopic, and (4) robotic, were taken into consideration. LCA was used to quantify the GHG emissions for these approaches in the ORs of Magee-Women's Hospital of the University of Pittsburgh Medical Center with one hysterectomy procedure being considered as the functional unit for this study. The boundaries encompassed the raw material extraction, production, use and end-of-life of the processes and products required to perform each type of hysterectomy from the moment the patient entered the OR to the moment she left the OR. Waste, both raw and disposable as also the amount of insufflating gas and anesthetic gases, were measured. Robotic hysterectomy was found to have the largest environmental CO_2e footprint over other types of hysterectomies in terms of generating medical waste and anesthetic gases.[15]

Inhalational anesthetic agents are halogenated fluorocarbons. They undergo minimal in-vivo metabolism and are powerful GHGs, as indicated by their global warming potential. This is a relative measure of how much heat is trapped by a given gas in the atmosphere compared with a similar mass of CO_2. Most inhalational anesthetic agents remain in the atmosphere for 1–15 years and are significant heat trapping gases.[16] N_2O, mostly used as a carrier gas, has a much longer atmospheric lifetime of 114 years with a heat trapping potential 310 times that of CO_2. Sevoflurane has 130 times heat trapping potential of CO_2 on a 100-year time scale whereas, desflurane is 2,500 times more potent.[3] Therefore, sevoflurane is preferable as compared to desflurane. Most of developed countries now avoid using N_2O, although it is still widely used in India.

In a study on carbon footprint in a 150 minute duration laparoscopic surgery, use of desflurane alone resulted in 762 kg CO_2e GHG whereas, desflurane with N_2O resulted in 757 kg CO_2e GHG per case. In contrast, sevoflurane alone resulted in 410 kg CO_2e GHG, whereas sevoflurane with N_2O resulted in 416 kg CO_2e GHG per case. Propofol use, on the other hand, was found to have limited GHG emissions; 402 kg CO_2e GHG per case. Therefore, it was suggested that propofol can be used as primary anesthetic without inhalational agents.[17]

Alexander et al.[18] undertook a quality assurance project from 2012–2016, to assess the volume of volatile anesthetics used in seven hospital pharmacies. In 2012, the amount of desflurane used was 1,318 L whereas for sevoflurane, it was 385 L. This resulted in a calculated CO_2 equivalent over 20 year period (CDE20) for desflurane and sevoflurane of 13,190,098 kg and 257,655 kg, respectively (total of 13.4 million kg of CO_2e). In subsequent years, there was a steady decline in use of desflurane and increased usage of sevoflurane. In 2016, the amount of desflurane used was 401 L and sevoflurane used was 772 L. Thus, the calculated CDE20 of 4,009,886 kg for desflurane and 515,979 kg for sevoflurane combined for a total carbon footprint of 4.5 million kg of CO_2e. The total volume of volatile anesthetics used decreased from 1,703 L to 1,173 L during this interval. The difference in total CDE20 between 2012 and 2016 was 8.9 million kg, representing a 66% reduction in GHG emissions which was equivalent to annual emissions produced by 1,700 personal vehicles driving an average of 22,000 km per year.[18]

A comparative LCA of disposable and reusable laryngeal mask airways (LMAs) observed that reusable LMA contributes 7.4 kg CO_2e of GHGs over its life cycle and the equivalent 40 disposable LMAs (reusable LMA being recommended for 40 times reuse) contribute 11.3 kg CO_2e, or approximately the equivalent to burning a gallon (4 L) of gasoline.[19]

ADVERSE EFFECTS OF CARBON FOOTPRINT

Perioperative carbon footprint can have serious adverse impact of global environment and human health **(Box 2)**. Pollution can result in climate changes resulting into overall global increase in atmospheric temperature, melting of glaciers, ozone layer depletion, decreased rainfall, increased incidence of acid rains, smog, fires, and rise in carcinogenic toxins. Melting of ice releases CH_4. Increase in water levels and global rise of temperature raises the risk of plant and animal species extinction. Fish stocks depletion occurs with adverse effect on marine ecosystem. Frequent floods, storms and tornedos lead to economic crises. Ozone layer depletion can lead to increased incidence of skin burns and cancers. The pattern of infectious diseases may get altered.[19-22]

REDUCTION OF PERIOPERATIVE CO_2 FOOTPRINT: STRATEGIES

Although climate impacts of surgical procedures are generally considered acceptable as necessary for providing quality care but it is possible to reduce CO_2 footprint of perioperative medicine. Still, it is desirable that this sector should contribute to the reduction in GHG emission as much as possible. This will not only reduce its impact on world environment but also reduce costs without compromising patient care.

McGain et al. presented an audit report of estimated practical and financial feasibility of an OR recycling program in six ORs in Melbourne, Australia. It was observed that a total of 1,265 kg waste was produced over 1 week during 237 operations: 570 kg (45%) of general waste and 410 kg (32%) infectious waste whereas recyclables reportedly amounted to 285 kg (23%) without any infectious contamination. The rate of achieved recycling/potential recycling rate was 285 kg/517 kg (55%). It was observed that the average waste disposal costs were similar for general waste and recycling and concluded that, OR recycling rates of 20–25% of the total waste in ORs can be achieved without compromising on infection control or financial constraints.[23]

A study on orthopedic ORs, provided a multicenter quality improvement report for reducing the carbon footprint. It was observed that these ORs are one of the major producers of waste because of large numbers of instrumentation

---

BOX 2: Adverse effects of carbon footprint.

Climate change
- Global increase in temperature
- Melting of glaciers and rise in water level
- Ozone layer depletion
- Decreased rainfall and increased acid rain
- Carcinogenic potential

and implants required. Selecting three major procedures, i.e., total hip replacement (THR), total knee replacement (TKR) and facet joint injections (FJI); the waste from these procedures was collected and weighed. It was observed that over a 2-week period, average waste from a THR was 12.1 kg (± 0.25 SD) and from TKR was 11.6 kg (± 0.18 SD) whereas, FJI created a waste of 1.8 kg (± 0.17 SD) on an average. After waste separation, 5.8 kg (± 0.17 SD) of THR waste, 5.3 kg (± 0.18 SD) of TKR waste, and 0.8 kg (± 0.2 SD) of waste from the FJI was of domestic waste nature. However, important point highlighted by this study was that, 47% of this waste was recyclable dry paper and card, a further 47% was potentially recyclable plastic and only 6% was definitely not recyclable (wet paper or card, nonrecyclable plastic).[24]

A pattern of utilization of disposable supply in 58 neurosurgical cases showed an average unused supply cost to the extent of $653 (range $89–$3640), or 13.1% of total surgical supply cost. It was further observed that the types of surgery (cranial/spinal, vascular, tumor, instrumentation of spine, etc.) as well as the surgeon were important predictors of the extent of unused disposable surgical supply in a particular case. However, duration of surgery and years of surgical training did not affect the percentage of unused supply cost. Based on their findings the authors calculated an approximately expenditure of $968 of OR waste per case, $242,968 per month and $2.9 million per year toward in neurosurgical department.[25]

Thus, the overall available evidence from various studies indicates that the impact of perioperative care on carbon footprint is huge. This is not only associated with environmental pollution, but it also imposes a great burden on healthcare expenses as well.

A survey was carried out through American Society of Anesthesiologists regarding the attitude of anesthesiologists toward environmental pollution and also, their knowledge about sustainability programs toward environmental protection in any of their institutions. A questionnaire was sent to 5,200 members of the American Society of Anesthesiologists of which 2,189 responded (42% response rate). Recycling was reported in 27.7% of ORs with 80.1% of respondents indicating an interest in recycling. 67% of the respondents reported that there was inadequate information about methods of intraoperative recycling. A sizeable number of respondents supported the incorporation of sustainability practices such as reprocessing equipment, using prefilled syringes and donating unused equipment and supplies with an affirmative response by 48.4% for reprocessing equipment, 56.6% for using prefilled syringes, and 65.1% for donating discarded equipment and supplies. However, only 12.6% of responders indicated that there was a mandate from hospital leadership to promote such sustainability programs in their institutions. It was concluded from the survey data that there was a lack of both adequate information on recycling as well as organization of sustainability programs in general.[26]

As a result of different studies in literature to reduce GHG emission in perioperative care following recommendations can be considered without any adverse impact on patient care.

Minimum materials in OR should be used with an emphasis on using reusable linens and towels. Recycling and regulated medical waste should be maximized. Single use devices should be reprocessed wherever possible. Occupancy sensors can be installed for off-hours. Hospital building should maximize the use of renewable energy sources available on existing grid system.[27] To improve environmental health, harmful medications should be substituted with safer alternatives. Pharmaceuticals should be safely managed and disposed off. Safer and more sustainable products should be purchased. Reduction in water consumption can also contribute to a large extent. Another possibility is to avoid unnecessary or harmful interventions or misallocation of patients. Unnecessary ICU admissions should be avoided.[28] Telemedicine should be used wherever appropriate.[29] Provision for ambulatory health care can reduce unnecessary transport.[20] WHO recommends ensuring the following elements to establish climate friendly hospitals:[30]

- Increase hospital energy efficiency.
- Green building design of hospital suited to local climate.
- Onsite renewable alternative energy generation.
- Use of alternative fuels for hospital vehicles, encourage walking, cycling, and use of public transport among staff.
- Provision of sustainably grown local food for staff/patients.
- Reduce, reuse, and recycle inventory.
- Water conservation, avoidance of bottled water.

ROLE OF ANESTHESIOLOGIST

Anesthesiologist, being a key figure among OR personnel, can contribute significantly toward reduction of GHG emissions and environmental pollution. They can reduce gaseous waste by using low fresh gas flows and avoiding high impact inhaled anesthetics, e.g., desflurane and N_2O. Further, it is worthwhile investing in waste anesthetic gas (WAG) trapping or WAG destruction technology for the anesthesia machines. They can also increase the use of intravenous and regional techniques thereby, reducing the requirement for inhaled anesthetics. Intravenous pharmaceutical waste can also be reduced by using prefilled syringes and appropriate size vials according to required dosages. It will also result in reducing the problem of disposing off unused medications. Similarly, anesthesia equipment waste can also be reduced by opening minimum required equipment and preferring procurement of reusable/reprocess of equipment over disposables. Stock inventory should be adjusted to minimum required levels thereby resulting in reduction of expired items. Solid waste segregation should be implemented carefully according to the type of waste (pharmaceuticals, solids, biohazards, etc.). It is particularly important to avoid putting all the waste into single bin which makes the recycling programs (especially useful for clean plastics, paper, cardboards, etc.) extremely difficult. Similarly, instead of using disposable towels, gowns, blankets, etc., they should seriously consider reusable linen.

Electronics constitute a significant component of OR and anesthesiologists can play an important role in avoiding use of electronics which have no proven benefit in a particular case, as also by using a qualified electronics recycling vendor for disposal of old equipment. While negotiating for upgradation of equipment in OR, suppliers and distributors should also be impressed upon to take back old equipment for refurbishment, reuse or even possible donation.

Anesthesiologists are expected to play a leadership role in establishing a sustainability committee at their workplaces thereby making prevention of pollution by perioperative health care an important mission. They should also be proactive in educating other staff members regarding cost benefit ratio of various environmental projects. All these measures will not only result in remarkable reduction in GHG emissions and environmental pollution in healthcare sector but will also result in substantial financial savings for hospitals.[28]

Anesthesiologists should re-examine and assess the impact of their clinical practice toward development of a safer environment. They can contribute in reduction of perioperative carbon footprint by reducing inhaled anesthetic waste, intravenous unused medications and old discarded anesthesia equipment. Appropriate segregation of solid waste should be carried out. Reusable linen can be used to minimize the amount of disposable linen. Most importantly anesthesiologist should develop or join a sustainability committee which can cater to issues related to reduction of carbon footprint. The comprehensive suggestions by the American Society of Anesthesiologists and WHO for adopting green ORs should be followed.[31]

All these practices may effectively reduce perioperative carbon footprint without compromising the level of health care provided. The government should also be amenable to suggestions from healthcare providers regarding safe and effective patient centered health services. There is a large scope for future research in this area with respect to mitigation of climatic changes and improvement of public health care.

CONCLUSION

Perioperative health care is associated with generation of considerable amount of hospital waste leading to generation of GHG. The resultant carbon footprint has potentially devastating impact on environment and human health. Providing a quality perioperative care to the patient without generating a significant carbon footprint is one of the increasingly challenging concerns. Carbon footprint of perioperative care cannot be reduced by miracle or magic, though a combination of various available approaches may be useful.

KEY POINTS

- Greenhouse gas (GHG) emission leading to global warming is one of the challenging public health issues.
- Carbon footprint is generated because of carbon dioxide, methane, nitrous oxide and chlorofluorocarbons.
- Perioperative healthcare service generates a considerable amount of GHGs.
- All inhalational anesthetic agents generate GHGs.
- Anesthesiologists can reduce inhaled anesthetic atmospheric waste by switching from inhalational to total intravenous anesthetics and using regional techniques wherever possible.

Contd...

Contd...

- Use of prefilled syringes, appropriately sized vials and disposal of vials having residual medications as per guidelines, can result in reduction of pharmaceutical waste.
- Carbon footprint during perioperative care can be significantly reduced by meticulous planning of hospital buildings, substituting harmful chemicals with safer alternatives, reducing and safely disposing wastes, switching to renewable energy, reducing water consumption, and using reusable linen and instruments.
- Adoption of comprehensive suggestions by the American Society of Anesthesiologists and WHO for green ORs should be followed to reduce perioperative GHG emission.

REFERENCES

1. Carbon Trust. "What is a carbon footprint?" [online] Available form http://www.carbontrust.co.uk/solutions/CarbonFootprinting/what_is_a_carbon_footprint.htm. [Last accessed October, 2020].
2. Yvon-Durocher G, Allen A, Bastviken D, Conrad R, Gudasz C, St-Pierre A, et al. Methane fluxes show consistent temperature dependence across microbial to ecosystem scales. Nature. 2014;507(7493):488-91.
3. Carnegie Mellon University Green Design Institute. Economic input-output life cycle assessment (EIO-LCA) US 2002 (428) model. [online] Available from http://www.eiolca.net. [Last accessed October, 2020].
4. Chung JW, Meltzer, DO. Estimate of the carbon footprint of the US health care sector. JAMA. 2009;302(18):1970-2.
5. Eckelman MJ, Sherman J. Environmental Impacts of the U.S. Health Care System and Effects on Public Health. PLoS One. 2016;11(6):e0157014.
6. Pichler PP, Jaccard IS, Weisz Um Weisz H. International comparison of health care carbon footprints. Environ Res Lett. 2019;14:064004.
7. Pandey D, Agrawal M, Pandey JS. Carbon footprint: current methods of estimation. Environ Monit Assess. 2011;178(1-4):135-60.
8. Matthews SC, Hendrickson CT, Weber CL. Estimating carbon footprints with input out-put models. In International Input Output meeting on managing the environment. Seville: IIOMME; 2008.
9. Wiedmann T, Minx J. A definition of carbon footprint. ISAUK Research Report 07-01. Durham: ISAUK Research and Consulting; 2007.
10. WRI/WBCSD. The greenhouse gas protocol: A corporate accounting and reporting standard revised edition. Geneva: World Business Council for Sustainable Development and World Resource Institute; 2004.
11. Carbon Trust. (2007). Carbon footprint measurement methodology, version 1.1. [online] Available from: http://www.carbontrust.co.uk. [Last accessed October, 2020].
12. Carbon Trust. Carbon foot printing. An introduction for organizations. [online] Available from http://www. carbontrust.co.uk/publications/publicationdetail.htm? [Last accessed October, 2020].
13. BSI. Publicly available specification 2050. Specification for the assessment of the life cycle greenhouse gas emissions of goods and services. London: British Standards Institute; 2008.
14. MacNeill AJ, Lillywhite R, Brown CJ. The impact of surgery on global climate: a carbon footprinting study of operating theatres in three health systems. Lancet Planet Health. 2017;1(9):e381-8.
15. Thiel CL, Eckelman M, Guido R, Huddleston M, Landis AE, Sherman J, et al. Environmental impacts of surgical procedures: life cycle assessment of hysterectomy in the United States. Environ Sci Technol. 2015;49(3):1779-86.

16. Sulbaek Andersen MP, Nielsen OJ, Wallington TJ, Karpichev B, Sander SP. Medical intelligence article: assessing the impact on global climate from general anesthetic gases. Anesth Analg. 2012;114(5):1081-5.
17. Thiel CL, Woods NC, Bilec MM. Strategies to Reduce Greenhouse Gas Emissions from Laparoscopic Surgery. Am J Public Health. 2018;108(S2):S158-S164.
18. Alexander R, Poznikoff A, Malherbe S. Greenhouse gases: the choice of volatile anesthetic does matter. Can J Anaesth. 2018;65(2):221-2.
19. Eckelman M, Mosher M, Gonzalez A, Sherman J. Comparative life cycle assessment of disposable and reusable laryngeal mask airways. Anesth Analg. 2012;114(5):1067-72.
20. McMichael AJ, Lindgren. Climate change: present and future risks to health, and necessary responses. J Intern Med. 2011;270(5):401-13.
21. Smith KR, Woodward A, Campbell-Lendrum D, Chadee D, Honda Y, Liu Q, et al. 2014 Human health: impacts, adaptation, and co-benefits. In: Climate Change 2014: Impacts, Adaptation, and Vulnerability. Part A: Global and Sectoral Aspects. Contribution of Working Group II to the Fifth Assessment Report of the Intergovernmental Panel on Climate Change. Cambridge: Cambridge University Press; 2014. pp. 709-54.
22. Watts N, Adger WN, Ayeb-Karlsson S, Bai Y, Byass P, Campbell-Lendrum DC, et al. The Lancet Countdown: tracking progress on health and climate change. Lancet. 2017;389(10074):1151-64.
23. McGain F, Jarosz KM, Nguyen MN, Bates S, O'Shea CJ. Auditing operating room recycling: a management case report. AA Case Rep. 2015;5(3):47-50.
24. Southorn T, Norrish AR, Gardner K, Baxandall R. Reducing the carbon footprint of the operating theatre: a multicentre quality improvement report. J Perioper Pract. 2013;23(6):144-6.
25. Zygourakis CC, Yoon S, Valencia V, Boscardin C, Moriates C, Gonzales R, et al. Operating room waste: disposable supply utilization in neurosurgical procedures. J Neurosurg. 2017;126(2):620-5.
26. Ard JL Jr, Tobin K, Huncke T, Kline R, Ryan SM, Bell C, et al. A survey of the American Society of Anesthesiologists regarding environmental attitudes, knowledge, and organization. AA Case Rep. 2016;6(7):208-16.
27. Grubler A, Wilson C, Bento N, Boza-Kiss B, Krey V, McCollum DL, et al. A low energy demand scenario for meeting the 1.5°C target and sustainable development goals without negative emission technologies. Nat Energy. 2018;3(6):517-25.
28. Weisz U, Haas W, Pelikan JM, Schmied H. Sustainable Hospitals: A Socio-Ecological Approach. GAIA. 2011;20(3):191-8.
29. Holmner A, Ebi KL, Lazuardi L, Nilsson M 2014. Carbon footprint of telemedicine solutions--unexplored opportunity for reducing carbon emissions in the health sector. PLoS One. 2014;9(9):e105040.
30. World Health Organization, Health Care without Harm. Healthy hospitals, healthy planet, healthy people: Addressing climate change in healthcare settings. Geneva: WHO; 2009.
31. American Society of Anesthesiologists; Task Force on Environmental Sustainability Committee on Equipment and Facilities. (2014). Greening the Operating Room and Perioperative Arena: Environmental Sustainability for Anesthesia Practice. [online] Available from https://www.asahq.org/resources/resources-from-asa-committees/environmental-sustainability/greening-the-operating-room. [Last accessed October, 2020].

CHAPTER 19

Colloids: An Overview

Sanjay Agrawal, Veena Asthana

INTRODUCTION

Critically ill patients lose fluids due to infections, trauma or burns and require fluid supplementation to prevent dehydration and maintenance of hemodynamic stability. Colloids solutions provide swifter volume expansion of the intravascular space, cannot permeate healthy capillary membranes and remain in the intravascular compartment for longer time thereby, retaining solvent (normal saline or ringer lactate) before moving to interstitial space.[1,2] Colloids can be naturally occurring (albumin or fresh frozen plasma) or synthetic (starches, dextrans, or gelatins).

ALBUMIN

Human albumin (HA) is a plasma substitute used to treat hypovolemia. It is the most abundant protein in plasma naturally synthetized in the liver.[3] Albumin maintains colloid osmotic pressure, hormones and drugs binding and transportation, modulation of nitric oxide, antioxidant and buffer capabilities. The mean half-life of albumin is 18–19 days. HA is prepared by alcoholic precipitation of pooled human plasma, pasteurized for 10 hours at +60°C for pathogen inactivation.[4] Prepared solution contains sodium octanoate and acetyltryptophan as stabilizers. It can be administered to all irrespective of their blood group, as there are no isoagglutinins or blood group substances present in solution rendering it safe for administration.[4,5]

Albumin is available as 5 and 25% solutions for intravenous administration. The 5% formulation have chloride content of 120–130 mEq/L, while 25% solution have chloride content of 20 mEq/L. Albumin 25% is a therapeutic choice when either sodium or fluid intake is restricted or in cases of oncotic deficiencies. Albumin 5% is more commonly used for volume replacement.[6,7]

Albumin is used for volume replacement in the perioperative period, in the intensive care unit (ICU) patients, burn patients, trauma patients, in pregnant women, and children. It is also used during hepatic surgery and for correction of hypoalbuminemia.

Albumin can cause allergic reactions resulting in skin ash, itching, fever, chills, and nausea vomiting. Hyperoncotic 20% HA is associated with adverse renal effects.

Albumin is absolutely contraindicated when there is established allergy to it. It is also contraindicated hypervolemic state, patients with restricted cardiac function, congestive heart failure (CHF) with pulmonary edema, and hypocoagulopathy.

SEMISYNTHETIC COLLOIDS

Semisynthetic colloids are a group of solutions with varying compositions utilized for fluid replacement therapy. Compositions includes bovine collagen, glucose polymer or amylopectin (maize derived).

Dextrans

Dextrans are branched polysaccharide molecules, produced from sucrose by enzyme degradation of dextran sucrase. It is a glucose polymer with alpha linkages at 1,6 or 1,3 positions. It is commercially available as dextran 70 and dextran 40 solutions with molecular weight of 70 kDa or 40 kDa respectively. The 6% solutions are isotonic while 10% solutions may be hypertonic compared to plasma.[6] Dextrans are indicated for volume restoration and duration of stay in circulation is 3–5 hours depending on molecular weight of the preparation. Increase in plasma volume varies between 100% (6% dextran) and 175% (10% dextran) of administered volume.[1] Smaller molecules of dextrans (<60 kDa) are rapidly excreted by kidney while larger molecular weight solutions remain in the bloodstream for longer duration. Dextrans may be present in tissue fluids, lymph or taken up by the reticuloendothelial cells. Higher the molecular weight, more is their circulation time in blood and their clinical effect.

Main use of dextrans is to improve microcirculation (microsurgical implant surgery) and in extracorporeal circulation (cardiopulmonary bypass). It improves microcirculation by reducing blood viscosity and inhibiting erythrocytes aggregation. Dextran-hypertonic saline preparations have a volume enhancing effect of up to 400% of the administered volume and may be beneficial in management of traumatic hemorrhagic shock.[1,6]

The recommended dosage of administration is 1.5 g/kg/day.

Dextrans can cause *anaphylactic reactions*. Lower the molecular weight of dextrans less is the incidence. They are triggered by release of vasoactive mediators produced by dextran reactive antibodies. Pretreatment with a hapten decreases the incidence of anaphylactic reactions.[8,9] Other complications associated with dextrans include:
- *Coagulation abnormalities*: Dose-dependent adverse effects on hemostasis are reported after dextran use. They are associated with platelet adhesiveness, decreased factor VIII levels and increased fibrinolysis.[10,11]
- *Interference with blood cross-matching:* Coating of red blood cell (RBC) surface by dextran interferes with cross-matching of blood.
- *Precipitation of acute renal failure:* Low molecular dextrans may accumulate in tissues and in renal tubules causing tubular plugging and induce hyperoncotic renal dysfunction.[12] This is especially seen with dextran 40.

They are seldom used for volume expansion these days because of availability of better, more suitable alternatives with lesser side effects like HES.

Gelatins

Gelatins are group of solutions formed from collagen derived by boiling animal connective tissues. The early solutions contained suspended gelatine of high molecular weight (about 100,000), produced prominent oncotic effect with the tendency to produce high viscosity and propensity to form gel at low temperatures.[6]

Types of gelatins available for clinical use are chemically classified as:
- Urea cross-linked gelatins (Polygeline).
- Succinylated gelatins (Gelofusine).
- Oxypolygelatins (Gelifundol).

Polygeline is obtained by thermal degradation of collagen from bovine bones using an alkali. The resultant polypeptides obtained after alkali treatment (molecular weight 12,000–15,000) are urea cross-linked utilizing hexamethyl di-isocyanate. The branching of the molecules by cross-linking lowers the gel melting point. Molecular weight of constituent molecules ranges from 5,000 to 50,000 with a weight-average of 35,000 and a number-average molecular weight of 24,500.[13]

Succinylated gelatins solutions consists of polypeptides with higher molecular weight (20,000) and modified by addition of succinic acid. Increased osmotic activity at physiological pH is a resultant of Donnan effect.

Physiochemical Properties

Succinylated and urea-linked gelatins are available as sterile preservative-free solutions in sodium chloride. Polygeline is available as 3.5% solution with electrolytes (Na^+ 145, K^+ 5.1, Ca^{++} 6.25 and Cl^- 145 mmoL/L). Large volume resuscitation with polygeline may theoretically increases the risk of increase serum calcium concentration. Shelf life of polygeline is up to 3 years at room temperature.

Succinylated gelatins are dispensed as 4% solution with electrolytes (Na^+ 154, K^+ 0.4, Ca^{++} 0.4 and Cl^- 120 mmoL/L). Lower chloride content of gelofusine is helpful in patients with hyperchloremic acidosis. Presence of lower calcium content makes it compatible with blood transfusions.

Gelatins have limited half-life of about 2.5 hours. Rapid elimination by the kidney results in peak plasma concentration falling to half in 2.5 hours. Only 13% of total volume administered remains in plasma after 24 hours, around 71% is excreted in the urine while 16% may be present in the extravascular compartment.[14] Only 3% is metabolized in body. Volume expansion by gelatins is about 70–80%. There is no upper limit of volume of solution that can be transfused.[15]

Indications of gelatin administration include hypovolemia secondary to hemorrhage, acute normovolemic hemodilution (ANH), extracorporeal circulation during cardiopulmonary bypass, and for preloading prior to spinal anesthesia.

They have the advantage of being cost effective compared to albumin and synthetic colloids. Moreover, they do not have an upper limit of volume transfusion and have no/minimal deleterious effects on renal system with large volume transfusion.[12]

However, gelatins also have certain disadvantages. They have higher incidence of anaphylactoid reactions, increase the bleeding time and impair platelet adhesiveness. Increased plasma renin activity and aldosterone secretion has also been reported.

Hydroxyethyl Starches

Hydroxyethyl starches (HES) are amylopectin derivatives, which are branched compound of starch. Natural amylopectin is rapidly hydrolyzed in about 20 minutes. HES are produced by hydroxyethyl substitution in amylopectin molecule mainly at positions C_2 and C_6. This substitution with hydroxyethyl reduces hydrolysis of starch by amylases in blood.[16,17]

Hespan was the first HES product in United States, introduced in 1970. Since then, newer preparations of HES are produced, differing in molecular weight, molar substitution (MS), and C2/C6 ratio. HES for clinical use are available as (6% HES 450/0.7, 10% HES 200/0.5 or 6% HES 130/0.4). The first number indicates concentration of HES in solution (6% vs. 10%), second denotes mean molecular weight (kilo Dalton) of HES (450 vs. 200 vs. 130) and the third MS (0.7 vs. 0.5 vs. 0.4). These parameters are important for pharmacokinetics of HES.

Physiochemical Properties

- *Concentration* (6% vs. 10%): Concentration of HES in solution influences the osmolarity of solution as well as propensity to increase in plasma volume after infusion. The 6% HES solutions are iso-oncotic with volume of expansion of about 100% (volume of expansion 1:1 to blood loss) whereas, 10% solutions are hyper-oncotic, with a volume effect exceeding the infused volume (about 145%, i.e., 1 mL for approximately 1.5 mL blood loss).[18]
- *Average molecular weight:* It is available as low molecular weight (70 kDa), medium molecular weight (200 kDa), and high molecular weight (450 kDa). Hydroxyethyl starches are polydisperse systems containing particles of variable molecular weight in solutions and ranging between 60 and 450 kDa. On transfusion, small molecules (<60 kDa) are rapidly excreted by kidneys while larger molecules (>70 kDa) are retained within the intravascular compartment. The number of active particles in solutions are responsible for osmotic effectiveness of solution at a given period. Excretion of the smaller particles (<60 Da) reduces the osmotic effectiveness of the infused solution while degradation of larger molecule into oncotically active particles helps in maintaining the pharmacological effects.[14]
- *Molar substitution (MS):* Low (0.45–0.58) or high (0.62–0.70). The degree of substitution by hydroxyethyl groups in the original amylopectin molecule is termed as MS. Higher the substitution, lesser is the degradation of amylopectin and longer the intravascular presence of osmotically active product.

Molar substitution is calculated as the average number of hydroxyethyl groups present per anhydrous glucose residue in amylopectin. MS is thus the average number of hydroxyethyl residues per glucose subunit. MS of 0.7 indicates presence of seven hydroxyethyl residues on average per 10 glucose subunits.

On basis of MS starches are classified as hetastarches (MS 0.7), pentastarches (MS 0.5), and tetrastarches (MS 0.4).

- *C2/C6 ratio:* This can be low (<8) or high (>8). It refers to the site of substitution with hydroxyethyl group on initial glucose molecule. Hydroxyethylation of the glucose subunits is guided predominantly toward the C2 and C6 carbon atoms. Hydroxyethyl groups at C2 atom inhibits the access of alpha-amylase to the substrate more effectively than at C6 position, prolonging its half-life. HES with high C2/C6 ratios degrades slowly.

Hydroxyethyl starches increases the colloid osmotic pressure similar to albumin. Volume of expansion is also similar to albumin but greater than gelatins. Duration of volume expansion ranges between 8 and 12 hours.[17,19] HES are mainly indicated for hypovolemic shock, but there is some evidence of anti-inflammatory properties which was demonstrated in the intestine during sepsis.

They are cost effective being cheaper than albumin with a comparable volume of expansion. The maximum allowable volume which can be transfused is 20 mL/kg for hetastarches, 33 mL/kg for pentastarches and up to 50 mL/kg with tetrastarches. HES have certain disadvantages too which are as follows:

- *Coagulation:* Reduction in factor VIII and von Willebrand factor, platelet function impairment, increase coagulation abnormalities, and bleeding complications.[20]
- *Accumulation:* HES can accumulate in the interstitial spaces and reticuloendothelial system. They may also deposit in tissues of skin, liver, muscle, spleen, intestine, trophoblast, and placental stroma. High molecular weight HES are more responsible for deposition. Such depositions are associated with pruritus.
- *Anaphylactoid reactions:* Incidence of anaphylactoid reactions is high with HES especially hetastarches.
- *Renal impairment*: Increase in creatinine, oliguria and acute renal failure are reported in patients admitted in critical care unit, those with pre-existing renal impairment and with the use of high molecular weight HES. Tetrastarch with lower molecular weight and MS (HES 130/0.4) have reduced effect on renal function despite large volume transfusion.[21]
- *Increase in amylase levels:* HES infusion may be associated with increase serum amylase levels.

Third Generation Hydroxyethyl Starches (Tetrastarch)

Reductions of molecular weight (450–130 kDa) and MS (0.7–0.4) leads to solutions with shorter half-life, better pharmacokinetics, and pharmacodynamics and reduction in side effects. Such starches may be derived from waxy maize or potato.[16]

Tetrastarches are safer than the earlier generation HES solutions in the following ways:
- *Effects on coagulation and platelet function:* Tetrastarches produce least effect on coagulation compared to older products.[20]
- *Accumulation and tissue storage:* Older HES molecules had tendency to accumulate, for tissue storage and slower metabolism. Rapid clearance of tetrastarch from body decreases tissue accumulation and its clinical manifestations.
- *Effects on plasma bilirubin:* Potato-derived HES 130/0.42 is associated with increased incidence of postoperative hyperbilirubinemia and is contraindicated in patients with severe hepatic impairment. Such effects on liver functions are not observed with maize derived starches.[16,19]
- *Effects on renal function:* Tetrastarch have little adverse renal effects owing to lower tendency to accumulate in tissue.
- *Special patient groups:* It is used cautiously in high-risk group of patients such as the elderly, children, and those with pre-existing renal impairment. The waxy maize-derived tetrastarch HES 130/0.4 has a well-documented safety profile. It is safe for use in pediatric age group.[6]

CRYSTALLOIDS VERSUS COLLOIDS

Despite the use of both crystalloids and colloids as effective means of fluid resuscitation, controversy persists over the efficacy and benefits of their use. Velanovich was the first to question the safety of colloids in fluid resuscitation. A number of systematic reviews have questioned the safety of colloids. Studies have reported significant increase in the risk of death with use of colloids for fluid resuscitation.[21,22]

CLINICAL EFFICACY OF VARIOUS COLLOIDS

Besides restoration of intravascular volume, HES administration improves microcirculation and tissue oxygenation. HES 130/0.4 improves tissue oxygenation faster and to higher values compared with other HES solutions.[17] The extent and duration of increase in intravascular volume depends on type of solution, patient's physical status, rate and volume of blood loss, colloid volume infused, and speed of administration. Longer intravascular persistence of HES was initially regarded as favorable due to its prolonged volume effect. A large number of studies demonstrate that this belief is not justified. A double-blind study investigated the efficacy and safety of HES 130/0.4 and HES 670/0.75 in patients undergoing major orthopedic surgery and demonstrated that both colloids were equally effective in the stabilization of hemodynamic.[21]

Infusion of colloids or crystalloids for initial hemodynamic stabilization in shock is debatable. As the stay of crystalloids in intravascular compartment is less and with larger volume of distribution, resuscitation with crystalloids requires more fluid and results in interstitial edema and may be inferior to combination therapy with colloids.[21]

Comparison of different colloids usage in intensive care demonstrated dextrans had unfavorable risk/benefit ratio. This is due to their propensity to cause anaphylactoid reaction, renal dysfunction, and major impact on hemostasis. Disadvantages of gelatins includes higher anaphylactoid potential, limited volume expansion compared to dextran and HES. Modern HES preparations have the least risk of anaphylactic reactions among the synthetic colloids. Use of older HES preparations (hetastarch, hexastarch, and pentastarch) is associated with impaired renal function and hemostasis, especially when used in large volumes.

CONCLUSION

Natural colloids such as albumin or synthetic colloids such as gelatins, dextrans or HES effectively expand the intravascular volume with minimal risk of edema. As compared to crystalloids, colloids probably makes little or no difference to mortality. Starches factors to be considered for use includes type of solution, volume of intravascular expansion, intravascular half-life, safe limit of volume to be transfused, and adverse effects produced by each might increase the need for blood transfusion, and renal replacement therapy. Albumin may make little or no difference to the need for renal replacement therapy.

ACKNOWLEDGMENT

The authors wishes to acknowledge the contributions of Dr Sharmishtha Pathak during preparation of the chapter.

KEY POINTS

- Intravascular volume expansion during intraoperative period is required to compensate for acute blood loss. Available options include use of crystalloids or colloids.
- Albumin a natural occurring colloid acts by increasing colloid osmotic pressure. It has a half-life of 25–35 days.
- Dextrans are branched polysaccharides with molecular weight ranging 40–110 kDa. T1/2 is 3–5 hours. Associated with high incidence of coagulation abnormalities, and renal dysfunction.
- Gelatins are formed from collagen of animal origin and increase the blood volume by 70–80% of volume infused. High dosage of infusion is not associated with renal dysfunction.
- Hydroxyethyl starches are amylopectin with hydroxyethyl substitution and are classified as hetastarch, pentastarch, and tetrastarch.
- Tetrastarches are newest generation of starches. Can be transfused to a volume of 50 mL/kg, less chances of renal dysfunction and coagulation abnormality.
- Factors to be considered for use includes type of solution, volume of intravascular expansion, intravascular half-life, safe limit of volume to be transfused and adverse effects produced by each.

REFERENCES

1. Niemi TT, Miyashita R, Yamakage M. Colloid solutions: a clinical update. J Anesth. 2010;24(6):913-25.

2. Lewis SR, Pritchard MW, Evans DJ, Butler AR, Alderson P, Smith AF, et al. Colloids versus crystalloids for fluid resuscitation in critically ill people. Cochrane Database Syst Rev. 2018;8(8):1-182.
3. Campos MA, Jain N, Gupta M. Albumin Colloid. Treasure Island (FL): StatPearls Publishing; 2020.
4. Vincent JL, Russell JA, Jacob M, Martin G, Guidet B, Wernerman J, et al. Albumin administration in the acutely ill: what is new and where next? Crit Care. 2014;18(4):231.
5. Matejtschuk P, Dash CH, Gascoigne EW. Production of human albumin solution: a continually developing colloid. Br J Anaesth. 2000;85(6):887-95.
6. Mitra S, Khandelwal P. Are all colloids same? How to select the right colloid? Indian J Anaesth. 2009;53(5):592-607.
7. Fanali G, di Masi A, Trezza V, Marino M, Fasano M, Ascenzi P. Human serum albumin: from bench to bedside. Mol Aspects Med. 2012;33(3):209-90.
8. Barron ME, Wilkes MM, Navickis RJ. A systematic review of the comparative safety of colloids. Arch Surg. 2004;139(5):552-63.
9. Kaye A, Kucera I. Intravascular fluid and electrolyte physiology, 6th edition. Miller R (Ed). Philadelphia: Churchill Livingstone; 2005. pp. 1763-98.
10. Martino P. Colloid and Crystalloid resuscitation, 3rd edition. Marino P (Ed). Philadelphia: Churchill Livingstone; 2007. pp. 233-54.
11. Van der Linden P, Ickx BE. The effects of colloid solutions on hemostasis. Can J Anesth. 2006;53(6 Suppl):S30-9.
12. Davidson IJ. Renal impact of fluid management with colloids: a comparative review. Eur J Anaesthesiol. 2006;23(9):721-38.
13. Dubois MJ, Vincent JL. Perioperative Fluid Therapy. New York: Wiley; 2007. pp. 153-611.
14. Persson J, Grände PO. Volume expansion of albumin, gelatin, hydroxyethyl starch, saline and erythrocytes after haemorrhage in the rat. Intensive Care Med. 2005;31(2):296-301.
15. Marino PL. Marino's the ICU Book. Baltimore: Lippincott Williams and Wilkins; 2013.
16. Westphal M, James MF, Kozek-Langenecker S, Stocker R, Guidet B, Van Aken H. Hydroxyethyl Starches different products--different effects. Anesthesiology. 2009;111(1):187-202.
17. Datta R, Nair R, Pandey A, Gupta N, Sahoo T. Hydroxyethyl starch: Controversies revisited. J Anaesthesiol Clin Pharmacol. 2014;30(4):472-80.
18. Glover PA, Rudloff E, Kirby R. Hydroxyethyl starch: a review of pharmacokinetics, pharmacodynamics, current products, and potential clinical risks, benefits, and use. J Vet Emerg Crit Care (San Antonio). 2014;24(6):642-61.
19. Yacobi A, Stoll RG, Sum CY, Lai C, Gupta SD, Hulse JD. Pharmacokinetics of hydroxyethyl starch in normal subjects. J Clin Pharmacol. 1982;22(4):206-12.
20. Kumar S. Clinical use of hydroxyethyl starch and serious adverse effects: need for awareness amongst the medical fraternity. Med J Armed Forces India. 2014;70(3):209-10.
21. Malbrain MLNG, Langer T, Annane D, Gattinoni L, Elbers P, Hahn RG, et al. Intravenous fluid therapy in the perioperative and critical care setting: executive summary of the International Fluid Academy (IFA). Ann Intensive Care. 2020;10(1):64.
22. Gandhi SD, Weiskopf RB, Jungheinrich C, Koorn R, Miller D, Shangraw RE, et al. Volume replacement therapy during major orthopedic surgery using voluven (hydroxyethyl starch 130/0.4) or hetastarch. Anesthesiology. 2007;106(6):1120-7.

CHAPTER 20

Newer Modes of Ventilation

PL Gautam, Gunchan Paul

INTRODUCTION

The aim of mechanical ventilation is to achieve adequate gas exchange while maintaining patient safety and comfort, and early liberation from ventilation. The conventional modes of ventilation are well understood, commonly used and fulfill the goals of adequate gas exchange. But these are accompanied by ventilator-induced lung injury (VILI) and delayed weaning.[1] In recent years, there has been much advancement in mechanical ventilation with the introduction of computerized control and artificial intelligence into the critical care ventilators. Introduction of small innovations and algorithms in the conventional volume control and pressure control modes has led to variety of newer modes and combinations of these modes in the market. New ventilators have incorporated assessment of patient's respiratory mechanics to deliver personalized ventilation.[2] The technological advances improve patient synchronization, comfort, and safety and also decrease the work of breathing (WOB) as these have feedback systems to respond to patient's dynamic ventilator requirements.

There is growing evidence in literature that newer modes have physiological and clinical benefits **(Box 1)**, but the lack of standard nomenclature for these new modes leads to lot of confusion even among the experienced critical care physicians.[3] This article briefly discusses the working principles, advantages, and limitations of the newer ventilator modes to help the practicing clinicians. However, any mode is as good as the intensivist who uses it. More important than the mode is the ventilator strategy as ventilator is just a means of support and not a cure for any condition. Current ventilator strategy has paradigm shift from limiting barotrauma (stress) or volutrauma (strain) to minimizing

---

BOX 1: Advantages of newer modes as compared to conventional modes.

- To achieve a desired tidal volume in pressure limited ventilation
- To provide lung protection in ARDS
- To allow more spontaneous ventilation
- For automation of ventilation to the weaning process

(ARDS: acute respiratory distress syndrome)

the ergotrauma, i.e., the energy expenditure associated with mechanical ventilation. Although conceptual, concerns are same and the difference lies in viewing the problem from different dimension and applying new strategies. Limiting ergotrauma is based on the concept that volume, pressure, rate, and flow, i.e., the mechanical factors should be considered as a part of a single physical entity: "the mechanical power" and hence, minimizing ergotrauma means prevention of generation of excessive transpulmonary pressure and excessive variation of pleural pressure.[4]

The classification of any ventilator mode depends on the:
Types of control: The set of operating characteristics that control any mechanical breath are classified as—trigger, control/limit and cycling variables.
- *Trigger variable*: It is that variable which starts inspiration. It may be ventilator initiated as in control modes or patient initiated as in assisted modes. Patient trigger may be flow or change in pressure in the ventilator circuit generated by the patient's effort or may be neural driven as seen in neurally adjusted ventilatory assist (NAVA).
- *Limit variable*: Limit variable is the maximum value that is achieved and maintained during inspiration. It may be pressure preset (pressure controlled) or volume preset (volume controlled) or dual control (e.g., pressure limited volume controlled). If the physician chooses the tidal volume (TV) to be the independent variable or limit, the mode is called volume control (VC), as the airway pressure varies according to the lung characteristics. If the driving pressure (change in pressure during the delivered breath) is the independent variable that is chosen by the operator, the mode is called pressure control (PC) and now, the TV varies as the compliance improves or worsens.
- *Cycling variable*: This variable is the one which ends inspiration. It may be time, volume or flow or pressure cycled. Hence, a volume-controlled breath is triggered by the machine (VC) or by the patient (volume assist-control), limited by flow, and cycled by volume while a pressure-controlled breath is triggered by the machine (PC) or the patient (pressure assist-control), limited by pressure, and cycled by time (PC) or flow (pressure support). **Table 1** describes the characteristics of mechanical breaths in conventional modes.

Level of support: It depends whether the ventilator allows mandatory breath or spontaneous breath. A controlled breath is triggered, delivered and cycled

TABLE 1: Key characteristics of various phases of breath in conventional modes*

Mode	Trigger	Target	Cyde
Volume control	Timer	Flow	Volume
Volume assist	Patient	Flow	Volume
Pressure control	Timer	Pressure	Time
Pressure assist	Patient	Pressure	Time
Pressure support	Patient	Pressure	Flow

*Trigger by patient means sensing by flow or pressure trigger, whichever has been set by the operator.

by ventilator. An assisted breath is triggered by patient, delivered and cycled as per preset mode settings. Mechanical ventilation is usually initiated in the control mode when the ventilator takes control of all the breaths but as the disease process starts recovering, the patient participates in the process of ventilation. This is then referred to as the assisted mode. Finally, as the patient gains control over his ventilation and breathes spontaneously, he is ready to be weaned from the ventilator.

Targeting scheme: It is referred to the way ventilator is triggered into inspiration, cycled into expiration and variables that limit inspiration. Most conventional modes deliver fixed parameters and take no feedback from the patient. Thus, they have open loop mechanism such that the ventilator settings at the initial point of time may not be appropriate when the patient condition improves or worsens. However, this limitation is overcome by the newer modes that are based on the closed loop mechanism. They make alterations in the control, cycle and limit variables with the feedback from the changes in the patient's lung characteristics, thus completing the loop.

Thus, the simple classification of the newer modes can be as **(Table 2)**:

- *Dual modes*: These modes have the capacity to switch between different modes (PC and VC) within a breath or between breaths and hence, combining the advantages of both volume as well as pressure control, e.g., volume support (VS), volume assured pressure support (VAPS), pressure regulated volume controlled (PRVC), etc.
- *Bilevel modes [spontaneous breathing + higher functional residual capacity (FRC)]*: Bilevel modes are the modes based on the augmented pressure ventilation where tidal exchange occurs between the two levels of pressure applied. They also allow unrestricted spontaneous breathing at any part of respiratory cycle, e.g., bilevel, biphasic positive airway pressure (BiPAP), airway pressure release ventilation (APRV). All these modes can be put in one category based on time controlled adaptive ventilation (TCAV) strategy. This Bilevel pressure support is different from bilevel inspiratory positive airway pressure (IPAP) used for noninvasive ventilation (NIV), where one level is continuous positive airway pressure (CPAP) and another is pressure assist.
- *Modes which adapt to lung characteristics*: Pressure augment, proportional assist ventilation (PAV), adaptive support ventilation (ASV).
- *Knowledge-based weaning modes*: These are automatic tube or resistance compensation (ATC and ARC), PAV, ASV and SmartCare. There are combined modes such as synchronized intermittent mandatory ventilation (SIMV) + pressure support ventilation (PSV) where synchronized intermittent mandatory breaths are combined with pressure support. Mandatory breath can be preset volume or pressure. Minimum mandatory ventilation (MMV) where minute ventilation is set and patient is allowed to breath but if patient hypoventilates then ventilator supports as back up and helps in weaning.
- *Better triggering mechanism*: Neural adjusted ventilator assist (NAVA).

TABLE 2: Classification of newer modes

Conventional modes

- Volume control, VC-A/C, CMV, assist/control
- Pressure control, PC-A/C, AC PCV
- SIMV-VC, SIMV-PC
- Continuous positive airway pressure (CPAP)
- Pressure support

Bilevel modes (Time controlled adaptive ventilation)

• Bilevel	(Puritan Bennett)
• Bi PAP	(Dräger Europe)
• Bi Vent	(Siemens)
• Bi Phasic	(Avea, Cardinal Health)
• APRV	
• PCV +	(Dräger Medical)
• Duo PAP	(Hamilton)

Dual modes

• Within a breath	• Volume assured pressure support (VAPS) • Pressure augment	VIASYS
• Breath to breath • (Pressure limited flow cycled)	• Volume support • VPS	
• Breath to breath • (Pressure limited time cycled)	• Pressure-regulated volume control (PRVC) • AutoFlow • Adaptive pressure ventilation • Volume control+ (VC+) • Volume targeted pressure control/pressure controlled volume guaranteed	Macquet Servo-i Evita, Dräger Medical Hamilton Galileo Puritan Bennett, Engström, GE
• Breath to breath	• Adaptive pressure ventilation	Hamilton

Smart modes (closed loop systems)

	• Mandatory minute volume (MMV)	Drager
	• Adaptive support ventilation/ AVM2	Hamilton
	• Mid frequency ventilation (MFV)	
	• Proportional assist ventilation (PAV)	Puritan Bennett™ 840

Knowledge-based weaning modes

- Automatic tube compensation (ATC)
- ASV
- PAV
- SmartCare
- NAVA

(CM: controlled mandatory ventilation; PCV: pressure-controlled ventilation; APRV: airway pressure release ventilation; AVM: adaptive ventilation mode; SIMV: synchronized intermittent mandatory ventilation; ASV: adaptive support ventilation; NAVA: neurally adjusted ventilatory assist; VPS: variable pressure support)

DUAL CONTROL WITHIN A BREATH

Volume assured pressure support: It is also called *pressure augmentation*. This mode assures a minimal TV by combining pressure support and volume control modes within a single breath.[5] Ventilator settings include pressure support/limit, peak flow rate, and respiratory rate, target TV, FiO_2 and positive end-expiratory pressure (PEEP). At first, pressure support breath is delivered with the set peak flow and if target TV is delivered it is flow cycled. If the computer senses that the delivered TV falls short of the desired TV, then the peak flow is maintained, i.e., it switches to constant-flow volume control **(Fig. 1)**. It uses a longer inspiratory time and the flow and duration is determined by the remaining TV to be delivered. Set flow rates must not be too low which can cause delayed change over from pressure control to volume control, thus leading to unwanted prolongation of inspiratory time.

This mode is used to ventilate a patient who requires substantial ventilator support and has a vigorous drive. VAPS reduces WOB by 50% over volume-control ventilation, improves dynamic compliance, reduces auto-PEEP, improves gas exchange and hence, there is less need of sedation.[6] It can be safely used in a patient being weaned from ventilator having unstable drive to supply back up TV in case patients efforts or mechanics alter. By assuring the TV, it maintains minimum minute ventilation and prevents rise of pCO_2 levels in the blood.

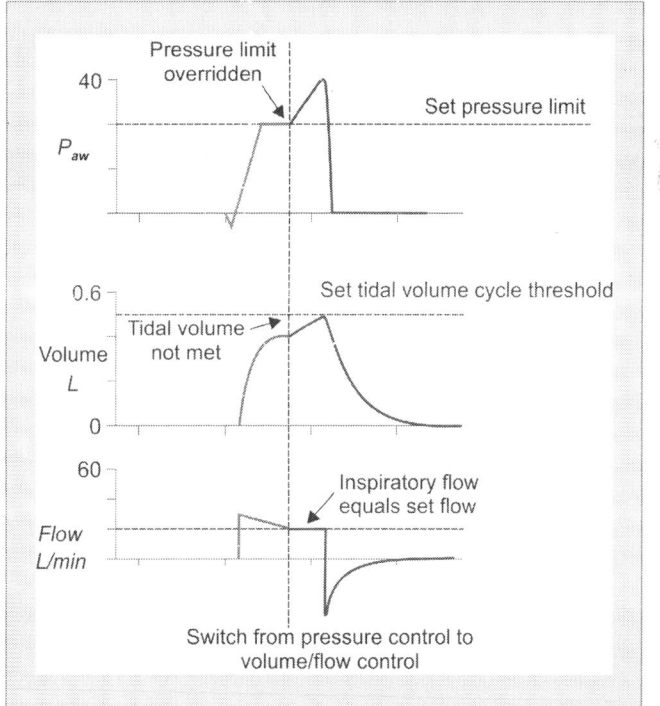

Fig. 1: Ventilatory graphics in VAPS show that when target TV is not delivered, pressure limit is over-ridden, decelerating flow changes to constant flow, i.e., switch from pressure control to volume control mode.
(VAPS: volume assured pressure support; TV: tidal volume)

DUAL CONTROL IN SUBSEQUENT BREATHS

Volume support: It is a closed loop type of PSV mode that takes feedback control for continuously adjusting the pressure support level from the delivered TV.[7] Initial test breath is delivered at 5 cmH$_2$O, pressure support is gradually increased until target TV is delivered. Maximum pressure support available is about 5 cmH$_2$O below the set pressure limit. If TV higher than the set TV is achieved, it results in lowering of pressure support. Patient can trigger a breath but in case of apnea, it switches to PRVC mode.[8]

Pressure-regulated volume control: It is known by various trade names; controlled mandatory ventilation (CMV) with autoflow, VC+, volume targeted pressure control/pressure controlled volume guaranteed. All of them basically deliver a volume targeted breath with decelerating flow. Ventilator settings to be adjusted include target TV, respiratory rate, inspiratory time, FiO$_2$ and PEEP. It is not a volume control mode because in volume-controlled ventilation (VCV) mode delivered volume is fixed, but in this mode minimum TV is guaranteed but not the maximal TV.[9]

It delivers a characteristic pressure control type of breath with decelerating flow so that the airway pressure remains constant. This varying flow allows the patient who can generate an inspiratory flow to receive flow according to his demand and thus, making him comfortable. In the initial breath the ventilator delivers the pressure control breath and measures the delivered TV. If patient's effort is large enough, the ventilator decreases the inspiratory pressure to deliver the minimum guaranteed TV and if the patients efforts is weak the vice versa changes occur in the inspiratory pressure **(Fig. 2)**. The adjustments in the

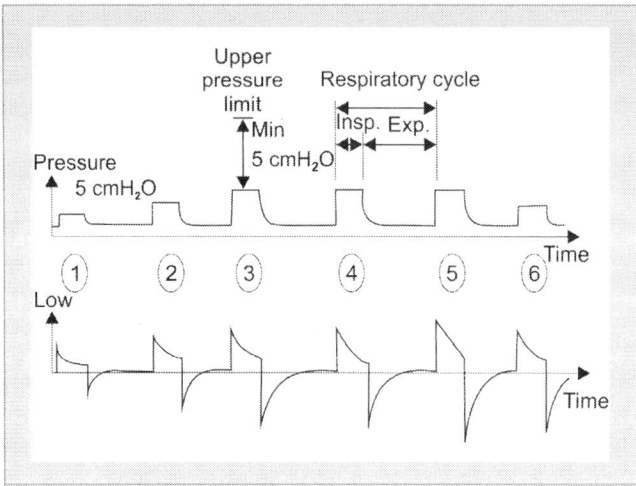

Fig. 2: Graphics on ventilator screen during PRVC mode (1) Breaths in PRVC deliver TV starting with minimal pressure, (2) Gradually the inspiratory pressure increases to achieve the target volume, (3) Maximum inspiratory pressure achieved is 5 cm below the set pressure limit, (4) Mandatory breaths are time cycled into expiration with decelerating flows, (5) and (6) When lung compliance improves such that higher TV is delivered with same inspiratory pressure, the inspiratory pressure decreases. (PRVC: pressure regulated volume controlled; TV: tidal volume).

Flowchart 1: Flowchart to describe the control mechanism of PRVC.

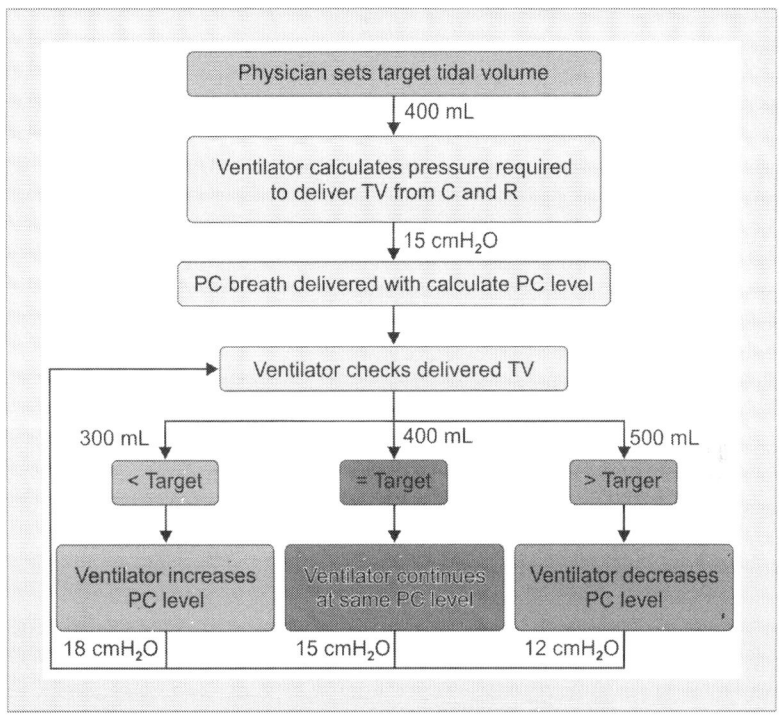

(PRVC: pressure regulated volume controlled; PC: pressure control; C: compliance; R: resistance of airway)

machine occur after the TV offsets the target value in a number of breaths, i.e., changes in pressure as a result of feedback of last 4–6 breaths. As in a pressure control mode, time ends inspiration and cycles into expiration. **Flowchart 1** shows the flowchart of the control mechanism of PRVC.

Pressure regulated volume controlled was designed to overcome the limitation of pressure control mode and deliver fixed TV with varying compliance with minimum P_{peak}. It is reported that the peak inspiratory pressures with this mode are lesser than volume control ventilation.[10] Hence, it limits volutrauma and prevents hypoventilation also. Also, the varying flows improve patient flow synchrony. It allows less operator manipulations and spontaneous weaning by reducing the inspiratory pressure when patient's efforts or compliance improves.[11]

This mode may not be ideal for patients with high respiratory drive such as in severe respiratory acidosis because the inspiratory pressure required to deliver the target TV will decrease and hence, the WOB is shifted on to the patient.[12] Similarly, it may not be suitable for patients with asthma and chronic obstructive pulmonary disease (COPD). Also, intermittent or variable patient's efforts may lead to variable TV which may be visualized on the bed side as asynchrony and paradoxically lead to increase in sedation. **Table 3** gives a comparison of the characteristics of the dual modes among each other.

TABLE 3: Comparison of the key characteristics of breaths in dual modes

Mode	VAPS	VS	PRVC
Trigger	Pressure/Flow	Pressure/Flow	Pressure/Flow
Control/Limit	Pressure → volume	Pressure	Pressure
Cycling	Flow → Time	Flow	Time

(VAPS: volume assured pressure support; VS: volume support; PRVC: pressure regulated volume controlled)

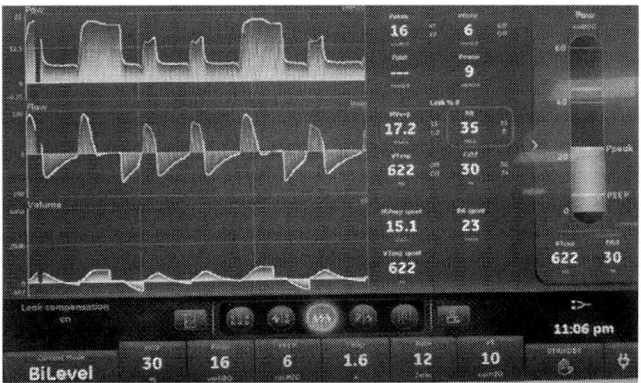

Fig. 3: Ventilator graphics in BiLevel + PS mode. P_{high} or P_{insp} is set to 16 cm and P_{low} or PEEP is set to 6 cm, RR set is 12 but total RR shown on the screen is 35, i.e., patient is allowed to take spontaneous breaths in between the mandatory breath with a pressure support of 10 cm that is set on the ventilator.
(PEEP: positive end-expiratory pressure; RR: respiratory rate; PS: pressure support).

TIME CONTROLLED ADAPTIVE VENTILATION STRATEGY (BiLevel, BIPAP, Bi Vent, BiPhasic, APRV, DuoPAP)

Bilevel positive airway pressure: It works by switching between the two airway pressures (a higher-pressure maintained in inspiration and a lower-pressure maintained in expiration) with provision to breath spontaneously.[13] By alternating the inhalation and exhalation pressures, the Bilevel allows the gas exchange to occur more efficiently, even during apnea. These deliver time triggered, pressure controlled, time cycled breath (i.e., constant pressure for constant period of time) along with the liberty of spontaneous breath at any point of respiratory cycle. Ventilator settings to be adjusted include P_{high} as inspiratory pressure, P_{low} as PEEP, time spent in P_{high} and P_{low} are T_{high} and T_{low}, respectively. **Figure 3** depicts the graphics in BiPAP mode. For a paralyzed patient, biphasic ventilation is identical to pressure control mandatory ventilation where TV is determined by lung compliance and the difference between P_{high} and P_{low} levels.[14]

By convention the main difference in Biphasic modes and APRV is the time spent in T_{high} and T_{low} or inspiratory:expiratory ratio (I:E ratio). Biphasic modes have an I:E ratio of 1:1–1:4 while T_{low} <1.5 seconds in APRV or I:E ratio is 4:1. **Figures 4A and B** compare the ventilator graphics of Bilevel with APRV. In

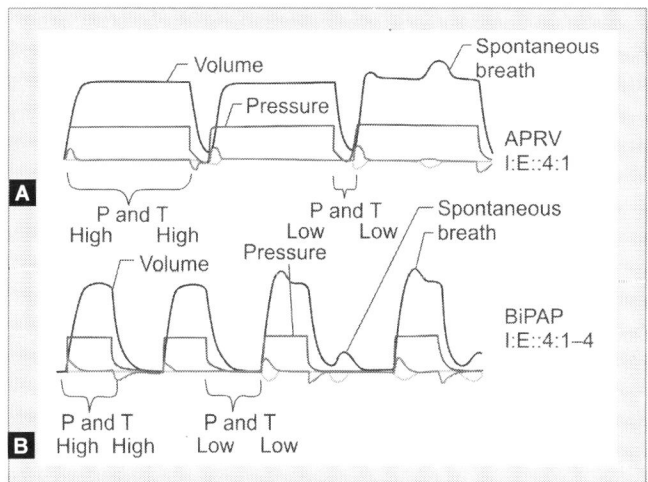

Figs. 4A and B: (A) Airway pressure release ventilation; and (B) Bilevel positive airway pressure are pressure controlled intermittent mandatory ventilation modes with spontaneous breaths allowed at any point without altering the ventilator delivered breaths. The main difference between the two is the time spend in high pressure or I:E ratio.
(APRV: airway pressure release ventilation; BiPAP: biphasic positive airway pressure)

TABLE 4: Various modifications if Bilevel ventilator modes	
Mode	Key features
BiPAP	Time cycled, pressure controlled, spontaneous breaths at both pressures allowed, T_{high} : T_{low}::1:1-4
BiPAP + PS	Pressure supported spontaneous breaths at P_{low}, weaning mode with increased T_{high}
APRV	Time cycled, pressure controlled, $T_{high} >>> T_{low}$ (4:1), spontaneous breaths P_{high} allowed, (Inverse ratio PCV)

(BiPAP: bilevel positive airway pressure; PS: pressure support; APRV: airway pressure release ventilation; PCV: pressure-controlled ventilation)

both, APRV and Biphasic modes, the pressure set for inspiration and expiration is delivered at set time intervals for mandatory breaths, and spontaneous ventilation is possible at any point during inspiration or expiration, i.e., patients breaths do not trigger a mechanical breath. Any ventilator capable of delivering Biphasic mode can deliver APRV or vice versa with main difference in these modes being extremes of I:E settings. **Table 4** compares the characteristics of breaths delivered by combination of Bilevel modes.

Biphasic modes are both for ventilation and weaning. As there is unrestricted spontaneous breathing, it improves synchrony, reduces the need of sedation and promotes weaning.[15] As spontaneous respiration is preserved, there is better distribution of ventilation to dependent areas of the lung hence, improving ventilation/perfusion ratio and gas exchange. Any positive pressure ventilation increases the intrathoracic pressure, thus, reducing the venous return. This in turn leads to decrease in right and left ventricular filling, low stroke volume, and cardiac output, especially in hypovolemic patients. But Bilevel modes reduce the mechanical ventilation to a level that is sufficient to support spontaneous breathing and this helps to reduce effects of ventilation on hemodynamics.[16]

Airway pressure release ventilation: This mode was first described for providing adequate ventilation in acute lung injury patients while avoiding high airway pressures.[17] In acute respiratory distress syndrome (ARDS), the alveoli are flooded or collapsed, so there is high shunt fraction leading to difficulty in oxygenation. Providing a high CPAP of 35 cmH_2O at FiO_2 of 100% will open the alveoli, oxygen will diffuse across into the pulmonary capillaries and the problem of oxygenation will be solved but without tidal breathing the pCO_2 will rise. If TV is generated by allowing the patient to breathe above this baseline CPAP (or PEEP) of 35, the distending pressures will drastically rise, even if the TV is very low. On the other hand, TV can be provided by suddenly decompressing the airway by lowering the pressure to zero. APRV is based on this concept of ventilating the lung at high mean airway pressure (P_{high}) and depressurize the airway long enough for gas to escape but short enough to prevent them from collapsing, i.e., adjusting T_{low} <1.5 seconds.

Initial settings include FiO_2 of 100%, P_{high} of 30–35 cmH_2O and P_{low} of 0 cm of H_2O, T_{high} is usually kept to 4 seconds and T_{low} of 0.8 seconds. Mean airway pressure and FiO_2 determine oxygenation and frequency of releases, time spent in T_{low} and gradient from P_{high} to P_{low} determine ventilation. If oxygenation is low, T_{low} can be shortened but if ventilation is concerning, T_{low} can be lengthened. This will allow CO_2 to be ventilated but may result in alveolar derecruitment which can affect oxygenation.

The main goal of APRV is to maximize lung recruitment by maintaining a higher mean airway pressure and hence, improve oxygenation; whereas the main aim of biphasic mode is to improve patient-ventilator synchrony.[18] APRV is based on the "open lung approach, and benefits depend on judicious selection of P_{high} and P_{low}". By ventilating within the steep portion of the curve, it avoids over-distention during inspiration and collapse during expiration thus, providing lung-protective ventilation **(Fig. 5)**. Its other advantages include preservation of spontaneous ventilation at any point of the respiratory cycle during APRV, which accounts for about 30% of minute volume.[19] This results in improved V/Q matching, decreased dead space and shunt. Lastly, maintenance of relatively long inflation time helps to improve functional residual capacity and oxygenation.

Mandatory minute volume: This mode guarantees a predetermined (expired) minute volume (VE), to the patient. If the patient breathes spontaneously to achieve the preset VE, no mechanical breath is delivered. If the patient's VE is less than the preset, mechanical breaths are delivered so that the remainder minute volume is provided and total VE is equal to the preset value.[20] The ventilator settings include preset minute volume (VE) and TV of the mechanical breaths. In this mode, as the spontaneous breath rate of the patient changes,

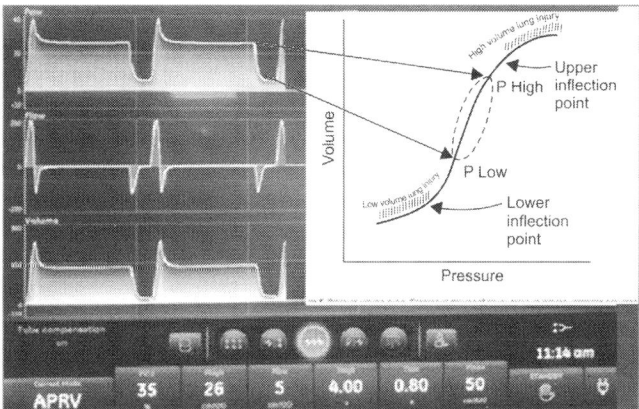

Fig. 5: Ventilator graphics in APRV. Pressure-volume curve show that high pressure ("P high") is set below the upper inflection point (UIP) and low pressure is set above the low inflection point (LIP). Corresponding flow curves depict that the flow curve goes back to zero at the end of inflation, indicating full lung inflation; and also goes back to zero during the release period before inflation starts, indicating complete gas exhalation with no intrinsic PEEP.
(APRV: airway pressure release ventilation; PEEP: positive end-expiratory pressure)

the rate of breaths delivered by the ventilator changes automatically, i.e., if spontaneous ventilation results in minute volume greater than the preset value, the rate of mandatory breaths progressively decreases and may even become zero. If spontaneous ventilation results in minute volume less than the preset minute volume value, the rate of mandatory breaths progressively increases but if patient has no spontaneous efforts at all, then all the breaths are machine triggered, volume or pressure controlled.

This ventilatory mode is similar to intermittent mandatory ventilation (IMV) where TV and rate of mechanical breaths is predetermined and patient is permitted to take spontaneous breaths in between these mechanical breaths. But if in IMV the predetermined respiratory rate is low, depression of spontaneous breathing due to any reason (e.g., sedation) leads to alveolar hypoventilation. However, this will not occur with MMV because the minute volume is predetermined not the respiratory rate, even if spontaneous ventilation is markedly depressed ensured VE is delivered. In spite of this, MMV is not a popular mode because fast and ineffective breathing with low TV to achieve the minute volume can result in auto-PEEP.[21] On the other hand, dead space may increase due to combination of delivering dangerously high-TVs and low respiratory rate.

SMART MODES (CLOSED-LOOP SYSTEMS)

The closed loop systems include ASV, PAV, NAVA, and knowledge-based systems (KBSs). PAV, NAVA, and KBS are basically advanced modifications of PSV **(Table 5)**.

TABLE 5: Comparison of the key characteristics of breaths of newer modes that adapt to changing lung characteristics

	PAV	NAVA	KBS	ASV
Principle	P_{insp} proportional to $Flow_{insp}$	P_{insp} proportional to EAdi	P_{insp} to maintain RR in comfort zone	P_{insp} and RR to minimize the WOB
Breath type	PSV	PSV	PSV	PSV/PCV/P-SIMV
Passive patient	No	No	No	Yes
Active patient	Yes	Yes	Yes	Yes
Automatic weaning	No	No	Yes	Yes

(PAV: proportional assist ventilation; NAVA: neurally adjusted ventilatory assist; KBS: knowledge-based systems; ASV: adaptive support ventilation; PSV: pressure support ventilation; PCV: pressure-controlled ventilation; RR: respiratory rate; WOB: work of breathing; SIMV: synchronized intermittent mandatory ventilation)

Adaptive support ventilation/adaptive ventilation mode 2: The next step in evolution from MMV is the ASV as it uses a closed loop feedback mechanism to achieve "Optimal" strategy to decrease the WOB. The machine selects the rate and TV according to the patient's respiratory mechanics that the brain would opt for if the patient was not on a ventilator. Hence, this mode provides specific minute ventilation and breathing pattern in a tailor-made fashion so that the total energy expenditure is minimal.[22] Thus, ASV is distinct from other modes that it provides both, total ventilatory support during the initiation and maintenance of mechanical ventilation and partial support during weaning. ASV works as PSV if the patient's respiratory rate is higher than the target, but works as pressure controlled mode if there is no spontaneous effort; and lastly when patient's respiratory rate (RR) is lower than target it works as synchronized IMV. Hence, the criteria for cycling off are flow in case of pressure support mode or time based for mandatory breaths in PCV or SIMV. As ASV is a combination of various modes is regarded as either "no mode", "integrated mode" or "three in one".

The automatic calculation of the minute ventilation by the ventilator in ASV is based on patient's ideal weight and the dead space (Vd = 2.2 mL/kg). This represents 100% of minute ventilation. The intensivist then sets a target percent of minute ventilation that the ventilator will support i.e. 100% support of minute ventilation in the patient of sepsis or ARDS (who have increased requirements) or 10–25% during weaning. Thus, minute ventilation (VE) delivered is actually the ratio between the minute ventilation calculated from ideal body weight (IBW) and percentage of minute ventilation (% VM) set by the operator. Then based on the inputs from the respiratory mechanics, i.e., resistance, compliance, auto-PEEP, the ventilator system selects the target ventilatory pattern. The concept of ASV is based on the *Otis equation* which states that for any given level of alveolar ventilation, there is a particular RR which achieves a lower WOB. From the data of respiratory mechanics, ASV logarithm calculates the ideal rate and volume combination which results in lowest WOB **(Fig. 6)**.

$$\text{Otis equation} = f = \frac{1 + 2a \times RC \times \dfrac{\text{Min Vol} - (f \times V_d)}{V_d} - 1}{a \times RC}$$

It also adjusts the I:E ratio and inspiratory pressure from the analysis of flow-volume curve and expiratory time constants so that the target volume is within the safety limit. The only ventilator settings in ASV include patient's sex and height for calculation of IBW, percentage of predicted minute ventilation (% MV), PEEP, FiO_2 and maximum pressure alarm (P_{max}).

Any change in the respiratory mechanics and spontaneous efforts of the patient are accompanied by alteration in the breathing pattern that results in higher energy efficiency and minimal effort. Thus, it ensures effective alveolar ventilation, minimizes WOB, optimal ventilation to reduce the risk of complications such as air trapping, barotrauma and volutrauma.[23]

Automatic tube compensation or automatic resistance compensation: Weaning is feasible with all modes which allow spontaneous efforts and delivery of breaths. PSV as sole mode or with various controlled mode combinations is often used as weaning mode. The real challenge following initiation of mechanical ventilation is successful weaning from mechanical ventilation and tracheal extubation. Increase in workload and preload may result in

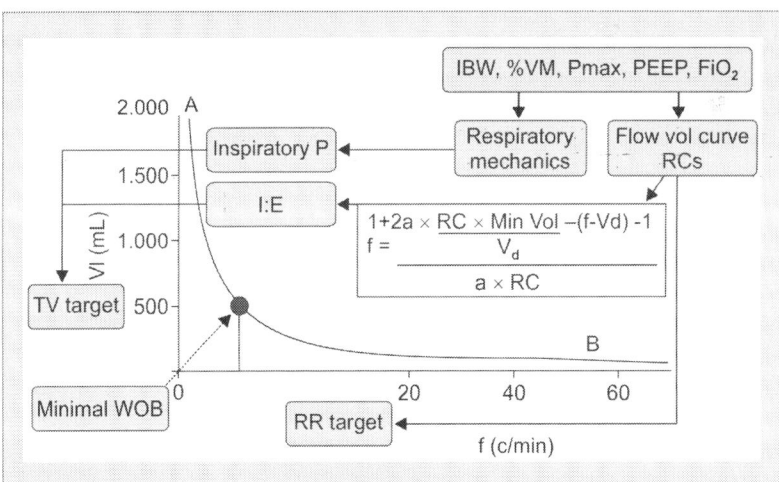

Fig. 6: Describes the operating principles of ASV. "A" shows the point of high WOB with low RR and high TV to overcome elastic pulmonary and thoracic forces. "B" point shows high WOB with high RR and low TV to overcome the resistance of flow. The ideal RR and TV is calculated by the Otis equation where f = RR, RC = airway resistance × respiratory compliance = time constant, Min Vol = minute volume, V_d = dead space, a = $(2\pi^2)/60$ = 0.33 (constant for sinusoidal flow).
(ASV: adaptive support ventilation; RR: respiratory rate; TV: tidal volume; WOB: work of breathing; IBW: ideal body weight; RC: resistance-compliance)

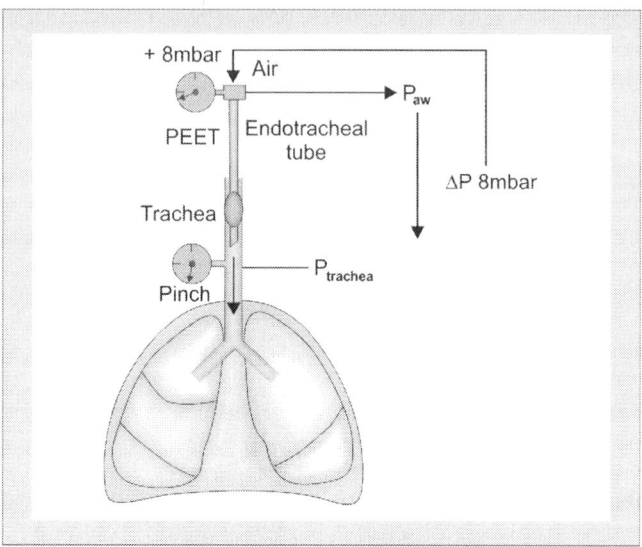

Fig. 7: $\Delta P = P_{aw}/P_{ETT} - P_{trachea}$ is measured to be 8mbar, a pressure support of 8 is added to the inspiration in ATC.
(ATC: automatic tube compensation)

failure despite successful spontaneous breathing trial (SBT) on T-piece or low support PSV. Another issue is delayed or failed weaning secondary to increased airway resistance imposed by the presence of endotracheal tube (ETT) leading to increased WOB. ATC overcomes these problems by transferring the work done by the patient (without ATC) to the ventilator (with ATC on).[24] Nowadays some ventilators have an in-built ATC facility (e.g., Evita XL, Drager Medical, PuritanBennett, 840).

Automatic tube compensation uses a closed loop mechanism to continuously calculate tracheal pressure ($P_{trachea}$). The pressure difference between the proximal end of the ETT and the tracheal pressure is then provided by the ventilator to overcome the resistance offered by the ETT ($\Delta P = P_{ETT} - P_{TRAC}$) **(Fig. 7)**. This means that ventilator with ATC provides variable pressure support to compensate for any variation in flow depending on whether patients are sleep or awake, calm or agitated. ATC simulates spontaneous breathing without ETT, hence also called "electronic extubation".

The P_{ETT} depends on flow rate and tube specifications—diameter and length [ETT/tracheal tube (TT) size has to be entered in the ventilator]. Tube factors are fixed (diameter and length), however, external factors like partial obstruction of the tube with secretions or kinking may lead to uncompensated resistance of the ETT even in ATC mode on.

As ATC decreases the WOB by overcoming the resistance of the tube, in theory it can enhance the weaning process more effectively than other common modes as CPAP or PSV **(Figs. 8A and B)**. But many trials have not shown superiority of ATC to other SBT methods because extubation failure and re-intubation rates in ICUs are low (10–20% of all extubations) and many are due to excessive secretions, inadequate cough, or abnormal mental status.[25]

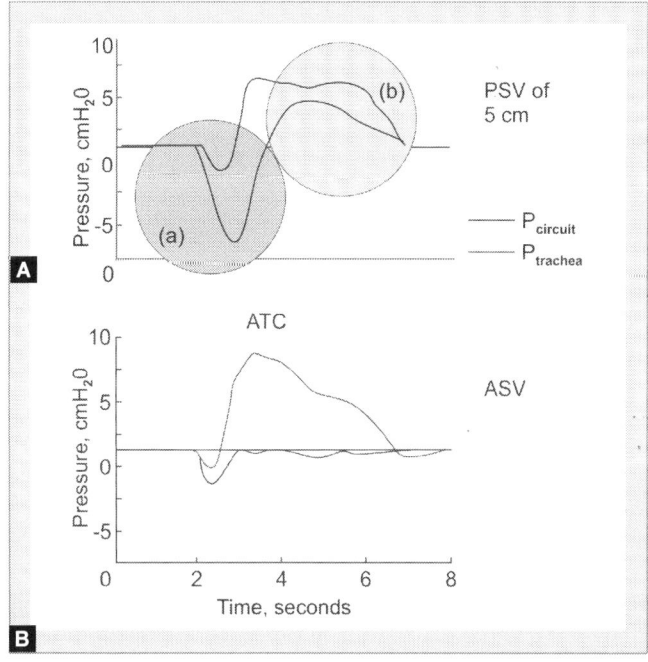

Figs. 8A and B: (A) Comparison of fixed PS and ATC. Airway resistance depends upon current gas flow, if PS is fixed (5 cmH₂O) throughout inspiration it may lead to under compensation as flow rate is high but PS is low (a) so patients will have to do more work to overcome resistance of ETT. At end of inspiration flow rate is low, fixed PS of 5 cm may be more than what is required therefore overcompensating for artificial airway resistance (b); (B) In ATC, PS is high at the beginning of breath and low at end of inspiration as flow rate decreases.
(PSV: pressure support ventilation; ATC: automatic tube compensation; PS: pressure support; ETT: endotracheal tube)

For ATC to be proven superior, re-intubation should only be contributed by increased WOB rather than other causes. Hence, although ATC is a safe, its use in routine clinical advantage is still controversial.

Proportional-assist ventilation: As the name suggests this mode provides assistance to each breath proportional to the instantaneous effort of the patient.[26] When the patient generates a breath by muscle contraction; the changes in the gas flow and volume from the ventilator toward the patient are detected by the ventilator as the inspiratory effort of the patient. This flow and volume are then amplified by the ventilator by respective gain controls such that their sum generates the control signal which is equal to the pressure support response of the ventilator. Automatic adjustments of flow, volume, and pressure occur in each breath. It is different from PSV, where a constant level of pressure support is generated by the ventilator throughout inspiration, independent of the patient's effort. While in PAV, the pressure applied is dependent on the effort of the patient, where the percentage of support to be delivered is preset: greater the inspiratory effort by the patient, the greater the increase in pressure applied by the ventilator **(Box 2)**.

> **BOX 2:** PAV: Algorithm.
> - Four initial breaths are delivered
> - An end-inspiratory maneuver is performed at end of each breath that yields patient's compliance and resistance
> - The first breath delivered uses the predicted value of resistance (according to the size of artificial airway) and estimation for compliance is based on patient's ideal body weight
> - Each valid measurement is then factored in until the 5th breath, which is first PAV breath
> - Measurements for respirator mechanics (compliance and resistance) are then intermittently repeated every 4–10 breaths
> - Flow and volume are also assessed after every 5 milliseconds
>
> (PAV: proportional assist ventilation)

Proportional-assist ventilation is similar to pressure support mode as all breaths are spontaneous and the RR as well as TV of each breath are controlled by the patient. Ventilator settings to be done include: airway type (ETT, TT), airway size (inner diameter), percentage of assist (ranging from 5 to 95%), limit of TV and pressure as safety measures.

According to equation of motion, pressure is required to generate a flow and deliver a given TV. In order to do so, the pressure must overcome the resistance (flow × resistance) and elastance (volume × elastance) of the respiratory system. It is calculated by P_{total} = flow × resistance + volume × elastance. During assisted ventilation, this pressure is partially generated by the patient and partially by the ventilator. In PAV, mechanical characteristics of the patient, i.e., the resistance and elastance are estimated in the first breath and then intermittently and the pressure assistance is provided by the ventilator by altering flow and volume according to the formula, P_{vent} = % flow assist × Resistance + % volume assist × elastance.

It does the real time assessment of WOB. This mode increases patient comfort by improving synchrony between neural and machine inflation time (neuro-ventilatory coupling). Hence, the need of paralysis and/or sedation decreases. As it automatically adapts to the changes in the lung mechanics and patient's efforts, the need for ventilator intervention and manipulation decreases.[27] Noninvasive use of PAV in Kyphoscoliosis and chronic obstructive pulmonary disease patients improves dyspnea score also.

Neurally Adjusted Ventilator Assist

It is a new assisted mode of ventilation that delivers a synchronized breath in proportion to the patient's effort. This mode is distinct from other modes in not being dependent on pressure, volume or flow sensing as trigger, rather it uses electrical activity of the diaphragm (EAdi) as a signal for controlling inspiratory and expiratory cycling by the ventilator[28] **(Flowchart 2)**. A modified nasogastric tube with microelectrodes at the distal tip is placed at the level of the diaphragm to record the EAdi. The EAdi signal is a direct measure of the impulses from the respiratory control center that result in activation of the diaphragm. The amplitude of this signal depends on the intensity and frequency of the involved

Flowchart 2: NAVA delivers ventilator assist in proportion to the neural inspiratory effort, a new approach to mechanical ventilation based on neural respiratory output which is different from the convention and much closer to the ideal technology.

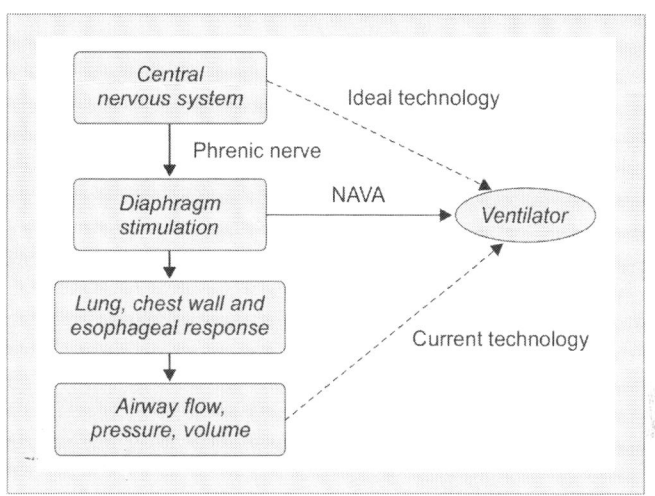

(NAVA: neural adjusted ventilator assist)

motor units of the diaphragm and hence is a measure of the strength of the breath taken by the patient. The inspiration begins when the EAdi rises above the expiratory level to the threshold level that has been set as, inspiratory cycling = EAdi exp + 0.5–2 µV, i.e., set threshold level. When the signal from the diaphragm EAdi falls to 70% of the maximum inspiratory value, expiration is cycled. As in PAV, inspiratory support is always in direct proportion to the efforts of the patient and proportionality constant, also known as the NAVA level, is set by the operator. All the ventilatory settings such as inspiratory time, I:E ratio, frequency are self-determined by the patient and the only setting done by the operator is the gain above the electrographic diaphragmatic potential (EAdi) to trigger inspiration.

Neurally adjusted ventilator assist is said to offer the greatest level of patient ventilator synchrony because the duration of inspiration and expiration delivered by the ventilator is adjusted by the neural signals from the respiratory control center.[29] Mechanical response of the diaphragm is triggered 20 ms after the signal originates in the brain, and this is four times more rapid as compared to the response time of other ventilators based on pneumatic trigger **(Fig. 9)**. Studies have shown significantly enhanced patient ventilator synchrony, greater variability in breathing pattern and lesser over-assistance by the ventilator with NAVA. As NAVA is independent of the physical properties of the circuit, the problems arising from leak of the circuit and auto PEEP do not affect the ventilatory cycle.[30] Leakage in the circuit can falsely trigger the ventilator in conventional modes and lead to dys-synchrony which is not seen in NAVA. The inspiratory efforts that do not trigger the ventilator (ineffective effort) virtually disappear with NAVA.

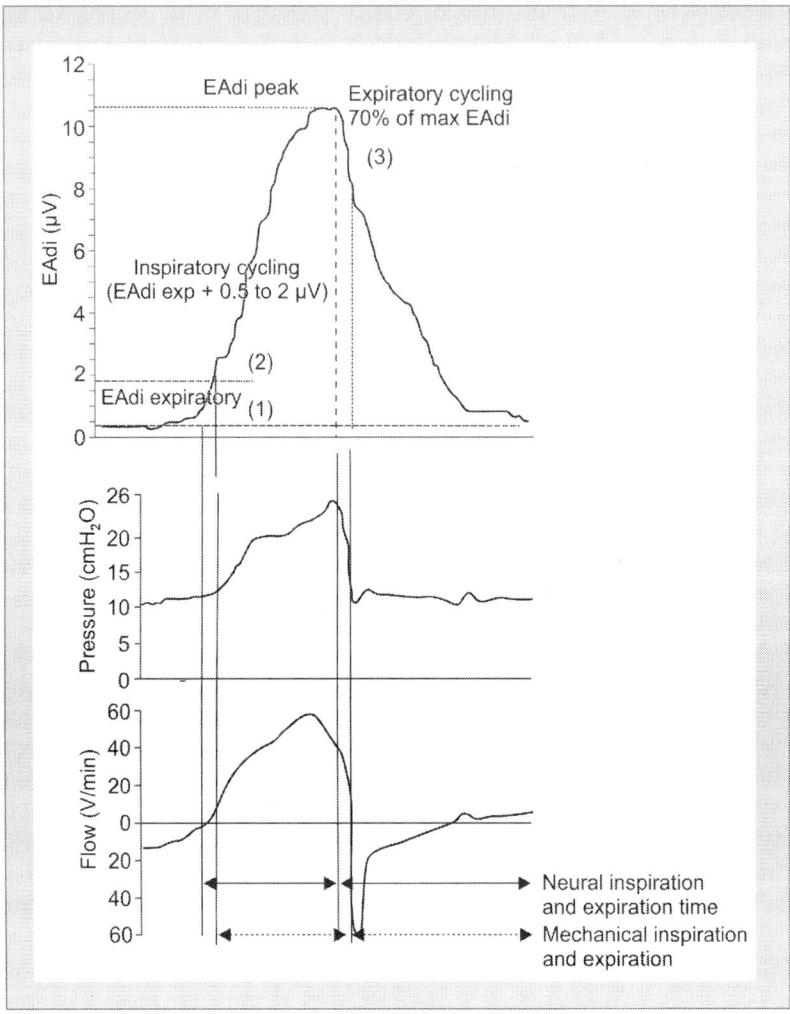

Fig. 9: Electrical activity of the diaphragm (EAdi) signal during ventilation in NAVA. The start of inspiration is marked by the increase in EAdi activity (1) from the expiratory value which is usually 0, under normal conditions. At the point where EAdi reaches a threshold value (2) the ventilator starts to assist, till the EAdi drops to 70% of the maximum value (3). The neural and mechanical inspiratory and expiratory times are also shown.

PHYSIOLOGICAL CLOSED-LOOP VENTILATION AND HIGHLY AUTOMATED SYSTEMS—NEOGANESH SMARTCARE

Automation is evolving day by day to target the set variable through closed loops. The current strategy for choosing mode of ventilation and parameter setting is very complex and based on the clinician's knowledge and experience. In addition to clinical parameters, intensivists consider the protective guidelines, hemodynamic status, transpulmonary pressure along with mechanical power etc. The INTELLiVENT®®-ASV®® (commercially available from Hamilton Medical AG, Bonaduz, Switzerland) is one such system which takes input of patient characteristics and settings of the control targets (EtCO$_2$ and SpO$_2$) to adjust ventilator support to meet the targets.[31] Another example of closed loop automation was GANESH system (using the EtCO$_2$, RR, and TV as inputs for their controller to adjust the level of PSV) which was later improved to a new level called NéoGanesh, which is equipped with not only sophisticated knowledge but also, temporal reasoning controller for a *"zone of comfort"*.

This is available as SmartCare®®/PS from Dräger (Drägerwerk AG, Lübeck, Germany).

NeoGanesh-SmartCare (Automated Adjustment of Pressure Support)

It is a closed loop modification of the PSV that is based on artificial intelligence. It is an automated knowledge-based weaning system that stabilizes the

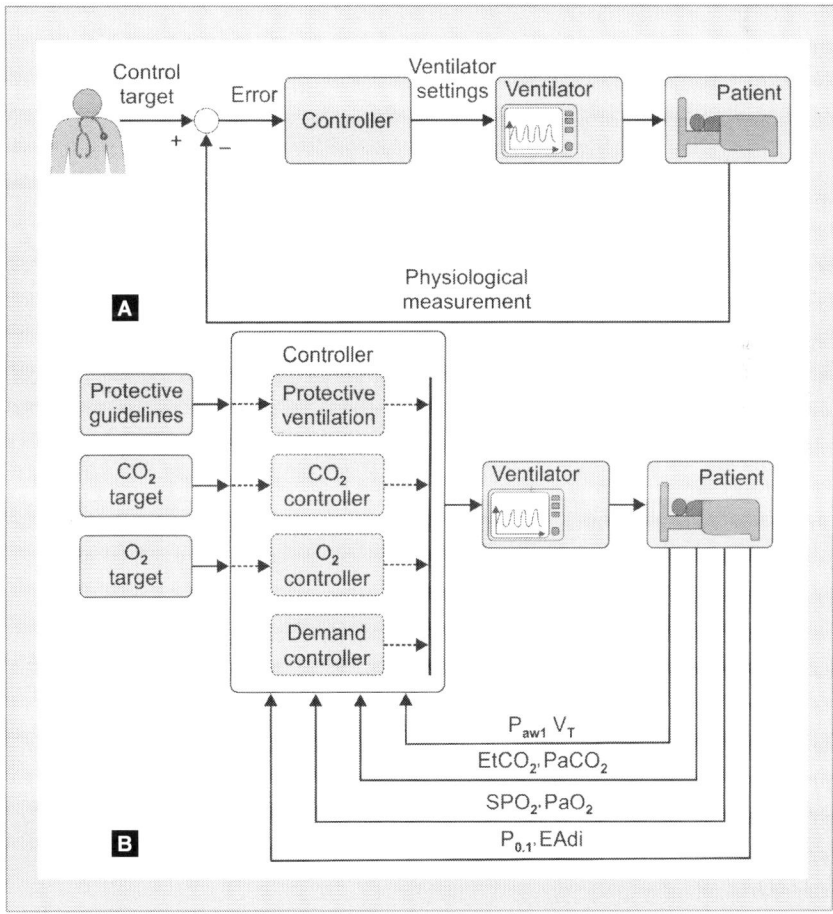

Figs. 10A and B: (A) Physiological closed-loop control (PCLC) for mechanical ventilation system; (B) The physiological measurements like RR, EtCO$_2$, tidal volume from the patient give feed back to the controller in the presented PCLC systems.

patient's spontaneous breathing in the comfort zone and reduces inspiratory support until the patient can be extubated.[32] The algorithm incorporated is based on patient's respiratory pattern and evidence from weaning protocols which adjusts the level of PS. The level of PS is elevated, if insufficient assist is the diagnosis based on increasing RR and other factors, or level of PS is reduced, if diagnosis is over assist based on the feedback from the TV, RR, and $EtCO_2$ values. In case of normal ventilation, the ventilator can gradually wean off PS and can self-initiate SBT based on pre-recorded clinical protocols. Literature shows evidence that it can significantly reduce the duration of weaning as well as incidence of weaning failures **(Figs. 10A and B)**.

CONCLUSION

The newer modes no doubt improve patient-ventilator synchrony, safety, oxygenation, and hasten the weaning process but there is lack of good quality of evidence for better patient outcome with their use. Man and machine interface play a major role. Further, any potential of harm with these modes has not been reported. Hence, better gas exchange and synchrony may not necessarily improve survival, new may not necessarily be better. Conventional modes being user friendly continue to be used most commonly in the intensive care while better understanding, training and long-term studies will prove the efficacy of newer modes.

KEY POINTS

- Newer ventilatory modes are targeted to achieve safety goals in addition to oxygenation and carbon dioxide wash out with minimal stress and strain.
- These modes and strategies focus on lung protective ventilation using plateau pressure less than 30 cmH_2O, but future is marching to include transpulmonary pressure as standard and ventilation targeting driving pressure. This will use minimal energy and protects right ventricular function also in addition to lung protection.
- Dual ventilation modes incorporate merits of both volume and pressure preset modes such as volume assured pressure support (VAPS), and PRVS. With assurance of volume and pressure limitation, these improve safety as well as ensure adequate ventilation.
- Modes adapting to lung characteristics use microprocessors to vary support within the same breath or from breath to breath, such as proportional assist ventilation (PAV), neurally adjusted ventilatory assistance (NAVA), adaptive support ventilation (ASV), etc. to improve the patient ventilator synchrony.
- Time controlled modes such as biphasic intermittent positive airway pressure (BIPAP), airway pressure release ventilation (APRV) are combinations of pressure-controlled ventilation (PCV) and spontaneous pressure support ventilation (PSV), and help ventilating the heterogenous alveoli in hypoxemic respiratory failure [acute respiratory distress syndrome (ARDS)] with lower mean airway pressures, also facilitating spontaneous ventilation.
- Physiological closed-loop ventilation (PCLC) and highly automated systems—NeoGanesh SmartCare are the upcoming technology, may help to ventilate difficult patients in near future.

REFERENCES

1. Mireles-Cabodevila E, Hatipoglu U, Chatburn RL. A rational framework for selecting modes of ventilation. Respir Care. 2013;58(2):348-66.
2. Mireles-Cabodevila E, Diaz-Guzman E, Heresi GA, Chatburn RL. Alternative modes of mechanical ventilation: a review for the hospitalist. Cleve Clin J Med. 2009;76(7):417-30.
3. van der Staay M, Chatburn RL. Advanced modes of mechanical ventilation and optimal targeting schemes. Intensive Care Med Exp. 2018;6(1):30.
4. Marini JJ. Evolving concepts for safer ventilation. Crit Care. 2019;23(Suppl 1):114.
5. Oscroft NS, Smith IE. A bench test to confirm the core features of volume-assured non-invasive ventilation. Respirology. 2010;15(2):361-4.
6. Okuda M, Kashio M, Tanaka N, Fujii T, Okuda Y. Positive outcome of average volume-assured pressure support mode of a Respironics V60 Ventilator in acute exacerbation of chronic obstructive pulmonary disease: a case report. J Med Case Rep. 2012;6:284.
7. Sottiaux TM. Patient-ventilator interactions during volume-support ventilation: asynchrony and tidal volume instability—a report of three cases. Respir Care. 2001;46(3):255-62.
8. Donn SM, Sinha SK. Newer modes of mechanical ventilation for the neonate. Curr Opin Pediatr. 2001;13(2):99-103.
9. Singh G, Chien C, Patel S. Pressure Regulated Volume Control (PRVC): set it and forget it? Respir Med Case Rep. 2019;29:100822.
10. Guldager H, Nielsen SL, Carl P, Soerensen MB. A comparison of volume control and pressure-regulated volume control ventilation in acute respiratory failure. Crit Care. 1997;1(2):75-7.
11. Betensley AD, Khalid I, Crawford J, Pensler RA, DiGiovine B. Patient comfort during pressure support and volume controlled continuous mandatory ventilation. Respir Care. 2008;53(7):897-902.
12. Kallet RH, Campbell AR, Dicker RA, Katz JA, Mackersie RC. Work of breathing during lung-protective ventilation in patients with acute lung injury and acute respiratory distress syndrome: a comparison between volume and pressure-regulated breathing modes. Respir Care. 2005;50(12):1623-31.
13. Putensen C, Wrigge H. Clinical review: Biphasic positive airway pressure and airway pressure release ventilation. Crit Care. 2004;8(6):492-7.
14. Rose L, Hawkins M. Airway pressure release ventilation and biphasic positive airway pressure: a systematic review of definitional criteria. Intensive Care Med. 2008;34(10):1766-73.
15. Rathgeber J, Schorn B, Falk V, Kazmaier S, Spiegel T, Burchardi H. The influence of controlled mandatory ventilation (CMV), intermittent mandatory ventilation (IMV) and biphasic intermittent positive airway pressure (BIPAP) on duration of intubation and consumption of analgesics and sedatives. A prospective analysis in 596 patients following adult cardiac surgery. Eur J Anaesthesiol. 1997;14(6):576-82.
16. Räsänen J, Downs JB, Stock MC. Cardiovascular effects of conventional positive pressure ventilation and airway pressure release ventilation. Chest. 1988;93(5):911-5.
17. Baum M, Benzer H, Putensen C, Koller W, Putz G. [Biphasic positive airway pressure (BIPAP)—a new form of augmented ventilation]. Anaesthesist. 1989;38(9):452-8.
18. Varpula T, Valta P, Niemi R, Takkunen O, Hynynen M, Pettilä VV. Airway pressure release ventilation as a primary ventilatory mode in acute respiratory distress syndrome. Acta Anaesthesiol Scand. 2004;48(6):722-31.

19. Myers TR, MacIntyre NR. Respiratory controversies in the critical care setting. Does airway pressure release ventilation offer important new advantages in mechanical ventilator support? Respir Care. 2007;52(4):452-8.
20. Guthrie SO, Lynn C, Lafleur BJ, Donn SM, Walsh WF. A crossover analysis of mandatory minute ventilation compared to synchronized intermittent mandatory ventilation in neonates. J Perinatol. 2005;25(10):643-6.
21. Singh PM, Borle A, Trikha A. Newer nonconventional modes of mechanical ventilation. J Emerg Trauma Shock. 2014;7(3):222-7.
22. Fernández J, Miguelena D, Mulett H, Godoy J, Martinón Torres F. Adaptive support ventilation: state of the art review. Indian J Crit Care Med. 2013;17(1):16-22.
23. Dongelmans DA, Veelo DP, Paulus F, de Mol BA, Korevaar JC, Kudoga A, et al. Weaning automation with adaptive support ventilation: a randomized controlled trial in cardiothoracic surgery patients. Anesth Analg. 2009;108(2):565-71.
24. Selek C, Ozcan PE, Orhun G, Şenturk E, Akinci IO, Cakar N. The comparison of automatic tube compensation (ATC) and T-piece during weaning. Turk J Anaesthesiol Reanim. 2014;42(2):91-5.
25. Cohen JD, Shapiro M, Grozovski E, Singer P. Automatic tube compensation-assisted respiratory rate to tidal volume ratio improves the prediction of weaning outcome. Chest. 2002;122(3):980-4.
26. Kondili E, Prinianakis G, Alexopoulou C, Vakouti E, Klimathianaki M, Georgopoulos D. Respiratory load compensation during mechanical ventilatio—proportional assist ventilation with load-adjustable gain factors versus pressure support. Intensive Care Med. 2006;32:692-9.
27. Bosma K, Ferreyra G, Ambrogio C, Pasero D, Mirabella L, Braghiroli A, et al. Patient ventilator interaction and sleep in mechanically ventilated patients: pressure support versus proportional assist ventilation. Crit Care Med. 2007;35(4):1048-54.
28. Verbrugghe W, Jorens PG. Neurally adjusted ventilatory assist: A ventilation tool or a ventilation toy? Respir Care. 2011;56:327-35.
29. Biban P, Serra A, Polese G, Soffiati M, Santuz P. Neurally adjusted ventilatory assist: A new approach to mechanically ventilated infants. J Matern Fetal Neonatal Med. 2010;23(Suppl 3):38-40.
30. Terzi N, Piquilloud L, Rozé H, Mercat A, Lofaso F, Delisle S, et al. Clinical review: Update on neurally adjusted ventilatory assist—report of a round table conference. Crit Care. 2012;16(3):225.
31. Lellouche F, Brochard L. Advanced closed loops during mechanical ventilation (PAV, NAVA, ASV, SmartCare). Best Pract Res Clin Anaesthesiol. 2009;23(1):81-93.
32. Platen PV, Pomprapa A, Lachmann B, Leonhardt S. The dawn of physiological closed-loop ventilation—a review. Crit Care. 2020;24(1):121.

CHAPTER 21

New Cardiac Drugs Anesthesia Implications

Neeti Makhija, Rohan Magoon

INTRODUCTION

Cardiovascular anesthesia practice involves the application of a wide range of pharmacological therapies belonging to diverse classes. Various indications range from symptomatic relief, preoperative cardiac stabilization for congestive heart failure (CHF) and angina, heart-rate and rhythm control, prevention of thromboembolic consequences, positive metabolic-modulation to systemic and pulmonary hemodynamic optimization. The pace of developments in the cardiovascular medicine has been rampant with the underlying impetus being largely driven by the ever-growing need for favorably modulating the adverse-effect profile of the existing drugs and to augment emphasis on recognizing newer agents that present the potential of treating the current cardiac pathologies with the aid of novel mechanistic pathways.[1] Alongside the approval of novel drugs and synergistic drug combinations, other evolving pharmacological developments include: novel indications, novel administration routes, consensus on the dosing regimen and efficacy and safety of the existing drugs in a new patient subset.

The attending anesthesiologist needs to be updated with the rapid drug developments in the field of cardiovascular medicine for an efficient management of both perioperative and intensive care scenarios. In addition, a sound knowledge of the drugs assist an anesthesiologist in formulation of pragmatic decisions on the preoperative continuation or discontinuation of drugs, comprehend the possible drug-drug interactions, consequential electrolyte alterations and the associated hemodynamic perturbations. This chapter reviews the pharmacological drug-classes that have witnessed considerable developments over the last decade and their implication in anesthesia practice.

ANTIARRHYTHMICS

Antiarrhythmic therapy is limited to a great extent by:
- Inadequate efficacy across the range of arrhythmias.
- Narrow safety-margin.
- Cardiac and extracardiac toxicity potential.

Amiodarone, though employed as a wide-spectrum antiarrhythmic, tends to accumulate in tissues on prolonged administration, culminating in significant organ toxicity. Several new compounds premised on the structural and electrophysiological characteristics of amiodarone have been recently developed.

Dronedarone such as amiodarone, is a deiodinated benzofuran with a potentially attenuated iodine-associated toxicity. The side-chain amendment results in diminished lipophilicity and considerably shortened half-life with a declined tissue-accumulation in contrast to amiodarone.[1] This moderately effective Vaughan William (VW) class III drug was approved by the Food and Drug Administration (FDA) for paroxysmal or persistent atrial fibrillation (AF) or flutter treatment in 2009 primarily premised on the report of ATHENA (A Trial with Dronedarone to Prevent Hospitalization or Death in Patients With Atrial Fibrillation) trial. The aforementioned placebo-controlled trial evaluated 400 mg twice a day dronedarone dose in patients with AF or flutter, outlining a substantial mortality reduction.[2] However, reports of hepatic toxicity necessitates concomitant liver-function monitoring.[3] In addition, ANDROMEDA (Antiarrhythmic trial with Dronedarone in Moderate to severe congestive heart failure Evaluating morbidity Decrease) trial suggested a worsened CHF with dronedarone treatment in patients with pre-existent moderate-severe failure, contraindicating the drug in Class IV CHF patients or the cohort with a history of recent cardiac decompensation.[4] Nausea, diarrhea, abdominal cramps, QT interval prolongation and bradycardia include other drug side effects, along with remarkable interactions with verapamil and diltiazem which may increase dronedarone levels on concomitant administration while dronedarone therapy may increase beta-blocker, digoxin and simvastatin levels.[5]

An increasing recognition of the fact that AF emanates as a consequence of an altered atrial tissue structure or function has prompted the search for atrial-selective targets as AF management options. These include certain important ionic-current targets (IKACh, IKur) and connexins (Cx-40).[6]

Vernakalant, an atrial-selective agent is in advanced investigation stage for the treatment of AF.[7] It is an atrial repolarization-delaying therapeutic agent with primary target being IKur (sustained outward potassium current). As IKur manifests in a substantial proportion in the atria, the drug has a predominant effect in fibrillating atria and is consequently much less proarrhythmogenic. Furthermore, it has multichannel blocking properties affecting the sodium-channels and IK-Ach both demonstrating a predominant atrial expression. Subsequent to the inhibition of the potassium ionic currents, vernakalant results in atrial refractoriness, and frequency as well as voltage-dependent sodium-channel block causes a significant impact on the intra-atrial conduction, especially at fast rates. This is plausibly the relevant most electrophysiological effect with regards to the AF termination. The drug is contraindicated in subjects with systolic hypotension <100 mm Hg, significant aortic stenosis, New York Heart Association (NYHA) functional class III and IV CHF and QT interval prolongation.

Recently, efforts to validate "upstream" therapies for AF targeting atrial remodeling have gained popularity.[8] Therapies altering rennin-angiotensin axis, alongside the anti-inflammatory and antioxidative therapies, are under investigation as monotherapy and as combination therapies in conjunction with the conventional antiarrhythmics. These include: angiotensin-converting enzyme (ACE) inhibitors, angiotensin-receptor blockers, statins, w-3 polyunsaturated fatty acids, glucocorticoids, spironolactone and pirfenidone.

Ranolazine and ivabradine, currently approved as antianginals, (discussed later in the chapter) are being investigated as add-on therapy in recurrent ventricular tachycardia (VT) in view of effects on the late inward Na current (INaL) and If current respectively classifying these agents as VW class I. They increase the diastolic excitation threshold, reduce the conduction velocity, and prolong the effective refractory period (ERP) in atria; all the more induce a notable accentuation of the postrepolarization refractoriness (ERP prolonged further beyond the repolarization).[9-11]

Azimilide is primarily an investigational VW Class III antiarrhythmic agent that transpires with the aim of pharmacological management of both supraventricular and ventricular tachyarrhythmias. Akin to the Class III antiarrhythmics, azimilide results in prolongation of the myocardial repolarization in a dose-dependent fashion by blocking multiple potassium currents enhancing the action-potential duration, QT interval, and ERP. The drug has been studied quite extensively in the ALIVE trial with no consequent effect on survival. However, the reduction in the rate of AF in the participants coupled with the ability of the drug to maintain sinus rhythm emerged as a remarkable finding of the above-mentioned trial.[12]

Piboserod, a novel drug, blocks atrial serotonin in 5-hydroxytryptaine (5-HT4) receptors which are in preponderance in human atrial cells. The stimulation of these pathways in general potentiates atrial arrhythmias. Piboserod is being investigated for sinus rhythm maintenance in AF.[13]

Adenosine augments the termination of the supraventricular tachycardia (SVT) in subjects with atrioventricular (AV) nodal re-entry by stimulating the A1 receptor of the adenosine family. Simultaneous stimulation of the A2A, A2B, and A3 adenosine-receptors occurs in the background of a nonselective mechanistic action. The drug has a range of side-effects, which include dyspnea, flushing, and chest discomfort. Therefore, a more selective A1 receptor agonists have been developed for SVT termination.[14] These include *selodenoson, tecadenoson and PJ-875* which are currently under investigation.

ANTICOAGULANTS

The introduction of low-molecular weight heparin (LMWH) and fondaparinux has particularly simplified the drug-regime of arterial or venous thrombosis considering these agents can be administered subcutaneously without strict coagulation monitoring, and carry a lower potential for heparin-induced thrombocytopenia (HIT).[15] However, the long-term use of the agents is limited by the propensity for accumulation in renal failure, the absence of antidote, and the potential to result in catheter thrombosis. **Flowchart 1** illustrates the

Flowchart 1: Classification of anticoagulant drugs.

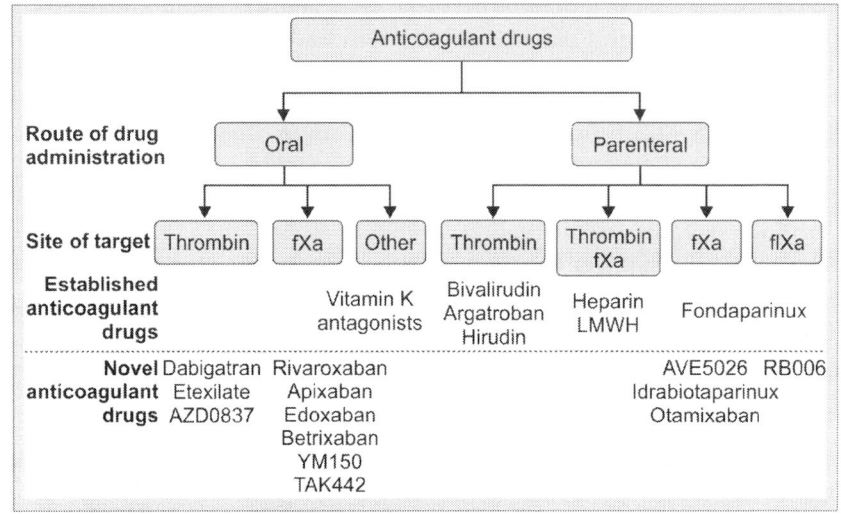

(fXa: factor Xa; fIXa: factor IX a; LMWH: low-molecular-weight heparin)

evolution of anticoagulant drugs and presents their mechanistic action and administrative routes.

Bivalirudin, (an engineered, bivalent 20-amino acid hirudin analog), is a parenteral direct thrombin inhibitor (DTI) which can also be used in patients with HIT, thus presenting an effective safe heparin alternative. The brevity of its half-life (25 minutes) precludes the need for an antidote therapy, albeit it can potentially accumulate in renal failure.[16] Interestingly, the dose-titration in accordance with the results of point-of-care coagulation tests (POCT) constitutes a practical advantage of heparin and bivalirudin over enoxaparin or fondaparinux, particularly in the clinical setting of percutaneous coronary intervention (PCI). Other parenteral DTIs include: *lepirudin, desirudin, and argatroban*.

Several new parenteral anticoagulant agents targeting factor Xa (fXa) in advanced developmental stages are: *AVE5026, idrabiotaparinux and otamixaban*. *RB006*, an anticoagulant ribonucleic acid (RNA) aptamer, has a highly specific target: factor IXa.[17,18] The new parenteral agents have a rampant onset of action with a more predictable anticoagulant effect, which in the context of idrabiotaparinux and RB006, can be offset by the neutralization augmented by intravenous (IV) avidin or RB007, respectively.

However, the greatest unmet need in the present times, is for the oral anticoagulants which can potentially replace vitamin K antagonists (VKAs). VKAs, such as the prototypical agent warfarin, despite being the traditional orally active agent for long-term anticoagulant therapy, present numerous inherent limitations. These include a slow and unpredictable onset of action, considerable variations in the dose-requirements, genetic and metabolic polymorphisms, regional dietary vitamin K intake differences, and a wide spectrum of drug-drug interactions.[19] Thus, a routine coagulation monitoring is necessary to ensure an optimal therapeutic range of international normalized ratio (INR). The new oral anticoagulants (NOACs), target either thrombin or fXa, representing viable alternatives to the conventional VKAs, gaining a recent widespread interest for the long-term anticoagulant therapy.

Oral Direct Factor Xa Inhibitors

Apixaban is absorbed rapidly, with the highest plasma concentration achieved 3 hours following oral administration. The drug is cleared with an 8–14 hours half-life and outlining multiple elimination pathways, including metabolism in the liver and, intestinal, and renal excretion. The drug was approved by the FDA in 2012 to minimize the risk of stroke and systemic embolism in nonvalvular AF (NVAF) [based on ARISTOTLE (Apixaban For Reduction In Stroke And Other Thromboembolic Events In Atrial Fibrillation) and AVERROES (Apixaban Versus Acetylsalicylic Acid to Prevent Stroke in Atrial Fibrillation Patients Who Have Failed or Are Unsuitable for Vitamin K Antagonist Treatment) clinical trials].[20] The dose recommended is 5 mg twice daily, with down-titration to 2.5 mg twice daily in patients depicting any two of the following: octogenarians, weight <60 kg and serum creatinine >1.5 mg/dL.

Edoxaban is an active compound that is absorbed rapidly, and has a half-life of 9–11 hours. The drug displays a dual elimination mechanism; approximately one-third is renally eliminated, and the rest is excreted in the feces. The drug was approved in 2015, by the FDA to reduce the risk of stroke and systemic embolism in NVAF [largely based on the ENGAGE AF-TIMI 48 (Effective Anticoagulation With Factor Xa Next GEneration in Atrial Fibrillation–Thrombolysis in Myocardial Infarction 48) study].[20] The dose recommended is 60 mg orally once daily with a diminished dose of 30 mg once daily in subjects with creatinine clearance (CrCl) of 15–50 mL/min.

Rivaroxaban manifests a rapid onset of action with a half-life of 7–11 hours and has 80% oral bioavailability. The drug displays a dual-elimination mode with both renal and hepatic contribution along with cytochrome P-450 (CYP)-3A4 dependent pathways. The FDA formally approved the drug for reducing the risk of stroke and systemic embolism associated with AF in 2011 (premised on RECORD 1, 2, and 3 trials).[14] The recommended dose is 10 mg to be taken orally once daily.

Oral Direct Thrombin Inhibitors

Dabigatran etexilate (approved in 2010 by the FDA) is a prodrug of active compound dabigatran which inhibits thrombin reversibly. The National Institute for Health and Care Excellence (NICE) approved the drug for stroke and systemic embolism prevention in NVAF with: former stroke history, transient ischemic attack (TIA) or systemic embolism, symptomatic CHF (NYHA functional class II or higher), left ventricle ejection fraction (LVEF) <40%, age ≥75 years, age ≥65 with one of the following: diabetes mellitus (DM), coronary artery disease (CAD) or systemic hypertension (HT). The drug is renally excreted with a 14–17 hours half-life. The daily recommended dose is 150 mg BD or 110 mg BD (>75 years) due to an enhanced risk of renal impairment.[20] Drugs that inhibit P-glycoprotein (P-gp) lead to an escalated drug bioavailability; therefore, a lesser dose is suggested for patients receiving P-gp inhibitors (e.g., amiodarone or verapamil). The RE-LY trial (Randomized Evaluation of Long-term Anticoagulation Therapy) has evaluated the comparison of 2 dabigatran doses (110 mg and 150 mg twice a day) with warfarin for noninferiority in the stroke or systemic embolus prevention in AF. When compared to the subjects "warfarinized" to an INR in a range of 2–3, both dabigatran dose regimes significantly reduced the annual rate of stroke or systemic embolism.[21]

REVERSAL AGENTS AGAINST NEW ORAL ANTICOAGULANTS

The development of reversal agents against NOACs is the pivotal breakthrough which can assist the expansion of the application of NOACs, particularly in emergency scenarios.

Idarucizumab is a humanized form of monoclonal antibody fragment (Fab) deduced from an immunoglobulin (IgG1) isotype against the dabigatran active compound. The recommended dose is 5 g and the 2015 FDA approval was based on a single-cohort based case-series trial wherein the dabigatran-treated patients who demonstrated uncontrolled life-threatening bleeding, or who required an emergency surgical intervention or an urgent procedure [RE-VERSE AD (A Study of the RE-VERSal Effects of Idarucizumab on Active Dabigatran)] were included.[22]

Andexanet is a recombinant, modified fXa molecular compound that is being actively evaluated as a direct reversal agent for subjects on a fXa inhibitor therapy, suffering from significant bleeding or requiring an emergency operative intervention.[23]

Aripazine is a small synthetic D-arginine molecule which has a broad spectrum of activity against the traditional and novel oral anticoagulants.[23]

ANTIPLATELET AGENTS

Antiplatelet drugs pharmacological repertoire has witnessed the inclusion of novel agents in the existing armamentarium **(Flowchart 2)**. *Ticagrelor and Prasugrel* constitute the antiplatelets that are pharmacological alternatives to clopidogrel in acute coronary syndrome (ACS). The major attributable advantages include diminished rates of ischemia and stent-thrombosis.[24,25] **Table 1** compares the three antiplatelet agents with regard to their pharmacokinetic and pharmacodynamics profile.

Vorapaxar: A novel oral protease activated receptor-1 (PAR-1) antagonist agent that inhibits the thrombin-mediated platelet activation. The drug rapidly results in more than 80% inhibition of the thrombin receptor-stimulating and peptide-induced platelet-aggregation in 2 hours. Given a considerable half-life (173–269 hours), steady-state drug concentration is reached in around 21 days following an initial dosing alongside a sustained platelet inhibition for more than 4 months. The agent has been approved by the FDA in 2014 for the

Flowchart 2: Classification of antiplatelet drugs.

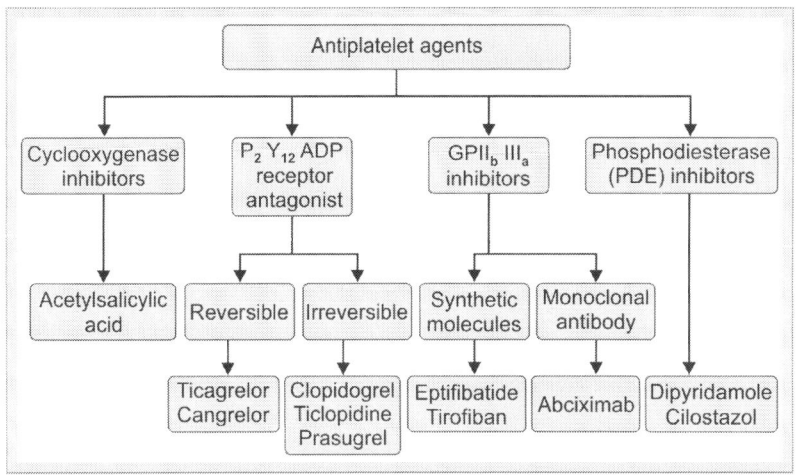

TABLE 1: Comparison of three common antiplatelet agents

Attributes	Clopidogrel	Ticagrelor	Prasugrel
Class	Second generation thienopyridine (Prodrug)	Cyto-pentyl-triazolopyrimidine	Third-generation thienopyridine (Prodrug)
Major comparative trial with clopidogrel		PLATO[25]	TRITON-TIMI 38[26]
FDA approval	2002 approved by the FDA for ACS treatment	2011 for thrombotic events reduction in patients with ACS	2009 for the prevention of thrombotic cardiovascular complications in ACS
Dose	*Load:* 300–600 mg *Maintenance:* 75 mg daily	*Load:* 180 mg *Maintenance:* 90 mg BID	*Load:* 60 mg *Maintenance:* 10 mg daily
Platelet inhibition mechanism	Irreversible inhibitor of P2Y12 component of ADP receptor (preventing ADP binding and activation of platelets)	Reversibly modifies P2Y12 component of ADP receptor (preventing ADP binding and activation of platelets)	Irreversible inhibitor of P2Y12 component of ADP receptor (preventing ADP binding and activation of platelets)
Oral bioavailability	>50% (active metabolite)	30–42%	>78% (active metabolite)
Elimination	*Esterases:* Metabolism by CYP-450 enzymes	Metabolism by CYP-450 enzymes	*Esterases:* Metabolism by CYP-450 enzymes
CYP metabolism	CYP2C19	CYP3A4/5	CYP3A4, CYP2B6

Contd...

Contd...

Attributes	Clopidogrel	Ticagrelor	Prasugrel
Time to onset of maximal platelet inhibition following loading dose	8 hours (300 mg) 2 hours (600 mg)	2 hours	30 minutes
Maintenances dose	75 mg OD	90 mg BD	10 mg OD
Time to recover platelet function after cessation	5 days	2–3 days	7 days

(ACS: acute coronary syndrome; ADP: adenosine diphosphate; CYP: cytochrome P enzyme; PLATO: platelet inhibition and patient outcomes trial; TRITON-TIMI: trial to assess improvement in therapeutic outcomes by optimizing platelet inhibition with prasugrel)

amelioration of the thrombotic cardiac and cardiovascular consequences in the subset with a positive history of myocardial infarction (MI) or peripheral atherosclerotic arterial disease (PAD).[27] CYP3A4 inducers or inhibitors can potentially impact the drug elimination. Therefore, strong enzyme inducers or inhibitors should be avoided with the drug therapy.[28]

Cangrelor: A potent IV nonthienopyridine, reversible $P2Y_{12}$-blocking agent is an adenosine-diphosphate (ADP) receptor antagonist that has a rapid onset of action with readily reversible effects. The drug has been approved by the FDA in 2015 for reducing the periprocedural thrombotic events.[29] Steady-state concentrations are attained after 18–24 hours of infusion in absence of a loading dose being recommended with a consequent platelet inhibition of >90%. Cangrelor is primarily inactivated by the plasma enzymes, and within 60 minutes of discontinuing the infusion, the platelet function potentially recovers to normal. These favorable pharmacokinetic properties render cangrelor a promising viable agent in the context of bridging the high-risk operative patients.[30]

METABOLIC MODULATORS

Metabolic modulators represent a pharmacological class that primarily act via optimization of the cardiac substrate metabolism.

Ranolazine is approved for the drug treatment of chronic stable angina which attenuates myocardial stunning, thereby limiting the infarct size. It acts through a subtle alteration in myocardial energy metabolism shifting from the fatty acid beta-oxidation toward the oxidation of glucose, thus increasing adenosine triphosphate (ATP) generation and, consequently, enhancing the contractile function. The pharmacological activity is not associated with any substantial reduction in the heart rate or blood pressure. Nevertheless, the drug is contraindicated in patients with pre-existing evidence of QT interval prolongation. The recommended initial dosing is 500 mg twice daily; which may be increased to a maximum of 1000 mg twice daily dose. The FDA approval in 2006 was primarily based on the combined findings of the Efficacy of Ranolazine in Chronic Agina (ERICA) and Combination Assessment of Ranolazine in Stable Angina (CARISA) trials.[31]

Trimetazidine (TMZ), a free fatty acid oxidation inhibitor that shifts the cardiac muscle metabolism from the free fatty acids dependency in favor of increased reliance on the glucose utilization, resulting into an enhanced generation of high-energy phosphates translating into a clinical anti-ischemic effect. There has been growing cumulative evidence that TMZ ameliorates ischemic injury and augments the human cardiac function. A randomized clinical trial has further substantiated the drug role in improving functional class, left ventricular ejection fraction (EF) in patients with CHF of diverse etiologies.[32]

ANTIHYPERTENSIVES

The major anti hypertensives which have been FDA approved as a monotherapy include the following:

Azilsartan medoxomil, is a prodrug, eventually hydrolyzed to azilsartan, which selectively acts as AT1 subtype angiotensin II receptor antagonist. The novel drug is indicated for hypertension treatment, either alone or in a combination with other agents.[33] The recommended initial dose is 80 mg taken orally once daily in adult patients.

Clevidipine, a calcium channel antagonist administered IV is a short-acting dihydropyridine. It selectively relaxes the smooth muscle cells that line the small arteries. It thus dilates the arterial lumen with resultant decrease in blood pressure as arterioles and small arteries primarily provide resistance to flow of blood. The drug is mainly indicated when oral therapy fails to control blood pressure elevations or when oral therapy is not desirable or feasible. As per recommendation the drug therapy is initiated with 1-2 mg/h till optimal reduction of blood pressure is achieved,[34] although in most patients, the desired therapeutic response usually manifests at doses of 4-6 mg/h.

Aliskiren[35] is a potent renin inhibitor and is active orally. The mechanism of action is by suppression of renin-angiotensin system resulting in reduction of blood pressure and cardiovascular events. The drug may be employed either alone or in combination with other agents. The initial recommended dose of the drug being 150 mg once daily which can be escalated up to 300 mg daily.

Nebivolol, being a third-generation beta blocker, is a racemic mixture of two enantiomersl-l and d-nebivolol. The drug has conventional beta-blocking effects, as well as nitric oxide (NO) mediated vasodilation resulting in reduction in blood pressure. The half-life of this drug varies between 10.3 and 31.9 hours depending on the rate of metabolism. The extensive first-pass metabolism is through the CYP-2D6 enzyme system, which has variable bioavailability (from 12% for extensive metabolizers up to 96% for poor metabolizers).[36] Starting dose of nebivolol is 5 mg once in a day and can go up to a maximum of 40 mg daily. Starting dose is reduced to 2.5 mg once daily in patients with hepatic or renal insufficiency. Nebivolol is better avoided in those with hepatic decompensation.

Various combinations of the novel and old calcium channel blockers (CCBs), beta-blockers, thiazide diuretics, angiotensin converting enzyme (ACE) inhibitors, renin inhibitors and angiotensin receptor blockers (ARBs) have been approved over the last decade by the US-FDA.

ANTIHEART FAILURE DRUGS

In those ailing from heart failure (HF) with reduced EF, the latest update on pharmacological management addresses two new classes of drugs (in addition to beta-blockers, ACE-inhibitors, aldosterone receptor antagonists or mineralocorticoid).
- A sinoatrial node modulator (generic: ivabradine, with brand name: Coralan, Coraxan, Corlanor, etc).
- An angiotensin receptor neprilysin inhibitor (ARNI) (generic name: sacubitril/valsartan, with brand name: Entresto).

Ivabradine basically reduces the heart rate. It is a hyperpolarization-activated cyclic nucleotide-gated channel blocker. The drug acts by reducing the spontaneous activity of the cardiac sinus node by selective inhibition of the If-current (If) or the cardiac pacemaker current, resulting in lowering of heart rate. The drug has no negative effect on myocardial contractility. The drug is particularly useful in patients who are on maximally tolerated doses of beta-blocker therapy or those with contraindication to beta-blocker therapy. The drug thus decreases the need of hospitalization in patients with chronic HF, LVEF ≤ 35%, with resting heart rate ≥70/min and in sinus rhythm.

The drug was approved by the FDA based on SHIFT (Systolic Heart failure treatment with the IF inhibiTor ivabradine) trial.[37] Starting dose of 5 mg twice a day is recommended. Maximum dose of up to 7.5 mg twice a day is acceptable. The major side effects are bradycardia, AF, hypotension, and sudden dizziness. Other side effects being tiredness, lack of energy, headache and blurred vision.

Entresto (ARNI) being a combination of *valsartan* which is an angiotensin II receptor blocker and *sacubitril*, a neprilysin inhibitor reduces the risk of cardiovascular death as well as hospitalization for patients with chronic HF (NYHA Class II–IV) with reduced EF. The drug was approved by the FDA based on PARADIGM-HF (Prospective Comparison of ARNI with ACEI to Determine Impact on Global Mortality and Morbidity in Heart Failure) randomized trial. This trial was a multinational, double-blind trial that compared entresto with enalapril in 8,442 adult patients who had symptomatic chronic HF (NYHA class II–IV) and systolic dysfunction (LVEF ≤ 40%). PARADIGM-HF trail demonstrated entresto being superior to enalapril for reduction in the risk of cardiovascular death and hospitalization.[38]

A starting dose of 49/51 mg of a combination drug (sacubitril/valsartan) is recommended twice-daily. The dose should be down-titrated to 24/26 mg (sacubitril/valsartan) twice-daily in patients with diseased liver and gross renal derangements. The major adverse effects include: hypotension, cough, dizziness, hyperkalemia or renal failure.

THERAPEUTICS IN PULMONARY ARTERIAL HYPERTENSION

Drug therapy for pulmonary arterial hypertension (PAH) initially relied on vasodilators lacking the specificity for pulmonary circulation and causing undesirable systemic vasodilation. The use of inhaled nitric oxide (i-NO) for PAH treatment (although well established) is doubtlessly cumbersome and expensive. Thus, there is search for less expensive and easily administrable oral and inhaled alternatives. The drug therapy for PAH is now directed toward control of PAH specifically rather than the etiologic. Rarely, CCBs such as nifedipine (starting dose 30 mg/kg) and diltiazem (starting dose 120 mg/kg) are administered to patients of PAH who demonstrates a positive vasoreactivity test.[39]

Flowchart 3: Drugs used for the treatment of pulmonary arterial hypertension targeting the various pathways for management.

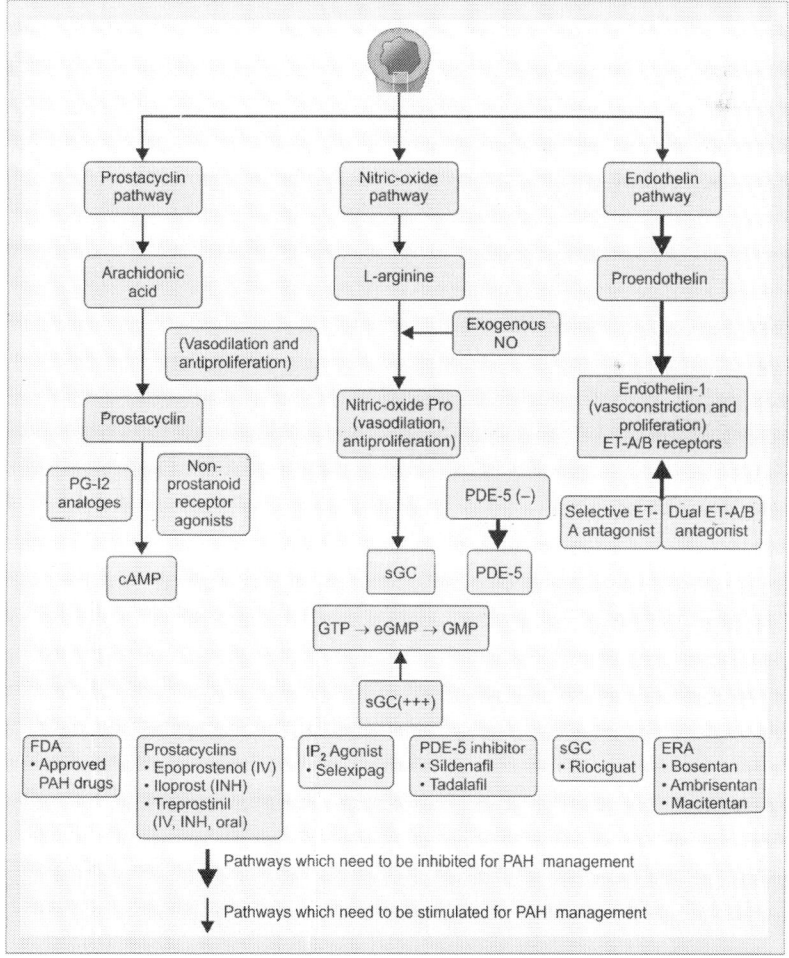

(cAMP: cyclic adenosine monophosphate; cGMP: cyclic guanosine monophosphate; ET: endothelin; ETA: endothelin receptor A; PDE: phosphodiesterase, sGC: soluble guanylyl cyclase; FDA: Food and Drug Administration; PAH: pulmonary arterial hypertension; GTP: guanosine triphosphate)

TABLE 2: Drugs for treatment of pulmonary arterial hypertension (PAH) approved by Food and Drug Association (FDA) over the last decade

Drug	Ambrisentan[40]	Tadalafil[41]	Treprostinil[42]	Riociguat[43]	Macitentan[44]	Selexipag[45]
Trial	ARIES 1,2	PHIRST	TRIUMPH FREEDOM C	CHEST-1 CTEPH PATENT-1 PAH	SERAPHIN	GRIPHON
FDA	2007	2009	2009	2013	2013	2015
MOA	Selective ETA receptor antagonist	PDE-5 inhibitor	Prostacyclin analog	sGC stimulator	dual ET-1 receptor antagonist	Nonprostanoid IP receptor agonist
Dose	5–10 mg OD	40 mg OD	3 breaths 18 µg per session, QID	1 mg TDS up to 2.5 mg TDS	10 mg OD	200 µg BD up to 1600 µg BD
Indication	Treatment of PAH	Treatment of PAH	Treatment of PAH	For CTEPH and PAH	Treatment of PAH	Treatment of PAH
Side Effects	• Peripheral edema • Nasal congestion • Sinusitis • Flushing • Palpitations	• Headache • Dyspepsia • Myalgia • Nausea • Back pain • Nasopharyngitis	• Cough • Headache • Throat irritation • Nausea • Flushing	• Headache • Dizziness • Dyspepsia/gastritis • Nausea • Diarrhea • Hypotension	• Anemia • Pharyngitis • Bronchitis • Headache • Influenza • Urinary infection	• Headache • Diarrhea • Jaw pain • Nausea • Myalgia • Vomiting

(CTEPH: chronic thromboembolic pulmonary hypertension; ET: endothelin; ETA: endothelin receptor A; MOA: mechanism of action; PDE: phosphodiesterase; sGC: soluble guanylyl cyclase).

Patients who do not respond to CCB therapy, are nonvasoreactive or do not undergo vasoreactivity testing are treated with PAH specific therapy. Cyclic guanine and adenine monophosphate (cGMP and cAMP) have an important role in modulating the vasomotor tone. The PAH specific drug therapy commonly targets one of the following three pathways **(Flowchart 3)**, many of these are approved by the FDA **(Table 2)**.

The three pathways are namely:
1. Prostacyclin pathway agonist (epoprostenol, treprostinil, iloprost, and selexipag).
2. Nitric-oxide-guanosine monophosphate (NO-GMP) enhancers [phosphodiesterase 5 inhibitors (PDE5s) the sildenafil, tadalafil], riociguat, and.
3. Endothelin receptor antagonists. That includes bosentan, ambrisentan, and macitentan.

The specific therapy for PAH is initiated with single drug therapy in case of World Health Organization (WHO) functional class I. However, in functional class II or III combination of drugs are administered either together from the beginning or as "add on" therapy. In patient with severe PAH or class IV functional status combination therapy including parenteral agent like prostanoid is administered. Epoprostenol (prostacyclin, PGI_2) is initiated with 1–2 ng/kg/min and increased every 1–2 days by 1–2 ng/kg/min up to maximum of 6–10 ng/kg/min. Thereafter, to sustain clinical effects, dose may have to be escalated by 1–2 ng/kg/min every 2–4 weeks. The doses may be further increased up to 20–40 ng/kg/min to attain a plateau.[46] Alternatively, IV or subcutaneous treprostinil may be administered. Inhaled trepostinil or iloprost can be administered where IV or subcutaneous are not possible.

Future Perspectives in Therapy of Pulmonary Arterial Hypertension

In addition to the novel drugs described in the **Table 2**, inhaled nitrite is currently being investigated in human PAH. It is to be noted that NO is also generated via NO synthase-independent pathway involving nitrite (NO_2). Multiple enzymes (aldehyde reductase, xanthine oxidoreductase, and deoxyhemoglobin) convert NO_2 to NO. Thus, therapy with inhaled NO_2 can possibly reverse PAH. NO_2 is more stable than NO with a half-life of 30 minutes, making intermittent dosing possible.[47]

In addition to enzymatic degradation of the cGMP and cAMP via PDEs, a transport system mediating active efflux also regulates the levels of these cyclic nucleotides. A multidrug resistance-associated protein-4 (MRP4), which is a member of ATP-binding cassette transporter family, helps in mediation of cyclic nucleotides efflux. In a recent research the overexpression of MRP4 in PAH patients is demonstrated. Inhibition of MRP4, thus represents a potential target for treatment of PAH in humans.[48]

ANESTHETIC IMPLICATIONS

Knowledge of preoperative drug therapy, duration of effects, side effects, adverse effects as well as optimization of patients prior to surgery forms an important part of anesthetic management in patients undergoing surgery. Of particular importance are the patients on anticoagulant and antiplatelet agents. Details of patients on anticoagulant therapy have already been described in the section on anticoagulants.

Patient on Dual Antiplatelet Therapy

Patients of acute coronary syndrome (ACS), and those following percutaneous intervention (PCI) with coronary artery stents are administered dual antiplatelet therapy (DAPT). DAPT therapy conventionally consists of cyclooxygenase inhibitor (aspirin) and $P2Y_{12}$ inhibitor clopidogrel. Around 5-10% are required to undergo noncardiac surgery during 1-year duration following PCI. Cessation of DAPT predisposes these patients to stent thrombosis. On the other extreme, the continuation of DAPT can potentially lead to bleeding. So, in these patients a tailored decision regarding the continuation or the discontinuation of DAPT should be in consensus with anesthesiologist, cardiologist, surgeon and the patient with the aim to minimize both ischemic and bleeding risk.[49]

Antiplatelet Therapy

The most commonly used antiplatelet agents clopidogrel and aspirin have variable platelet inhibitory effect and takes 5-7 days for reversal of effects.[50] The newer $P2Y_{12}$ inhibitors prasugrel and ticagrelor exhibit nearly 90% platelet inhibition, but recovery after discontinuation after prasugrel is 7-10 days which is more than that of clopidogrel; although the recovery for ticagrelor is 3-5 days. The cangrelor and glycoprotein IIB/IIIa inhibitors have immediate to early onset of action with almost 90-100% antiplatelet activity and advantage of recovery occurs within hours of discontinuation. Particularly with cangrelor recovery occurs within 3-5 minutes. Additionally, the short acting IV reversible antiplatelets have potential to provide bridge for oral agents to surgery.[30,51] Also, knowledge of recovery after last antiplatelet is of clinical relevance in situations of perioperative bleeding to understand whether transfusion of platelet concentrates would be beneficial.[52]

Bleeding versus Stent Thrombosis

Previously, patients with first generation drug eluting stent (DES) namely the sirolimus or paclitaxel, were administered DAPT up to 1 year. With the evolution of nonfirst-generation DESs, namely everolimus or zotarolimus, which are less thrombogenic with a shorter time to re-endothelialization, require DAPT for a period of 6 months only. As per updated 2016 American College of Cardiology/American Heart Association (ACC/AHA) guidelines, an elective noncardiac surgery should be performed after 6 months after placement of DES.[49] However, if the risk of delaying surgery is greater than stent thrombosis, then surgery could be considered 3 months post-DES placement.[49] Generally, after PCI during the initial re-endothelialization period cessation of DAPT carries a much greater risk of stent thrombosis than bleeding.

Bridge Therapy to Surgery

In a situation as above where surgery is inevitable, there is need to bridge DAPT to prevent stent thrombosis without added risk of perioperative bleeding. Bridging therapy involves the replacing long acting antiplatelet agents before surgery with an antiplatelet agent of short duration, rapid-onset, reversible and available in IV form. Both GPIIb/IIIa inhibitors and cangrelor have shown promise as a bridge to $P2Y_{12}$ inhibitor discontinuation in patients with DES. In the above trials, although, clopidogrel was discontinued, but aspirin was continued.[53] For bridging, aspirin treatment should be continued, and the other oral agent be stopped 5-7 days prior to the surgery. A short-acting IV agent ought to be started no more than 72 hours after the discontinuation of the DAPT. Approximately 4-6 hours (or 1 hour for cangrelor) prior to the surgery, the IV drug is discontinued and carefully restarted 6 hours following surgery. The patient's usual DAPT is cautiously reinitiated as soon as the involved risk of perioperative hemorrhage is negligible.

RECOMMENDATIONS

As per recommendations, elective surgery should be delayed for 14 days after balloon angioplasty, 30 days after bare metal stents, 6 months after DES preferably and a minimum of 3 months. In case of post re-endothelialization period, aspirin should be continued where possible except for intracranial surgery, where it should be discontinued for 3-4 days; $P2Y_{12}$ inhibitors to be discontinued, and platelet function tests considered. In case of emergent or urgent surgery occurring in the re-endothelialization period, DAPT continuation is considered. In surgeries with high bleeding risk, $P2Y_{12}$ inhibitors are stopped, aspirin is preferably continued or stopped if necessary, for only 3-4 days and bridge therapy with cangrelor, tirofiban or eptifibatide. In situation of nonsurgical bleed, test for platelet function may be performed. The DAPT is to be restarted as soon as possible.[49]

CONCLUSION

To conclude, over the last decade various newer cardiac drugs have been included in the armamentarium of cardiovascular drugs. The attending anesthesiologist needs to be updated with the rapid drug developments in the field of cardiovascular medicine for an efficient management of both perioperative and intensive care scenarios. Knowledge of preoperative drug therapy, duration of effects, side effects, adverse effects, drug interactions, associated electrolyte alterations, hemodynamic perturbations; as well as optimization of patients prior to surgery forms an important part of perioperative management in patients undergoing surgery. Of particular importance are the patients on anticoagulant and antiplatelet therapy with a need to undergo surgical intervention. Future trials are still required to be carried out in the field of various cardiovascular pharmacological categories in search of novel drugs with better efficacy, fewer side effects/adverse effects/interactions.

> **KEY POINTS**
>
> - Cardiac practice involves the application of a gamut of pharmacological agents where potency, efficacy and side-effects need to be most tenuously balanced as per the clinical context, alongside a sound categorization of the "Yin" and "Yang" of the associated therapies.
> - An anesthesiologist needs to keep pace with the ever-rampant drug developments in the dynamic field of cardiovascular medicine for staging an improved management of both perioperative and intensive care clinical scenarios, to strengthen his/her role as a perioperative physician.
> - Knowledge of preoperative drug therapy, duration of effects, side-effects, adverse effects as well as optimization of patients prior to surgery forms an important part of anesthetic management in patients undergoing surgery. Of particular importance are the patients on anticoagulant and antiplatelet agents and are scheduled for surgery.
> - The chapter highlights the evolving trends with a take on the future perspectives in the major cardiovascular pharmacological categories.

REFERENCES

1. Magoon R, Choudhury A, Malik V, Sharma R, Kapoor PM. Pharmacological update: New drugs in cardiac practice: a critical appraisal. Ann Card Anaesth. 2017;20(Suppl):S49-56.
2. Hohnloser SH, Crijns HJ, van Eickels M, Gaudin C, Page RL, Torp-Pedersen C, et al. Effect of dronedarone on cardiovascular events in atrial fibrillation. N Engl J Med. 2009;360(7):668-78.
3. FDA Warns about severe liver injury associated with Multaq (Dronedarone). 2011. US Food and Drug Administration. FDA drug safety communication: severe liver injury associated with the use of dronedarone (marketed as Multaq); 2011. [online] Available from: http://www.fda.gov/drugs/drugsafety/ucm240011.htm. [Last accessed October, 2020].
4. Kober L, Torp-Pedersen C, McMurray JJ, Gøtzsche O, Lévy S, Crijns H, et al. Increased mortality after dronedarone therapy for severe heart failure. N Engl J Med. 2008;358(25):2678-87.
5. ElMaghawry M, Farouk M. Dronedarone-digoxin interaction in PALLAS: a foxglove connection?. Glob Cardiol Sci Pract. 2015;2015:4.
6. Ehrlich JR, Biliczki P, Hohnloser SH, Nattel S. Atrial-selective approaches for the treatment of atrial fibrillation. J Am Coll Cardiol. 2008;51(8):787-92.
7. Cheng JWM, Rybak I. Pharmacotherapy options in atrial fibrillation: focus on vernakalant. Clin Med Therapeut. 2009;1:215-30.
8. Burstein B, Nattel S. Atrial fibrosis: mechanisms and clinical relevance in atrial fibrillation. J Am Coll Cardiol. 2008;51(8):802-9.
9. Ratte A, Wiedmann F, Kraft M, Katus HA, Schmidt C. Antiarrhythmic properties of ranolazine: inhibition of atrial fibrillation associated TASK-1 potassium channels. Front Pharmacol. 2019;10:1367.

10. Koncz I, Szel T, Bitay M, Cerbai E, Jaeger K, Fülöp F, et al. Electrophysiological effects of ivabradine in dog and human cardiac preparations: potential antiarrhythmic actions. Eur J Pharmacol. 2011;668(3):419-26.
11. Frommeyer G, Weller J, Ellermann C, Kaese S, Kochhäuser S, Lange PS, et al. Antiarrhythmic properties of ivabradine in an experimental model of short-QT-Syndrome. Clin Exp Pharmacol Physiol. 2017;44(9):941-5.
12. VerNooy RA, Mangrum JM. Azimilide, a novel oral class III anti-arrhythmic agent for both supraventricular and ventricular arrhythmias. Curr Drug Targets Cardiovasc Haematol Disord. 2005;5(1):75-84.
13. Singh S. Trials of new antiarrhythmic drugs for maintenance of sinus rhythm in patients with atrial fibrillation. J Interv Card Electrophysiol. 2004;10(Suppl 1):71-6.
14. Elzein E, Zablocki J. A1 adenosine receptor agonists and their potential therapeutic applications. Exp Opin Investig Drugs. 2008;17(12):1901-10.
15. Weitz JI, Hirsh J, Samama MM. New antithrombotic drugs: American College of Chest Physicians Evidence-based clinical practice guidelines (8th edition). Chest. 2008;133(6 Suppl):234S-56S.
16. Stone GW, Witzenbichler B, Guagliumi G, Peruga JZ, Brodie BR, Dudek D, et al. Bivalirudin during primary PCI in acute myocardial infarction. N Engl J Med. 2008;358(21):2218-30.
17. Savi P, Herault JP, Duchaussoy P, Millet L, Schaeffer P, Petitou M, et al. Reversible biotinylated oligosaccharides: a new approach for a better management of anticoagulant therapy. J Thromb Haemost. 2008;6(10):1697-706.
18. Sabatine MS, Antman EM, Widimsky P, Ebrahim IO, Kiss RG, Saaiman A, et al. Otamixaban for the treatment of patients with non-ST-elevation acute coronary syndromes (SEPIA-ACS1 TIMI 42): a randomised, double-blind, active-controlled, phase 2 trial. Lancet. 2009;374(9692):787-95.
19. Hirsh J. Oral anticoagulant drugs. N Engl J Med. 1991;324(26):1865-75.
20. Eriksson BI, Quinlan DJ, Weitz JI. Comparative pharmacodynamics and pharmacokinetics of oral direct thrombin and factor Xa inhibitors in development. Clin Pharmacokinet. 2009;48(1):1-22.
21. Ezekowitz MD, Connolly S, Parekh A, Reilly PA, Varrone J, Wang S, et al. Rationale and design of RE-LY: randomized evaluation of long-term anticoagulant therapy, warfarin, compared with dabigatran. Am Heart J. 2009;157(5):805-10.
22. Schiele F, van Ryn J, Canada K, Newsome C, Sepulveda E, Park J, et al. A specific antidote for dabigatran: functional and structural characterization. Blood. 2013;121(18):3554-62.
23. Lu G, DeGuzman FR, Hollenbach SJ, Karbarz MJ, Abe K, Lee G, et al. A specific antidote for reversal of anticoagulation by direct and indirect inhibitors of coagulation factor Xa. Nat Med. 2013;19(4):446-51.
24. Steg PG, Harrington RA, Emanuelsson H, Katus HA, Mahaffey KW, Meier B, et al. Stent thrombosis with ticagrelor versus clopidogrel in patients with acute coronary syndromes: an analysis from the prospective, randomized PLATO trial. Circulation. 2013;128(10):1055-65.
25. Held C, Asenblad N, Bassand JP, Becker RC, Cannon CP, Claeys MJ, et al. Ticagrelor versus clopidogrel in patients with acute coronary syndromes undergoing coronary artery bypass surgery: results from the PLATO (Platelet Inhibition and Patient Outcomes) trial. J Am Coll Cardiol. 2011;57(6):672-84.
26. Serebruany VL. Timing of thienopyridine loading and outcomes in the TRITON trial: the FDA Prasugrel Action Package outlook. Cardiovasc Revasc Med. 2011;12(2):94-8.

27. Morrow DA, Braunwald E, Bonaca MP, Ameriso SF, Dalby AJ, Fish MP, et al. Vorapaxar in the secondary prevention of atherothrombotic events. N Engl J Med. 2012;366(15):1404-13.
28. Merck. Vorapraxor (Zontivity). Whitehouse station, NJ; Merck & Co., Inc.; 2013.
29. Bhatt DL, Stone GW, Mahaffey KW, Gibson CM, Steg PG, Hamm CW, et al. Effect of platelet inhibition with cangrelor during PCI on ischemic events. N Engl J Med. 2013;368(14):1303-13.
30. Angiolillo DJ, Firstenberg MS, Price MJ, Tummala PE, Hutyra M, Welsby IJ, et al. Bridging antiplatelet therapy with cangrelor in patients undergoing cardiac surgery: a randomized controlled trial. JAMA. 2012;307(3):265-74.
31. Lopaschuk GD, Ussher JR, Folmes CD, Jaswal JS, Stanley WC. Myocardial fatty acid metabolism in health and disease. Physiol Rev. 2010;90(1):207-58.
32. Fragasso G, Palloshi A, Puccetti P, Silipigni C, Rossodivita A, Pala M, et al. A randomized clinical trial of trimetazidine, a partial free fatty acid oxidation inhibitor, in patients with heart failure. J Am Coll Cardiol. 2006;48(5):992-8.
33. Baker WL, White WB. Azilsartan medoxomil: a new angiotensin II receptor antagonist for treatment of hypertension. Ann Pharmacother. 2011;45(12):1506-15.
34. Deeks ED, Keating GM, Keam SJ. Clevidipine: a review of its use in management of acute hypertension. Am J Cardiovasc Drugs. 2009;9(2):117-34.
35. Sanoski CA. Aliskiren: an oral direct renin inhibitor for the treatment of hypertension. Pharmacotherapy. 2009;29(2):193-212.
36. Hilas O, Ezzo D. Nebivolol (bystolic), a novel beta-blocker for hypertension. P T. 2009;34(4):188-92.
37. Chaudhary R, Garg J, Krishnamoorthy P, Shah N, Lanier G, Martinez MW, et al. Ivabradine: heart failure and beyond. J Cardiovasc. Pharmacol Ther. 2016;21(4):335-43.
38. McMurray JJ, Packer M, Desai AS, Gong J, Lefkowitz MP, Rizkala AR, et al. Angiotensin-neprilysin inhibition versus enalapril in heart failure. N Engl J Med. 2014;371(11):993-1004.
39. Atz AM, Adatia I, Lock JE, Wessel DL. Combined effects of nitric oxide and oxygen during acute pulmonary vasodilator testing. J Am Coll Cardiol. 1999;33(3):813-9.
40. Galiè N, Olschewski H, Oudiz RJ, Torres F, Frost A, Ghofrani HA, et al. Ambrisentan for the treatment of pulmonary arterial hypertension: results of the ambrisentan in pulmonary arterial hypertension, randomized, double-blind, placebo-controlled, multicenter, efficacy (ARIES) study 1 and 2. Circulation. 2008;117(23):3010-9.
41. Galiè N, Brundage BH, Ghofrani HA, Oudiz RJ, Simonneau G, Safdar Z, et al. Tadalafil therapy for pulmonary arterial hypertension. Circulation. 2009;119(22):2894-903.
42. McLaughlin VV, Benza RL, Rubin LJ, Channick RN, Voswinckel R, Tapson VF, et al. Addition of inhaled treprostinil to oral therapy for pulmonary arterial hypertension: a randomized controlled clinical trial. J Am Coll Cardiol. 2010;55(18):1915-22.
43. Ghofrani HA, Galiè N, Grimminger F, Grünig E, Humbert M, Jing ZC, et al. PATENT-1 Study Group. Riociguat for the treatment of pulmonary arterial hypertension. N Engl J Med. 2013;369(4):330-40.
44. Pulido T, Adzerikho I, Channick RN, Delcroix M, Galiè N, Ghofrani HA, et al. Macitentan and morbidity and mortality in pulmonary arterial hypertension. N Engl J Med. 2013;369(9):809-18.
45. Simonneau G, Torbicki A, Hoeper MM, Delcroix M, Karlócai K, Galiè N, et al. Selexipag: an oral, selective prostacyclin receptor agonist for the treatment of pulmonary arterial hypertension. Eur Respir J. 2012;40(4):874-80.
46. Badesch DB, McLaughlin VV, Delcroix M, Vizza CD, Olschewski H, Sitbon O, et al. Prostanoid therapy for pulmonary arterial hypertension. J Am Coll Cardiol. 2004;43(12 Suppl S):56S-61S.

47. Zuckerbraun BS, George P, Gladwin MT. Nitrite in pulmonary arterial hypertension: therapeutic avenues in the setting of dysregulated arginine/nitric oxide synthase signalling. Cardiovasc Res. 2011;89(3):542-52.
48. Wielinga PR, van der Heijden I, Reid G, Beijnen JH, Wijnholds J, Borst P. Characterization of the MRP4- and MRP5-mediated transport of cyclic nucleotides from intact cells. J Biol Chem. 2003;278(20):17664-71.
49. Levine GN, Bates ER, Bittl JA, Brindis RG, Fihn SD, Fleisher LA, et al. 2016 ACC/AHA Guideline Focused Update on Duration of Dual Antiplatelet Therapy in Patients With Coronary Artery Disease: A Report of the American College of Cardiology/American Heart Association Task Force on Clinical Practice Guidelines: An Update of the 2011 ACCF/AHA/SCAI Guideline for Percutaneous Coronary Intervention, 2011 ACCF/AHA Guideline for Coronary Artery Bypass Graft Surgery, 2012 ACC/AHA/ACP/AATS/PCNA/SCAI/ STS Guideline for the Diagnosis and Management of Patients With Stable Ischemic Heart Disease, 2013 ACCF/AHA Guideline for the Management of ST-Elevation Myocardial Infarction, 2014 AHA/ACC Guideline for the Management of Patients With Non-ST-Elevation Online access in http://ekja.org Antiplatelet therapy and surgery VOL. 70, NO. 1, FEBRUARY 2017 20 Acute Coronary Syndromes, and 2014 ACC/AHA Guideline on Perioperative Cardiovascular Evaluation and Management of Patients Undergoing Noncardiac Surgery. Circulation. 2016;134(10):e123-55.
50. Angiolillo DJ, Fernandez-Ortiz A, Bernardo E, Alfonso F, Macaya C, Bass TA, et al. Variability in individual responsiveness to clopidogrel: clinical implications, management, and future perspectives. J Am Coll Cardiol. 2007;49(14):1505-16.
51. Savonitto S, D'Urbano M, Caracciolo M, Barlocco F, Mariani G, Nichelatti M, et al. Urgent surgery in patients with a recently implanted coronary drug-eluting stent: a phase II study of 'bridging' antiplatelet therapy with tirofiban during temporary withdrawal of clopidogrel. Br J Anaesth. 2010;104(3):285-91.
52. Song JW, Soh S, Shim JK. Dual antiplatelet therapy and non-cardiac surgery: evolving issues and anesthetic implications. Korean J Anesthesiol. 2017;70(1):13-21.
53. Morici N, Moja L, Rosato V, Sacco A, Mafrici A, Klugmann S, et al. Bridge with intravenous antiplatelet therapy during temporary withdrawal of oral agents for surgical procedures: a systematic review. Intern Emerg Med. 2014;9(2):225-35.

CHAPTER 22

Role of Extracorporeal Therapy in Sepsis

Prakash Shastri

INTRODUCTION

Sepsis evokes both pro- as well as anti-inflammatory responses, which is manifested by the release of inflammatory mediators such as interleukins and cytokines into the circulation. This response may get dysregulated in severe sepsis. Although, certain cytokines (e.g., tumor necrosis factor-α, interleukin-6, interleukin-1, and high mobility group proteins such as high mobility group box protein 1 (HMGB-1) have been implicated in this process,[1] no single mediator has been identified as having "the" critical role in the pathogenesis. In the past, studies have concentrated on suppression of a single cytokine which failed to show outcome benefits.[2,3] This was followed by the so called "peak concentration hypothesis" which proposed that very high concentrations of not one but several mediators may play a role in the evolution of the syndrome.[4] Based on this theoretical concept, extracorporeal therapies (ECTs) have been used to remove cytokines and endotoxins to ameliorate this response. However, studies done so far have revealed conflicting results and failed to demonstrate the beneficial effect of ECTs.[3]

BLOOD PURIFICATION DEVICES USED IN THE TREATMENT OF SEPTIC SHOCK

The first filter cartridges for ECTs were developed in Japan which consisted of polystrene fiber coated with polymyxin B (PMX). The polymyxin coating allowed adsorption of endotoxin such as lipopolysaccharide. It has been licensed in Japan more than 20 years back based on a meta-analysis which showed a survival benefit in patients with sepsis.[5] Two trials were done—one in Europe and the other in North America and were funded by the manufacturers of Toraymyxin ostensibly for approvals in these markets. The Italian trial, EUPHAS (Early Use of Polymyxin B Hemoperfusion in Abdominal Septic shock), an open-label study[6] had a sample size was 64 and the patient population consisted of patients in septic shock of abdominal origin. The primary end-point was achievement of hemodynamic stability in 48 hours. Secondary endpoints included 28-day mortality and changes in the severity scores. The authors reported improvement in hemodynamics (as indicated by reduced requirement of vasopressors) and decreased 28-day mortality in the study group. Based on these results the trial was stopped prematurely before the sample size was reached. The study has been criticized[7] on the ground that, even though PMX hemoperfusion appeared to achieve a decrease in vasopressor requirement it did not affect day 28 mortality for want of adequate sample size.

In 2015, the ABDOMIX study, a French multicenter trial was published in the same patient population but in a larger cohort[8] (222 patients) where adequacy of surgical source control was also factored in. The patients received two hemoperfusion treatment with a 24 hour gap. There was no improvement in organ function [as per the sequential organ failure assessment (SOFA score)] in the intervention group and the reduction in 28-day mortality in the intervention group was not statistically significant.

A follow-up trial EUPHRATES (Evaluating the Use of Polymyxin B Hemoperfusion in a Randomized controlled trial of Adults Treated for Endotoxemia and Septic shock), was conducted.[9,10] In this trial patients endotoxin activity assay (EAA) was done and only those whose EAA was more than 0.6 were enrolled. In this randomized multicentric trial, conducted in North America, the primary outcome was to see the effect on 28-day all-cause mortality. The intervention group received two sessions of PMX hemoperfusion of 90–120 minutes completed within 24 hours of enrollment. The design of the study allowed a more homogeneous patient selection and blinding was done by the use of a "façade" hemoperfusion filter. The trial enrolled 450 patients between 2010 and 2016. The study failed to show difference in outcome and there were serious adverse events in 65% of cases such as worsening of sepsis in the intervention arm. The publication of this study prompted the authors of a meta-analysis published in the same year to conclude that there is currently insufficient evidence to support the routine use of PMX hemoperfusion to treat patients with sepsis or septic shock. However, in a posthoc analysis of the EUPHRATES data only patients with specific endotoxin activity (EAA 0.6–0.89) were included. The patients with higher EAA were excluded. The 28-day survival in the PMX group was better in the intervention group [HR 0.56 (95% CI 0.33, 0.95) p = 0.03]. PMX treatment showed better hemodynamic stability and higher ventilator free days. There were no significant differences in other end points.[11]

On the basis of this subgroup analysis the US Food and Drug Administration (FDA) has granted approval for another trial (TIGRIS NCT 03901807) as an amendment in the protocol of EUPHRATES trial. The estimated enrollment is 150 patients and the study are likely to be completed in September 2022.

New developments in this technique continued. Another ECT for sepsis called the coupled plasma filtration adsorption which adsorbs both proinflammatory and anti-inflammatory mediators was introduced that has gained more acceptance among the ICU physicians. This device marketed as the "CytoSorb®" filter, is made up of polymer beads with pores to adsorb all cytokines, including HMGB-1, but not endotoxin. It has a large surface area to make it more efficient. The CytoSorb® is a standard whole blood perfusion cartridge that can be used with conventional hemodialysis machines. A standard therapy consists of hemoperfusion for 24 hours. Several case series have been published. It has found that treatment with CytoSorb® was associated with hemodynamic stabilization and a reduction in blood lactate levels. In a

German case series[12] (26 patients) hospital mortality was higher in postsurgical patients as compared to medical patients and also, if the therapy was started less than 24 hours of the recognition of septic shock. They did not observe any device-related adverse events. It was a hypothesis generating descriptive study and did not include 28-day mortality as the primary outcome. There is only one randomized control study in 37 patients who underwent cardiac surgery. In these patients, the addition of CytoSorb® on the cardiopulmonary bypass pump had no effect on the levels of cytokines postbypass or hemodynamic instability that accompanies cardiac surgery.[13]

The "oXiris®"-filter has been developed by Baxter to adsorb both endotoxins and cytokines during renal replacement therapy (RRT). It is a standard a polyacrylonitrile (AN69)-based membrane treated with polyethylenimine (which is positively charged). The polyethylenimine allows the adsorption of endotoxins (which are negatively charged) while the membrane proper removes the cytokines. This filter is designed for continuous renal replacement therapy (CRRT) only. However, due to lack of studies, there is little evidence that it is effective. Hence, no recommendation can be made for its clinical use. In a French case series 31 patients with septic shock underwent CRRT with the oXiris® membrane. Only in the sickest [as per simplified acute physiology score II (SAPS II)] the hospital mortality was lower than predicted. There was no significant improvement in organ function (as depicted by the SOFA score) but a significant decrease in norepinephrine requirement. Patients with gram-negative bacilli (GNB) infections, especially intra-abdominal sepsis benefited the most.[14]

A retrospective cohort study MOSAKI (The Membrane Adsorbing oXiris Filter in Septic Patients with AKI, NCT03914586) is underway in Italy and the results are expected in early 2021. So again, published evidence for this technique is not available, but Baxter has received FDA Emergency Use Authorization (EUA) status for oXiris® blood purification filter to treat COVID-19 patients admitted in the ICU with confirmed or imminent respiratory failure.

CONCLUSION

In this review we have described in brief all the blood purification devices used in the ICUs the world over and are still being used in the treatment of septic shock. ECTs have not been able to carve a niche for themselves in the management of sepsis, primarily because sepsis is described as a syndrome and not a disease entity. The stages and severity of the disease have not been well defined to allow a homogeneous cohort to be selected for controlled trials. In the absence of evidence or adequately powered randomized control trial they are used as rescue therapies in patients having severe sepsis or septic shock with hypotension refractory to vasopressors.

KEY POINTS

- Sepsis evokes both pro- as well as anti-inflammatory responses, manifested by the release of inflammatory mediators such as interleukins and cytokines into the circulation.
- "Peak concentration hypothesis" proposed that very high concentrations of several mediators may play a role in the evolution of the syndrome.

Contd...

Contd...

- Based on this theoretical concept, ECTs have been used to remove cytokines and endotoxins to ameliorate this response.
- Extracorporeal therapies have not been able to carve a niche for themselves in the management of sepsis primarily because sepsis is described as a syndrome and not a disease entity. The stages and severity of the disease have not been well defined to allow a homogeneous cohort to be selected for controlled trials.
- Due to lack of large well-designed randomized control trials especially in humans, ECTs remain as potential therapies whose efficacy does not have robust evidence to support it.

REFERENCES

1. Tetta C, Bellomo R, Inguaggiato P, Wratten ML, Ronco C. Endotoxin and cytokine removal in sepsis. Ther Apher. 2002;6(2):109-15.
2. Marshall JC. Such stuff as dreams are made on: mediator-directed therapy in sepsis. Nat Rev Drug Discov. 2003;2(5):391-405.
3. McMaster P, Shann F. The use of extracorporeal techniques to remove humoral factors in sepsis. Pediatr Crit Care Med. 2003;4(1):2-7.
4. Ronco C, Bonello M, Bordoni V, Ricci Z, D'Intini V, Bellomo R, et al. Extracorporeal therapies in non-renal disease: treatment of sepsis and the peak concentration hypothesis. Blood Purif. 2004;22(1):164-74.
5. Zhou F, Peng Z, Murugan R, Kellum JA. Blood purification and mortality in sepsis: a meta-analysis of randomized trials. Crit Care Med. 2013;41(9):2209-20.
6. Cruz DN, Antonelli M, Fumagalli R, Foltran F, Brienza N, Donati A, et al. Early use of polymyxin B hemoperfusion in abdominal septic shock: the EUPHAS randomized controlled trial. JAMA. 2009;301(23):2445-52.
7. Vincent JL. Polymyxin B hemoperfusion and mortality in abdominal septic shock. JAMA. 2009;302(18):1968-70.
8. Payen DM, Guilhot J, Launey Y, Lukaszewicz AC, Kaaki M, Veber B, et al. Early use of polymyxin B hemoperfusion in patients with septic shock due to peritonitis: a multicenter randomized control trial. Intensive Care Med. 2015;41(6):975-84.
9. Dellinger RP, Bagshaw SM, Antonelli M, Foster DM, Klein DJ, Marshall JC, et al. Targeted polymyxin-B hemoperfusion for the treatment of endotoxemia and septic shock: a multicenter randomized controlled trial (EUPHRATES). JAMA. 2018;320(14):1455-63.
10. Fujii T, Ganeko R, Kataoka Y, Furukawa TA, Featherstone R, Doi K, et al. Polymyxin B-immobilized hemoperfusion and mortality in critically ill adult patients with sepsis/septic shock: a systematic review with meta-analysis and trial sequential analysis. Intensive Care Med. 2018;44(2):167-78.
11. Klein DJ, Foster D, Walker PM, Bagshaw SM, Mekonnen H, Antonelli M. Polymyxin B hemoperfusion in endotoxemia septic shock patients without extreme endotoxemia: a post hoc analysis of the EUPHRATES trial. Intensive Care Med. 2018;44(12):2205-12.
12. Kogelmann K, Jarczak D, Scheller M, Drüner M. Hemoadsorption by CytoSorb in septic patients: a case series. Crit Care. 2017;21(1):74.
13. Bernardi MH, Rinoesl H, Dragosits K, Ristl R, Hoffelner F, Opfermann P, et al. Effect of hemoadsorption during cardiopulmonary bypass surgery-a blinded, randomized, controlled pilot study using a novel adsorbent. Crit Care. 2016;20:96.
14. Schwindenhammer V, Girardot T, Chaulier K, Grégoire A, Monard C, Huriaux L, et al. oXiris® use in septic shock: experience of two French centres. Blood Purif. 2019;47(Suppl 3):1-7.

CHAPTER 23

Recent Advances in the Management of Cancer Pain

PN Jain, RS Thota

INTRODUCTION

Over a million new cases of cancer are diagnosed annually in India, and it is estimated that the cancer burden will almost double during the approaching two decades.[1] Worldwide, the incidence of pain in advanced stages of cancer approaches 70–80%.[2] A study was conducted at four regional cancer centers in India, where nearly 88% of the patients reported experiencing pain for about 7 days, and approximately 60% reported that their worst pain was severe.[3] A recent meta-analysis, including studies published between 2005 and 2014, found that over half cancer patients receiving anticancer treatment and two-thirds of patients with advanced and metastatic cancer had pain.[4]

Cancer pain has been broadly divided into three types. Pain may be due to tumor, which is the most common presentation (70–80%), due to treatment (adverse effects from chemotherapy, surgery or radiotherapy) or pain could be unrelated to cancer (e.g., diabetic neuropathy, postherpetic neuralgia, anginal pain, joint pain or myofascial pain). A comprehensive history with a good physical examination unravels all components of pain to be addressed after an expeditious pain syndrome diagnosis. Cancer immunotherapy has evolved dramatically with improved understanding of immune microenvironment and immune-surveillance.[5] Treatment with immune checkpoint inhibitors (ICIs) in patients with advanced nonsmall cell lung cancer (NSCLC) has achieved landmark 3-year overall survival (OS) rates of 19% and 26.4% among previously treated and treatment-naive patients, respectively, and up to over 18 months of progression-free survival.[6] Various hormonal treatment therapies are successfully employed in the management of carcinoma. Antiestrogens (tamoxifen or toremifene), aromatase inhibitors (anastrozole and letrozole) still as progestins (megestrol and medroxyprogesterone) may all have roles in management.[7] These therapies may result in varieties of pain, e.g., aromatase inhibitors are commonly related to arthralgia.[8]

Worldwide, many guidelines and protocols are available for the management of cancer pain. Recently, Indian Society for Study of Pain (ISSP), cancer pain Special Interest Group (SIG) (2019), published seven guidelines on assessment, diagnosis, pharmacological, complimentary, interventional treatment, and palliative aspects of cancer pain in adults[9-15] after extensively discussing and searching the evidence-based cancer pain management with regard to Indian perspectives.

Who can prescribe opioids and how to prescribe opioids has been made clear, together with an amended Narcotic Drugs and Psychotropic Substances Act (NDPS Act).[11] The ISSP guidelines also integrate the palliative aspects into cancer pain management.[15] Striving to eliminate or minimize chronic pain through opioid therapy has led to the iatrogenic injury to the general population at large as happened during USA opioid epidemic. Therefore, physicians should not only aim to titrate pain but strive to enhance the quality of life. Using opioid therapy to titrate pain intensity may not improve quality of life automatically. It is unrealistic and potentially damaging expectation for patients as well as clinicians, especially so in noncancer pain setting. What matters ultimately is not whether the patient's pain intensity has reduced, but whether the patient's overall quality of life has improved.[16] Opioid therapy may be a cornerstone for the treatment of cancer pain. However, opioids are not panacea always. Previous studies have shown that about 20–40% of patients' pain was not relieved by application of the three step World Health Organization (WHO) analgesic **(Fig. 1)** ladder.[17] Few patients are having opioid resistant pain. Neuropathic or bone metastasis pains are typical examples. Pain arising due to muscle spasm, decubitus ulcer, fractures, epidural cord compression and headache due to raised intracranial pressure may not respond to opioids. Clinicians should adopt a multimodal approach to triage such patients to receive other suitable therapies. The long-term adverse effects of opioids on cognitive function and on the immune and endocrine systems are largely ignored in palliative care but pose significant issues in

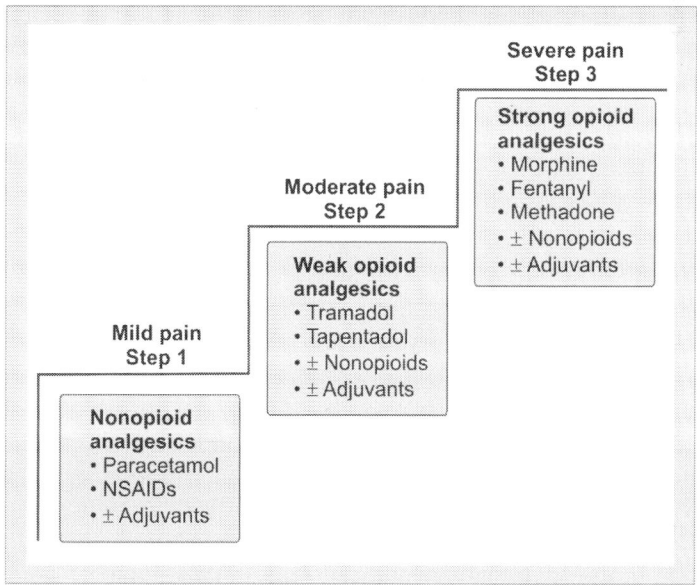

Fig. 1: Three step World Health Organization (WHO) analgesic ladder.
(NSAIDs: nonsteroidal anti-inflammatory drugs)

those who survive cancer.[18] During Covid era, aggressive opioid therapy may compromise the existing immune-compromised cancer patients to opioid-related inhibition of natural killer (NK) cell activity thereby, exposing to further infections and complications. There is a scarcity of randomized controlled trials (RCTs) for long-term use of opioids in cancer pain.[19] Nonetheless, opioids like codeine, morphine, oxycodone and fentanyl are often utilized in conjunction with paracetamol ± nonsteroidal anti-inflammatory drugs (NSAIDs) and coanalgesics (adjuvants) to manage cancer pain. Other treatment modalities outside the WHO analgesic ladder (including interventional techniques like nerve blocks or intrathecal analgesia delivery) are endorsed within the original WHO recommendations.[19] In this article, we are going to discuss about the recent updates in management of cancer pain.

All cancer pain guidelines including our ISSP cancer pain SIG guidelines acknowledge that analgesic therapy is the cornerstone of pain management. The goal of such therapy is to attain optimal pain relief with minimum or tolerable side effects with a minimal acceptable quality of life.

PHARMACOLOGICAL TREATMENT

Nonopioid Analgesics

Paracetamol

In a recent Cochrane review,[20] which assessed the role of oral paracetamol within the management of cancer pain, three small RCTs assessed paracetamol together with opioids. None assessed the use of paracetamol alone (first step). All studies used paracetamol as an add-on to be established treatment with strong opioids and other nonparacetamol medication. The paracetamol dose was apparently 1,500 mg daily, and it demonstrated less pain relief at that dose than NSAIDs or aspirin at the doses used. Overall, there was no high-quality evidence for or against using paracetamol (alone or with opioids) for cancer pain.[20] The ISSP cancer pain SIG guidelines provide a Grade B recommendation for the use of paracetamol alone or together with opioids for mild to moderate pain.[10]

Nonsteroidal Anti-inflammatory Drugs

The role of NSAIDs in cancer pain was assessed during a recent Cochrane review.[21] Nine of the 11 included studies had substantial risk of bias, being small and having incomplete outcome data. In four studies, NSAIDs initially reduced moderate or severe pain after 1 or 2 weeks (415 participants). Overall, there was no high-quality evidence for or against the utilization of NSAIDs (alone or with opioids). Thus, there is no high-quality evidence to support or refute the use of NSAIDs alone or together with opioids for the three steps of the three-step WHO cancer pain ladder. The ISSP cancer pain SIG guidelines provide a Grade B recommendation for the utilization of NSAIDs alone or together with opioids for mild to moderate pain.[10] NSAIDs can have gastrointestinal (GI), renal and cardiovascular (CV) toxicity.[22]

Based on individual risk of GI or CV toxicity, the subsequent recommendations are made about NSAID choice:[22-24]
- *No CV or GI risk:* Nonselective NSAID (ibuprofen, diclofenac).
- *Gastrointestinal risk +, no CV risk:* Avoid NSAIDs if possible; if essential celecoxib (200 mg/24 h).
- *Cardiovascular risk +/- GI risk:* Avoid if possible; naproxen (1 g/24 h) or low dose ibuprofen (<1200 mg/24 h).

Weak Opioid Analgesics

Tramadol

The role of tramadol with or without paracetamol in cancer pain management was assessed in an exceedingly recent Cochrane review.[25] Participants with chronic malignant tumor-related pain who were experiencing pain intensities described as moderate to severe, with most experiencing a minimum of 4/10 with current treatment were assessed in 10 studies. The daily oral dosage is typically up to 400 mg, although some guidelines suggest that 400 mg is the maximum dose. When combined with paracetamol, daily dosage is usually a maximum of eight tablets, each containing tramadol 37.5 mg and paracetamol 325 mg. There is a very low-quality evidence, that it is not as effective as morphine due to its mild mu receptor action. This review[25] does not provide a reliable indication of the likely effect. The place of tramadol in managing cancer pain and its exact role as step 2 of the WHO analgesic ladder is unclear. Many times, a substantial time is lost to titrate its dose, therefore many pain physicians prefer to use low dose morphine early on rather than using tramadol. Some trials are underway to clarify the real benefits of using one regime over the other in moderate pain. The ISSP cancer pain SIG guidelines provide a Grade B recommendation for the utilization of weak opioids like tramadol, tapentadol and codeine together with nonopioid analgesics for mild to moderate pain.[10]

Codeine

The role of codeine alone and with paracetamol for cancer pain because of diverse kinds of malignancy was assessed during a recent Cochrane review.[26] 12 studies used codeine as one agent and three combined it with paracetamol. Most studies investigated the effect of one dose of medication, while five used treatment periods of 1, 7 or 21 days. Most studies used codeine at doses of 30–120 mg. The available evidence indicates that codeine is not more effective than placebo, but has increased risk of nausea, vomiting, and constipation. This may also be possibly due to congenital deficiency of certain cytokines enzyme systems in some specific population. Uncertainty remains on the magnitude and time-course of its analgesic effect and therefore, the safety and tolerability in longer-term use data is not available for youngsters.[26] Codeine is converted to morphine (10:3) to exhibit its indirect therapeutic effect, having higher load of side effects and with better analgesics availability, it has gradually lost its place in cancer pain control armamentarium in modern practice. However, in absence other strong opioids, as in developing countries which is a perennial issue, this cheap drug can still relieve patients' suffering successfully till the end of life.

Tapentadol

The role of oral tapentadol in cancer pain management was assessed during a recent Cochrane review,[26] including four studies. All the studies used a parallel group design and included an initial titration phase to work out the most effective and tolerated dose, followed by a maintenance phase. Tapentadol medication was taken twice daily and doses ranged from 50 to 500 mg per day.[26] Information from RCTs on the effectiveness and tolerability of tapentadol was limited. The available studies were of moderate or small size and used different designs, which prevented pooling of information. Pain relief and adverse events were comparable between the tapentadol and morphine and oxycodone groups.

In all clinical studies with cancer pain patients, prolonged release (PR) tapentadol was well tolerated and provided adequate analgesia, which was noninferior to the quality opioids morphine-controlled release or oxycodone-controlled release.[27] Tapentadol PR are often considered a universal, strong, centrally acting analgesic drug for the management of moderate-to-severe cancer pain, both in opioid-naive and opioid-pretreated patients. Its good analgesic efficacy seems to result, partly due to the inherent synergistic mechanisms of tapentadol acting also on neuropathic components of cancer pain.[27]

As an alternative to weak opioids, low doses of strong opioids can be an option but is not included in WHO guidance (Grade B recommendation as per ISSP cancer pain SIG guidelines).[10]

Strong Opioids

Morphine

In a Cochrane review, all formulations of morphine were compared with one another and other opioids. 62 studies were included during this assessment. Morphine is an efficient analgesic for cancer pain. Pain relief did not differ between oral morphine modified release (Mm/r) and morphine immediate release (MIR). Modified release versions of morphine were effective for 12-or 24-hour dosing counting on the formulation. Daily doses in studies ranged from 25 mg to 2000 mg with a mean of between 100 and 250 mg. It was concluded that almost all patients will achieve a high level of pain relief within a minimum of 2 weeks. A little proportion of participants failed to achieve adequate analgesia with morphine and about 6% of participants discontinued treatment with morphine due to intolerable adverse events.[28] Oral route is the preferred route of administration. Intravenous or subcutaneous (SC) route of administered is suggested only, if rapid control of pain is needed.[10] The opioid of first choice for moderate to severe cancer pain is oral morphine (Grade A as per the ISSP cancer pain SIG guidelines).[10]

Amendment of the NDPS Act was done in 2014, and therefore, the relevant NDPS rules for essential narcotic drugs (ENDs) were announced by the Government of India in May 2015.[29] As per the amended NDPS Act 2015, any registered health professional (RMP) can prescribe opioids.[11] The prescription should be written in *Capital Letters*, with generic name of the opioid prescribed. It should have exact number of tablets/injection/patches to be dispatched with timings and route of the drug to be taken.

Adverse effects should be anticipated and managed appropriately in a very timely manner. Patients should be educated about the side effects and management of those side effects. Common side effects are constipation, nausea and vomiting, delirium, pruritus, central system toxicities such as motor and cognitive impairment and confusion, hallucination, somnolence, sedation, myoclonic jerks, and infrequently respiratory depression. Opioid-induced hyperalgesia could develop in patients on long-term opioids and may be identified early to optimize pain management.[11]

Methadone

In a Cochrane review,[30] six studies were assessed. There have been no studies in children. The included studies differed most in their methods and comparisons, so that no synthesis of results was feasible. Supported by low-quality evidence, methadone may be a drug that has similar analgesic benefits to morphine and incorporates a role within the management of cancer pain in adults. Due to its longer duration of action, its dose titration should be done judiciously. An electrocardiogram (ECG) and renal function test is required to be done prior to starting methadone medication. A pain and palliative care specialist have to be consulted if one is unfamiliar with methadone prescription, monitoring and equianalgesic dose rotation.[10,31]

Transdermal Opioids

Buprenorphine and fentanyl are strong opioids, often used as transdermal patches. They are especially indicated when there is a sustained pain which is moderate to severe in intensity and oral opioids are not effective or applicable like in a patient with vomiting, or unable to swallow or intestinal obstruction or when there is compliance issue. Effective systemic analgesic concentrations of transdermal fentanyl are generally reached within 3–23 hours, with steady state plasma concentrations achieved within 36–48 hours.[23] After 48 hours, if patients are requiring two or more rescue doses/day to effectively treat breakthrough pain, they ought to be assessed for a dose increase (by 12–25 µg/h).[23] Effective systemic analgesic concentrations of transdermal buprenorphine are generally reached within 11–24 hours, with steady state being reached after 1–3 days (depending on the preparation).[23] After 72 hours, if patients are requiring two or more rescue doses/day to effectively treat breakthrough pain, they must be assessed for a dose increase to the subsequent available higher strength.[23] ISSP cancer pain SIG guidelines a Grade D recommendation for transdermal fentanyl use when opioid requirements are stable.[10] Buprenorphine patches should be considered as a fourth-line option, other opioids are not found effective (Grade A).[10]

Adjuvant Analgesics

Adjuvant analgesics are drugs that are not primarily analgesics,[12] but in specific conditions can exhibit analgesic properties. Adjuvant analgesics are prescribed mainly in mixed cancer pain like neuropathic cancer pain,[32] chemotherapy-induced peripheral neuropathy, and metastatic bone pain. They are prescribed together with an opioid or by themselves.

Duloxetine is a serotonin-noradrenaline reuptake inhibitor and is licensed for treatment of diabetic peripheral neuropathic pain. In a multicenter randomized crossover trial of duloxetine versus placebo[33,34] it significantly reduced the typical pain score in patients with painful chemotherapy-induced peripheral neuropathy from platinum and taxane agents.

A double-blind RCT assessed the clinical efficacy of pregabalin, amitriptyline and gabapentin in neuropathic cancer pain compared to placebo.[35] All three drugs were found effective in relieving cancer-related neuropathic pain, with statistically and clinically significant morphine sparing effect. Pregabalin was reported effective in relieving neuropathic cancer pain and neuropathic symptoms compared to other antineuropathic medications.

A meta-analysis of four RCTs examined whether combining opioids with pregabalin or gabapentin, compared to opioid monotherapy improved cancer pain.[36] There was no significant difference in pain relief between groups; however, adverse events were more frequent in combination arms. Due to heterogeneity and also the relatively poor quality of RCTs, the real advantage of combination therapy in patients with neuropathic cancer pain could not be ascertained. Clinicians should balance potential benefits against the recognized adverse effects of combination therapy.[36]

WORLD HEALTH ORGANIZATION THREE-STEP ANALGESIC LADDER

Twenty-five studies were included for evaluating the effectiveness of the WHO cancer pain relief guidelines,[19] and concluded in an integrated review that WHO recommendations are effective for cancer pain relief in majority of patients. The best attribute of these guidelines is its simplicity to implement with safety even in a primary setting when patients' individual details are also incorporated. It dwells mainly on pain intensity suggesting a suitable oral analgesic. The conundrum of updating the WHO guidelines is to encompass the most recent pharmacologic and interventional innovations while maintaining its original simplicity. In one observational study,[37] it was found that only 48% of the pain prescriptions in cancer pain clinic were adherent to WHO three step analgesic ladder, which was due to undertreatment and underdosing of opioids.

There are many other cancer pain guidelines namely NCCN (National Cancer Care Network) and CDC (the Centers for Disease Control and Prevention) and ASCO (American Society for Clinical Oncology). NCCN recommends a flexible approach with simultaneous use of multiple therapies (analgesics, cancer therapy, physical and psychological therapy and interventional techniques, etc.) wherever and whenever applicable. CDC guidelines are mainly aimed for primary care physicians and have not included palliative care or end of life care. One of the major knowledge deficits remain to find out accumulated empirical evidence regarding the long-term opioid therapy in patients with persistent cancer or treatment-related pain. In response to CDC opioid guideline for chronic pain, ASCO opined that despite multiple cancer pain guidelines available, the solid evidence is lacking about the opioid use.

BONE PAIN

Bisphosphonates and denosumab are well-established therapies to scale back the frequency and severity of skeletal-related events in patients with bone metastasis. However, the analgesic effect of those medications on bone pain is uncertain.[38] Of the 43 studies which were assessed, evidence to support an analgesic role for bisphosphonates and denosumab was found weak. Bisphosphonates and denosumab appear to be beneficial in preventing pain by delaying the onset of bone pain instead of by producing an analgesic effect per se.[38] A Cochrane meta-analysis[39] reviewed 15 studies to see the efficacy and safety of radioisotopes in patients with bone metastases and observed a little advantage of radioisotopes for complete pain relief [risk ratio (RR): 2.10, 95% CI: 1.32–3.35; number needed to treat (NNT) to profit = 5] and complete/partial relief (RR: 1.72, 95% CI: 1.13–2.63; NNT = 4) within the short-and medium term and concluded that radioisotopes provide complete reduction in pain over a period of 1–6 months, but severe adverse effects like leukocytopenia and thrombocytopenia are frequently associated.[39] In a randomized placebo-controlled trial of SC salmon calcitonin[40] for analgesic effect in refractory metastatic bone pain, it was shown to have a significant reduction in pain after SC calcitonin injection therapy at 14th and 30th day assessment. However, this study could not reach a statistical significance which may be attributed to the small sample size of the study.

INTERVENTIONAL TREATMENT

There is a limited amount of high-quality evidence for interventional pain management techniques to manage cancer pain because of difficulties in performing RCTs in this therapeutic arena. The interventional treatment should be offered when conventional therapy fails to supply adequate benefit and/or causes undesirable side effects.[14]

Two recent meta-analyses have shown endoscopic-guided celiac ganglion neurolysis is effective in relieving pain in 80% and 72% of cancer patients, respectively.[41] Furthermore, the Cochrane review had demonstrated that celiac plexus neurolysis has fewer adverse effects as compared to opioids, therefore, may be considered for pain relief.[42]

Epidural, intrathecal, or intraventricular opioid infusions have been widely accepted as methods which provide good benefits to select group of patients in whom the pain is not controlled by medications given systemically. They do not have undesirable side effects at doses required to produce the analgesia. However, there is only limited number of high-quality studies on this. There are two randomized trials[43,44] showing both improved analgesia and prolonged survival in patients receiving neuraxial opioids as compared to traditional medical management. These neurolytic or neuromodulation techniques should be used in conjunction with medical management as part of interdisciplinary treatment. Early institution of analgesic interventions helps not only in effective pain management, but also in reduction in opioid doses, their side effects even have a better survival. Technical expertise, proper infrastructure, trained paramedical staff, and proper patient selection is of utmost importance for sustained safety and efficacy.[45]

The ISSP cancer pain SIG guidelines on interventional pain management for cancer pain in adults emphasize the importance of interventional pain management treatment as adjunct therapy for pharmacological cancer pain management.[14]

A systematic review[34] evaluating the effectiveness and safety of vertebral augmentation for malignant vertebral compression fractures (VCFs) was done assessing 87 studies between January 1, 2000 and January 3, 2018. This review showed clinically relevant improvements in pain, Oswestry Disability Index (ODI), Karnofsky Performance Score (KPS) in patients with VCFs because of malignancy treated with either percutaneous vertebroplasty (PVP) or kyphoplasty (KP). Cement leakage is common, but rarely symptomatic. PVP and KP are safe and effective palliative procedures for painful VCFs in patients with malignant spinal lesions.

CONCLUSION

Despite available effective analgesic agents, a majority of cancer patients do suffer moderate to severe pain worldwide. A thorough "total pain" assessment by a multidisciplinary team may fill the gap to chart out an adequate pain prescription which should be monitored time to time as the clinical conditions keep changing due to either ongoing disease process or due to the adverse effects of administered cancer therapies.

KEY POINTS

- Cancer pain can be caused due to the tumor, cancer treatment itself or may be unrelated to cancer.
- Cancer pain is often a mixed pain involving nociceptive as well as neuropathic pain components.
- Nociceptive components may arise from inflammation, tumor infiltration of soft tissues or stretching of periosteum or fascia, hollow viscus, occlusion of arteries and veins.
- Non-nociceptive (neuropathic) pain arises due to infiltration or compression of nerves by the tumor, raised intracranial pressure or spinal cord compression.
- Assessment of pain is paramount. "Total pain" concept should be adopted to decipher various components of pain.
- Cancer therapy also relieves pain. Radiotherapy reduces bone metastases pain.
- Treatment of cancer pain is multidisciplinary.
- Opioids are cornerstone for control of cancer pain of moderate or severe intensity.
- When analgesics fail or cause adverse effects, interventions are employed.
- Nonpharmacological options include cognitive behavioral therapy, yoga, and meditation/relaxation as part of multimodal treatment.

REFERENCES

1. Mallath MK, Taylor DG, Badwe RA, Rath GK, Shanta V, Pramesh CS, et al. The growing burden of cancer in India: epidemiology and social context. Lancet Oncol. 2014;15(6):e205-12.
2. Saini S, Bhatnagar S. Cancer pain management in developing countries. Indian J Palliat Care. 2016;22(4):373-7.
3. Doyle KE, El Nakib SK, Rajagopal MR, Babu S, Joshi G, Kumarasamy V, et al. Predictors and prevalence of pain and its management in four regional cancer hospitals in India. J Glob Oncol. 2018;4:1 9.
4. van den Beuken-van Everdingen MH, Hochstenbach LM, Joosten EA, Tjan Heijnen VC, Janssen DJ. Update on Prevalence of Pain in Patients With Cancer: Systematic Review and Meta-Analysis. J Pain Symptom Manage. 2016;51(6):1070-90.
5. Ayoub NM, Al-Shami KM, Yaghan RJ. Immunotherapy for HER2-positive breast cancer: recent advances and combination therapeutic approaches. Breast Cancer (Dove Med Press). 2019;11:53-69.
6. Remon, J, Reguart N, Auclin E, Besse B. Immune-related adverse events and outcomes in patients with advanced non-small cell lung cancer: a predictive marker of efficacy?. J Thorac Oncol. 2019;14(6):963-7.
7. Stebbing J, Slater S, Slevin M. Breast cancer (metastatic). BMJ Clin Evid. 2007;2007:0811.
8. Niravath P. Aromatase inhibitor-induced arthralgia: a review. Ann Oncol. 2013;24(6):1443-9.
9. Chatterjee A, Thota RS, Ramanjulu R, Ahmed A, Bhattacharya D, Salins N, et al. Indian Society for Study of Pain, Cancer Pain Special Interest Group Guidelines, for the Diagnosis and Assessment of Cancer Pain. Indian J Palliat Care. 2020;26:164-72.
10. Ramanjulu R, Thota RS, Ahmed A, Jain P, Salins N, Bhatnagar S, et al. Indian Society for Study of Pain, Cancer Pain Special Interest Group Guidelines on Pharmacological Management of Cancer Pain (Part I). Indian J Palliat Care. 2020;26(2):173-9.
11. Thota RS, Ramanjulu R, Ahmed A, Jain P, Salins N, Bhatnagar S, et al. Indian Society for Study of Pain, Cancer Pain Special Interest Group Guidelines on Pharmacological Management Of Cancer Pain (Part II). Indian J Palliat Care. 2020;26(2):180-90.
12. Ramanjulu R, Thota RS, Ahmed A, Jain P, Bhatnagar S, Salins N, et al. Indian Society for Study of Pain, Cancer Pain Special Interest Group Guidelines on Pharmacological Management of Cancer Pain (Part III). Indian J Palliat Care. 2020;26(2):191-97.
13. Ahmed A, Thota RS, Bhatnagar S, Jain P, Ramanjulu R, Salins N, et al. Indian Society for Study of Pain, Cancer Pain Special Interest Group Guidelines on Complementary Therapies for Cancer Pain. Indian J Palliat Care. 2020;26(2):198-202.
14. Ahmed A, Thota RS, Chatterjee A, Jain P, Ramanjulu R, Bhatnagar S, et al. Indian Society for Study of Pain, Cancer Pain Special Interest Group Guidelines on Interventional Management for Cancer Pain. Indian J Palliat Care. 2020;26(2):203-9.
15. Salins N, Thota RS, Bhatnagar S, Ramanjulu R, Ahmed A, Jain P, et al. Indian Society for Study of Pain, Cancer Pain Special Interest Group Guidelines on Palliative Care Aspects in Cancer Pain Management. Indian J Palliat Care. 2020;26(2):210-14.
16. Sullivan MD, Ballantyne JC. Must we reduce pain intensity to treat chronic pain; Pain. 2016;157(1):65-9.
17. Weiss SC, Emanuel LL, Fairclough DL, Emanuel EJ. Understanding the experience of pain in terminally ill patients. Lancet. 2001;357(9265):1311-5.
18. Seyfried O, Hester J. Opioids and endocrine dysfunction. Br J Pain. 2012;6(1):17-24.

19. Carlson CL. Effectiveness of the World Health Organization cancer pain relief guidelines: an integrative review. J Pain Res. 2016;9:515-34.
20. Wiffen PJ, Derry S, Moore RA, McNicol ED, Bell RF, Carr DB, et al. Oral paracetamol (acetaminophen) for cancer pain. Cochrane Database Syst Rev. 2017;7(7):CD012637.
21. Derry S, Wiffen PJ, Moore RA, McNicol ED, Bell RF, Carr DB, et al. Oral nonsteroidal anti-inflammatory drugs (NSAIDs) for cancer pain in adults. Cochrane Database Syst Rev. 2017;7(7):CD012638.
22. Bhala N, Emberson J, Merhi A, Abramson S, Arber N, Baron JA, et al. Vascular and upper gastrointestinal effects of non-steroidal anti-inflammatory drugs: meta-analyses of individual participant data from randomised trials. Lancet. 2013;382(9894):769-79.
23. Twycross R, Wilcock A, Howard P. Palliative Care Formulary, 6th edition. Nottingham: Palliative drugs.com Ltd., 2017.
24. Scarpignato C, Lanas A, Blandizzi C, Lems WF, Hermann M, Hunt RH, et al. Safe prescribing of nonsteroidal anti-inflammatory drugs in patients with osteoarthritis; an expert consensus addressing benefits as well as gastrointestinal and cardiovascular risks. BMC Med. 2015;13:55.
25. Wiffen PJ, Derry S, Moore R. Tramadol with or without paracetamol (acetaminophen) for cancer pain. Cochrane Database Syst Rev. 2017;5(5):CD012508.
26. Wiffen PJ, Derry S, Naessens K, Bell RF. Oral tapentadol for cancer pain. Cochrane Database Syst Rev. 2015;2015(9):CD011460.
27. Kress HG, Coluzzi F. Tapentadol in the management of cancer pain: current evidence and future perspectives. J Pain Res. 2019;12:1553-60.
28. Wiffen PJ, Wee B, Moore RA. Oral morphine for cancer pain. Cochrane Database Syst Rev. 2016;4(4):CD003868.
29. Government of India Gazette Notification GSR 359(E). Amending the Narcotic Drugs and Psychotropic Substances Rules, 1985, Namely Called the Narcotic Drugs and Psychotropic Substances (Third Amendment) Rules; 2015 (dated 5th May 2015 Issued).
30. Nicholson AB, Watson GR, Derry S, Wiffen PJ. Methadone for cancer pain. Cochrane Database Syst Rev. 2017;2(2):CD003971.
31. Ramkiran S, Thota RS. Methadone in cancer pain. Indian J Palliat Care. 2020;26(2):215-20.
32. Finnerup NB, Attal N, Haroutounian S, McNicol E, Baron R, Dworkin RH, et al. Pharmacotherapy for neuropathic pain in adults: a systematic review and meta-analysis. Lancet Neurol. 2015;14(2):162-73.
33. Smith EM, Pang H, Cirrincione C, Fleishman S, Paskett ED, Ahles T, et al. Effect of duloxetine on pain, function, and quality of life among patients with chemotherapy-induced painful peripheral neuropathy: a randomized clinical trial. JAMA. 2013;309:1359-67.
34. Sørensen ST, Kirkegaard AO, Carreon L, Rousing R, Andersen MØ. Vertebroplasty or kyphoplasty as palliative treatment for cancer-related vertebral compression fractures: a systematic review. Spine J. 2019;19(6):1067-75.
35. Mishra S, Bhatnagar S, Goyal GN, Rana SP, Upadhya SP. A comparative efficacy of amitriptyline, gabapentin, and pregabalin in neuropathic cancer pain: a prospective randomized double-blind placebo-controlled study. Am J Hosp Palliat Care. 2012;29(3):177-82.
36. Kane CM, Mulvey MR, Wright S, Craigs C, Wright JM, Bennett MI. Opioids combined with antidepressants or antiepileptic drugs for cancer pain: systematic review and meta-analysis. Palliat Med. 2018;32(1):276-86.

37. Thota RS, Jain PN, Bakshi SG, Dhanve CN. Opioid-prescribing in practices chronic cancer pain in a tertiary care pain clinic. Indian J Palliat Care. 2011;17(3):222-6.
38. Porta-Sales J, Garzón-Rodríguez C, Llorens-Torromé S, Brunelli C, Pigni A, Caraceni A. Evidence on the analgesic role of bisphosphonates and denosumab in the treatment of pain due to bone metastases: a systematic review within the European Association for Palliative Care guidelines project. Palliat Med. 2017;31(1):5-25.
39. Roqué I Figuls M, Martinez-Zapata MJ, Scott-Brown M, Alonso-Coello P. Radioisotopes for metastatic bone pain. Cochrane Database Syst Rev. 2011;(7):CD003347.
40. Jain PN, Chatterjee A. A randomized placebo-controlled trial evaluating the analgesic effect of salmon calcitonin in refractory bone metastasis pain. Indian J Palliat Care. 2020;26(1):4-8.
41. Puli SR, Reddy JB, Bechtold ML, Antillon MR, Brugge WR. EUS-guided celiac plexus neurolysis for pain due to chronic pancreatitis or pancreatic cancer pain: a meta-analysis and systematic review. Dig Dis Sci. 2009;54(11):2330-7.
42. Arcidiacono PG, Calori G, Carrara S, McNicol ED, Testoni PA. Celiac plexus block for pancreatic cancer pain in adults. Cochrane Database Syst Rev. 2011;2011(3):CD007519.
43. Smith TJ, Staats PS, Deer T, Stearns LJ, Rauck RL, Boortz-Marx RL, et al. Randomized clinical trial of an implantable drug delivery system compared with comprehensive medical management for refractory cancer pain: impact on pain, drug-related toxicity, and survival. J Clin Oncol. 2002;20(19):4040-9.
44. Smith TJ, Coyne PJ, Staats PS, Deer T, Stearns LJ, Rauck RL, et al. An implantable drug delivery system (IDDS) for refractory cancer pain provides sustained pain control, less drug-related toxicity, and possibly better survival compared with comprehensive medical management (CMM). Ann Oncol. 2005;16(5):825-33.
45. Bhatnagar S, Gupta M. Evidence-based clinical practice guidelines for interventional pain management in cancer pain. Indian J Palliat Care. 2015;21(2):137-47.

CHAPTER 24

Management of Head and Neck Neuralgia

Anoop Raj Gogia, Amita Gupta

INTRODUCTION

Head and neck neuralgias are common in clinical practice. Due to complex anatomy and specialized sensory innervation of the head, face, and neck, many of these neuralgias pose diagnostic challenges. Common head and neck neuralgias encountered in clinical practice are trigeminal neuralgia (TN), glossopharyngeal neuralgia (GPN), occipital neuralgia and postherpetic neuralgia (PHN). Other causes of head and neck pain which may mimic these neuralgias include constant pain caused by compression, irritation, or distortion of cranial nerves or upper cervical roots by structural lesions, head or facial pain attributed to herpes zoster (HZ), central poststroke pain and facial pain attributed to multiple sclerosis.

TRIGEMINAL NEURALGIA

Trigeminal neuralgia is the most common type of neuralgia encountered in clinical practice, with an estimated annual incidence of 4–8 per 100,000 individuals.[1] It primarily affects middle aged and elderly population, females being more affected than males. As per International Headache Society (HIS) Classification, International Classification of Headache Disorders (ICHD-3)[2] TN is described as a disorder characterized by recurrent unilateral brief electric shock-like pains, abrupt in onset and termination, restricted to one or more branches of trigeminal nerve, and triggered by innocuous stimuli. It may develop without apparent cause or be a result of another diagnosed disorder. Additionally, there may be concomitant continuous pain of moderate intensity within the distribution(s) of the affected nerve division(s). Maxillary and mandibular divisions are more commonly affected. The pain may be so intense that the patient winces, hence also called tic douloureux. Mild autonomic symptoms such as lacrimation and/or redness of the ipsilateral eye may be present. There is usually a refractive period following painful paroxysm. Onset is usually sudden, and bouts of pain tend to persist for weeks or months before remitting spontaneously. Trigger zones have been identified typically on face, lips or tongue, where even tactile stimuli like washing the face, brushing the teeth, or air breeze may trigger an attack of pain. The most common cause of TN, in about 95% of cases, is vascular compression near the root entry zone. Vascular compression leads to demyelination, which in turn leads to ectopic action potential generation that is suspected to allegedly drive the sharp lancinating episode.

Diagnosis of Trigeminal Neuralgia

Trigeminal neuralgia must be diagnosed on the basis of history and clinical examination. Investigations are designed to identify a likely cause. In case the patient shows sensory or motor deficit within the trigeminal distribution on neurological examination, neuroimaging investigations must be done to explore possible cause.

Classical TN is described as development of neuralgia without apparent cause other than neurovascular compression. Root entry zone is the most common site for compression of neurovascular bundle. In secondary TN an underlying disease (other than neurovascular compression) is present to explain the cause. Clinical examination in these patients usually, but not always, shows sensory changes. Recognized causes are tumor in the cerebellopontine angle, arteriovenous (AV)-malformation and multiple sclerosis.

Investigations

In typical case of TN, diagnosis is usually clinical and neuroimaging studies are not required. Magnetic resonance imaging (MRI) and magnetic resonance angiography (MGA) are done, if decompressive surgery is under consideration for vascular compression.

Treatment

The management strategies of pain should strive for improvements in pain as well as other functional elements such as sleep, mood, social, and spiritual consequences of pain. It is these factors that drive much of patients' quality of life. Various guidelines emphasize on multidisciplinary team approach for the management of neuropathic pain.[3,4] Besides pharmacological management of pain, nonpharmacological therapies such as psychotherapy, physiotherapy, exercise, and massage should be initiated early to avoid or control issues such as depression, anxiety, sleep disturbances, etc.

Pharmacological Management

Carbamazepine (CBZ), 200–1,200 mg/day, is the first line drug in medical management of TN as per the recent guidelines[5] and has been found to be effective in nearly 70% of the patients of TN. CBZ should be started as 100 mg twice daily dose taken with food and increased gradually (100 mg/day every 1–2 days) till substantial (>50%) pain relief is achieved which starts within 48 hours.[6] The effectiveness of CBZ was demonstrated in several studies.[6-8] CBZ reduces both the frequency and intensity of painful paroxysms and is equally effective on spontaneous and trigged attacks.[9] Diagnosis of TN should be reconsidered in case of failure of response to CBZ.[10] CBZ acts by suppression of spontaneous neuronal activity by binding to voltage gated sodium channels, and preventing repetitive, and sustained firing of action potential. Most important side-effects of CBZ are dizziness, sedation, imbalance, endocrine dysfunction and rarely agranulocytosis. Oxcarbazepine (300–1,200 mg BID), a structural analogue of CBZ, has fewer side-effects and can be substituted if patient is unable to tolerate or has become refractory to CBZ. Randomized controlled trials, comparing oxcarbazepine (600–1,800 mg/day) to CBZ in TN patients, have demonstrated reduction in painful episodes in more than 80% of patients.[11,12]

Few other drugs recommended in case CBZ, and oxcarbazepine are ineffective or are not well tolerated, include phenytoin 300–400 mg daily, lamotrigine 400 mg or duloxetine (20–90 mg/day) daily. Gabapentin (900–3600 mg/day) is another anticonvulsant drug frequently being used in the treatment of TN. Its mechanism of action as anticonvulsant is likely by inhibition of the alpha-2 delta subunit of voltage gated calcium channels. Gabapentin is effective in 80% of patients when used as first line drug and in 50% cases of failure due to CBZ. Pregabapin, a precursor of gabapentin can also be used. Baclofen may also be tried either alone or in combination with an anticonvulsant. The initial dose is 5–10 mg TID, gradually increasing to 20 mg QID if needed.

Carbamazepine or other first line drugs can be combined with local infiltrations and peripheral nerve blocks with local anesthetics and steroid injections at frequent intervals. According to a recent overview,[13] gabapentin in combination with ropivacaine injections into trigger sites benefited both pain control and quality of life, and pregabalin was effective at 1 year follow-up in TN patients.

Recently, Hu et al.[14] in a systematic review evaluated the efficacy and safety of injection of botulinum toxin type A (BTX-A) in TN. They elicited good response to treatment in approximately 70–100% of patients with reduced mean pain intensity and frequency in approximately 60–80% with no major adverse events reported.

Interventional Therapy

Various interventional techniques have been tried for the treatment of TN, but they should only be considered after failure of medical management.

Surgical Decompression

Long-term pain relief can only be achieved by open surgical craniectomy and microvascular decompression (MVD) by inserting a sponge between the compressing vessel and trigeminal nerve. The pain free period following MVD ranges from 0.5 to 10 years.[15] After 5 years, the percentage of pain free patients ranges from 58 to 78%.[16,17] The patients with immediate pain remissions in postoperative period have excellent or good outcomes.[17] Complications commonly seen with this procedure are infections, facial palsy, facial numbness, cerebrospinal fluid leak, and hearing deficit with a mortality in 0.1% patients.

Management of Head and Neck Neuralgia

Percutaneous Interventions

Radiofrequency ablation (RFA) is a technique in which there is controlled ablation of trigeminal ganglion and nerve roots using RF. Patients with TN having good pain relief with diagnostic trigeminal ganglion block may be considered for RFA. Approximately 88% and 61% of patients have been reported to have complete pain relief immediately and at 3 years respectively.[18,19] The reported side-effects are weakness of muscles of mastication, dysesthesia, and corneal numbness.

Glycerol rhizolysis is a technique in which 0.5 mL of glycerol is injected in trigeminal cistern. Hyperbaric glycerol sinks and produces discrete neurolysis of second and third division of TN. Pain relief is usually immediate. Approximately 84% of patients still have complete pain relief after 6 months.[18,19] Dysesthesias, masseter weakness, corneal anesthesia and herpes labialis have been reported as complications of this procedure.

Percutaneous balloon compression (PBC) was introduced by Mullan et al.[20,21] and has been extensively used in the treatment of TN due to its simplicity, and low cost. A balloon is guided into Meckle's cave under fluoroscopy and is then inflated with a small volume of contrast dye, compressing the trigeminal ganglion for 3–10 minutes. PBC has immediate postoperative pain relief ranging from 80 to 90%.[22,23]

Gamma knife surgery is a noninvasive stereotactic radiosurgery used in elderly patients or patients who have medical comorbidities and who refuse open surgery.[24] It uses computed tomography (CT) or MRI guided radiations at the root entry zone of the trigeminal nerve. It usually takes 1–2 months for response to be seen.[18,24] Following gamma knife surgery 55% patients remained pain free in a 3-year of follow-up.

Among the percutaneous treatment options for TN, RFA has the best long-term pain relief. However, adverse side effects are maximum (29%) with RFA, compared with glycerol rhizolysis (29%), PBC (16%), and gamma knife surgery (12%).[18,25,26] gamma knife surgery can be performed under local anesthetic only.

Two types of neuromodulation have been described as optional treatments for chronic pain, refractory to conventional medical and surgical treatment: motor cortex stimulation (MCS) and deep brain stimulation (DBS), but their efficacy is variable.

GLOSSOPHARYNGEAL NEURALGIA

Glossopharyngeal neuralgia is a rare condition compared to TN. The prevalence of GPN is estimated to be approximately 0.8 per 100,000 populations per year. Patients with GPN often describe pain in throat, tonsillar region, and posterior third of tongue, larynx, nasopharynx and pinna of the ear. GPN produces symptoms of severe, lancinating, paroxysmal pain that is triggered by tactile stimuli such as swallowing or coughing. GPN can result from vascular compression at the root entry zone of brain stem, tumors, infection, postsurgery or multiple sclerosis, but many cases are idiopathic. Eagle's syndrome or styalgia is glossopharyngeal nerve hyperexcitability syndrome due to an elongated styloid process or calcified stylohyoid ligament.

Diagnosis of GPN is based on detailed history and examination with special emphasis on throat examination and neck palpation.

Investigations

- *X-ray:* An orthopantomogram or lateral soft tissue X-ray helps to identify elongated and calcified styloid process.
- *CT scan with 3D reconstruction:* It is the gold standard for visualizing anatomically complex styloid process.[27]
- *Magnetic resonance imaging:* Contrast image helps identify neurovascular compression of the glossopharyngeal nerve, demyelinating disease or tumors, etc.
- *Magnetic resonance angiogram:* Helps to evaluate for a vascular loop compressing on the nerve root entry zone and is done if intervention is planned.[28]

Treatment

Pharmacotherapy

Since GPN has the same pathogenesis as of TN, pharmacological treatment strategies for GPN are on the same lines as of TN.

Additional measures which can be employed are cold and hot compresses, physical therapy, and psychological counseling.[29]

Interventional Therapy

A diagnostic block with a local anesthetic helps confirm the origin of the pain. If diagnostic blocks are successful, glossopharyngeal nerve block with a local anesthetic and a steroid serves as an excellent adjunct to the pharmacologic treatment of GPN. It helps in rapid palliation of pain while oral medications are titrated to effective levels. Glossopharyngeal nerve can be blocked via: the intraoral and extraoral approaches. Intraorally, it can be blocked by infiltration at the base of posterior tonsillar pillar by local anesthetics. The extraoral technique is safe and easy to perform. Complications include intravascular injection because of proximity of the glossopharyngeal nerve to internal jugular vein and carotid artery, hoarseness of voice due to concomitant block of the recurrent laryngeal nerve, tachycardia and hypertension via blockade of vagus nerve.[30,31] Bilateral glossopharyngeal nerve blocks must not be given simultaneously to avoid complete vocal cord paralysis.

Surgical Decompression

Resection of enlarged styloid process on the affected side is the best option for styloid-stylohyoid syndrome. Other causes of nerve compression must be ruled out first.

Microvascular decompression of the glossopharyngeal root (Jannetta technique) is safe and effective option in patients who do not respond to medical management. MVD shows symptomatic relief in 84.7% of patients, long-term pain relief in 64%, recurrence rates of 7%, and permanent complications in up to 5.5% of patients.[32,33]

Percutaneous Interventions

Radiofrequency ablation of the GPN root is performed at the jugular foramen to target inferior petrous ganglion of Andersch. Severe bradycardia and hypotension can occur due to vagal stimulation during the procedure. After RFA, pain relief in a study has been found to be 73.2% at 1 year, 63% at 3 years, 53.2% at 5 years, and 43.0% at 10 years.[34]

Stereotactic radiosurgery with gamma knife surgery can be tried in elderly patients or patients with comorbid conditions, but data on safety and efficacy is limited.[34-36]

Chemical neurolysis using absolute alcohol, glycerol or phenol can also be performed.

HERPES ZOSTER AND POSTHERPETIC NEURALGIA

Postherpetic neuralgia is a chronic neuropathic pain symptom complex, following HZ or shingles, defined as pain persisting for 3 months or more after the onset of rash in the same dermatome.[37] HZ occurs from the reactivation of the dormant varicella-zoster virus (VZV) from the geniculate, trigeminal or the dorsal root ganglion of the spinal cord.[38,39] Onset of the disease is accompanied by pain within the dermatome, preceding lesions by 48–72 hours; an erythematous maculopapular rash which evolves rapidly into vesicular lesions. The total course of the disease in normal persons is 7–10 days. This neuropathy is very severe and is characterized by significant allodynia, hyperalgesia, and burning dysesthesia. Changes in the sensation in the dermatome, resulting in either hypo- or hyperesthesia are common. First division of the trigeminal nerve (zoster ophthalmicus) is most common to be involved. Geniculate ganglion of the facial nerve may be affected causing pain and vesicles in the external auditory canal, loss of taste in anterior two-thirds of the tongue and ipsilateral facial palsy (Ramsay Hunt syndrome). In majority of cases there is progressive improvement in pain, but in 1–2% cases pain may persist for years. Clinical features of acute HZ such as prodromal pain, intense acute pain, severity of rash, and ophthalmic involvement with keratitis and other intraocular complications are associated with increased risk of PHN. Female sex, increased age and diabetes are other predisposing factors for PHN.[39-42] Incidence of HZ has been reported to be varying from 2.2 to 3.4/1,000 patients/year and PHN occurs in 9–19% of all HZ patients.[43,44]

Patients with HZ benefit from antiviral therapy, as evidenced by reduction of acute phase rash, duration of new lesion formation and resolution of zoster related pain.[45] Valacyclovir and famciclovir are superior to acyclovir in terms of pharmacokinetics and pharmacodynamics, and should be preferred. Studies and meta-analyses showed that oral corticosteroid therapy does not prevent PHN.[46,47]

For the management of pain of acute neuritis analgesics ranging from nonsteroidal anti-inflammatory drugs (NSAIDs) to narcotics and its derivatives, drugs such as gabapentin, pregabalin, tricyclic antidepressants (TCAs), lignocaine patches, calamine lotion, capsaicin cream and nerve blocks are beneficial. Stellate ganglion block helps in pain control and hastening of rash healing. Repeated injections of local anesthetics have been administered to treat acute shingles. According to Colding,[48] the pain relief started 10-15 minutes after the block and usually lasted for 8-12 hours. Additionally, the pain was less intense when it returned.

Treatment

Pharmacological Management

It is first line treatment for alleviation of pain symptoms in PHN. Even with adequate doses, up to 40-50% of patients with PHN do not get satisfactory relief from pain. Various classes of medications recommended as first-line agents for the treatment of PHN are TCAs, gabapentin, pregabalin, opioids, capsaicin and topical lignocaine.

Tricyclic antidepressants such as amitriptyline and nortriptyline) with or without anticonvulsants such as gabapentin or pregabalin should be started first. TCAs also help in relieving anxiety, and sleeplessness associated with PHN because of their anxiolytic and sedative properties. Nortriptyline is better tolerated with greater efficacy and fewer anticholinergic side-effects. Nortriptyline is started with low doses (10 mg at bedtime) and slowly titrated (10 mg every 3-5 days) as tolerated by the patient up to a maximum dose of 150 mg daily. After 1-2 weeks of the treatment with maximum tolerated dose TCAs should be tapered off over next 3-4 weeks.[49] Adverse effects of TCAs include weight gain, dizziness, blurring of vision, postural hypotension, urinary retention, constipation and sexual dysfunction.[50]

Antiepileptics (gabapentin and pregabalin) in combination with TCAs have been found to be superior to TCAs alone for PHN. Gabapentin is started at a low dose of 100 mg three times daily, with gradual increase every 5-7 days, to optimum dose providing adequate pain relief (usually, 300-400 mg TID). Side effects of gabapentin include dizziness, somnolence, and ataxia and peripheral edema. Tolerance to the side effects develops over 1-2 weeks and patient should be informed about this before starting the treatment. Limitation of gabapentin is its short half-life, thus requiring frequent dosing and low patient compliance. Gabapentin is equally efficacious to nortriptyline in treating PHN pain and improving sleep;[50] a combination of the two drugs was better than each one alone.[51]

Gastroretentive gabapentin and gabapentin encarbil are the two types of extended release formulations have been approved by the Food and Drug Administration (FDA) in 2011 and 2012.[52] These have better efficacy, and tolerability, avoid long titration period and permit single daily dosing.

The mechanism of action of pregabalin is similar to that of gabapentin, but it differs in its pharmacokinetics. Compared to gabapentin's less predictable zero-order absorption, pregabalin has first-order absorption with stable 90% bioavailability at different doses. In addition, the pain relief is usually noticed within 48 hours,[53] which is earlier than with gabapentin. Pregabalin should be started at 75 mg twice daily and may be increased to 150 mg twice daily after 1 week, if required.

Topical lignocaine can be combined with pregabalin for additive pain relief.[54] It is available in the form of gel or eutectic mixture of local anesthetics (EMLA), lignocaine 2.5% and prilocaine 2.5%, and lignocaine dermal patches. In a randomized, multicenter study, that compared the effectiveness of pregabalin and topical lignocaine, a larger percentage of patients receiving topical lignocaine 5% reported a 2-point or greater decrease in pain on a 0–10-point scale and fewer adverse effects at 4 weeks of therapy.[54] In a separate study, a novel 8% lignocaine spray with possible shorter latency was described as safe and effective for use as a rescue therapy for PHN pain.[55,56] The application of patch also protects the exacerbation of pain on allodynic skin.

Capsaicin is an alkaloid extracted from hot chili peppers and is available as 0.025% and 0.075% lotion or cream. Topical capsaicin acts in the skin to attenuate cutaneous hypersensitivity and reduce pain by a process best described as "defunctionalization" of nociceptor fibers defunctionalization is due to a number of effects that include temporary loss of membrane potential, inability to transport neurotrophic factors leading to altered phenotype, and reversible retraction of epidermal and dermal nerve fiber terminals. Capsaicin binds to vanilloid receptor subtype 1 [transient receptor potential vanilloid subtype 1 (TRPV1)], an ion channel-type receptor. TRPV1 can also be stimulated with heat, protons and physical abrasion. By binding to the TRPV1 receptor, the capsaicin molecule produces similar sensations to those of excessive heat or abrasive damage, explaining why the spiciness of capsaicin is described as a burning sensation.

Pain relief was achieved regardless of concomitant systemic antineuropathic pain medication use.[57] Topical lignocaine should be applied before application of capsaicin to minimize erythema and pain caused by capsaicin.

Opioids and tramadol: Due to their side-effects like dependence, addiction, and misuse, the use of opioids is controversial despite good analgesic properties. Opioids are used as second-line or third-line drugs for PHN.[58] Tramadol is a milder opioid with lesser addiction liability and can be administered orally. Tramadol has been found to be less effective in pain relief in PHN than other opioid, but it is better tolerated and a safer drug to use.

Interventional Therapy

Various peripheral nerve blocks and field blocks with local anesthetics and steroids have been reported to eliminate PHN pain for a prolonged period. Some nonrandomized trials assessing sympathetic blockade in PHN have failed to demonstrate benefit, and there is very little data to suggest a beneficial effect.[59,60] For superficial trigeminal nerve blocks, the local anesthetic solution should be injected in close proximity to the three individual terminal superficial branches of the trigeminal nerve divisions: frontal nerve (of the ophthalmic nerve, V1 division); infraorbital nerve (of the maxillary nerve, V2 division); and mental nerve (sensory terminal branch of the mandibular nerve, V3 division). Lingual and inferior alveolar branches of mandibular nerves can be blocked by intraoral approach, behind the third molar.

For a complete maxillary block, the maxillary nerve is accessible at the upper part of the pterygopalatine fossa. The suprazygomatic approach seems to be the safest and is easiest to perform. Nerve stimulation may help locate the pterygopalatine fossa: complications include cephalgia, facial paralysis, trismus, and hematoma.

Mandibular nerve is blocked where the nerve emerges through the foramen ovale. The risk of puncture of the internal maxillary or middle meningeal arteries can be high when the needle inserted too high in the space between the coronoid and condylar processes. After an injection of a large volume of local anesthetic solution, transient facial nerve block has been reported, which resolved spontaneously without sequelae. Steroids (triamcinolone) have been recommended along with local anesthetic for prolonged pain relief. The nerve blocks have to be repeated weekly or fortnightly for 3-4 times for complete relief.

Radiofrequency ablation using the heat lesioning at temperature 67°C or higher has been reported in literature for PHN. Common side effects of heat lesioning include dysesthesia, hypesthesia and paresis.[61]

Pulsed radiofrequency lesioning (PRF) is a safe, nondestructive, neuroablative modality, which obviates the complications of heat lesioning. It helps in pain modulation and can be performed multiple times, as needed.

Neuromodulation

Peripheral neuromodulation has been described by various authors for the management of intractable PHN, which is refractory to the commonly used regimes. After successful trial stimulation, a permanent stimulator is placed and patient medications are tapered off following onset of the effect. Upadhyay SP and Kouroukli I et al. reported management of a case of supraorbital PHN, where after trial stimulation, a permanent stimulator was placed and the patient had excellent pain relief 8 weeks poststimulation without any side effect.[62]

Trigeminal tractotomy (targeting the trigeminal descending tract in medulla and *trigeminal nucleotomy* (targeting nucleus caudalis) have been described in small case series.

Central nervous system lesions may involve thalamotomy, cingulotomy, prefrontal leukotomy and other central locations. *Gamma knife thalamotomy* resulted in 70% relief in pain by Young et al. *Prefrontal lobectomy* is now not considered because of effects on intellectual performance.

OCCIPITAL NEURALGIA

Occipital neuralgia is a condition where the occipital nerves, the nerves running through the scalp, are injured. Occipital neuralgia occurs result of pinched nerves or muscle tightness in the back of neck. It can also be caused by a head or neck injury or inflammation in that region. Many cases are as a result of chronic muscle tension. List of possible causes include osteoarthritis of the upper cervical spine, trauma, cervical disk degeneration, diabetes, gout, vasculitis or infection in local area.

Symptoms of occipital neuralgia are pain of continuous aching, burning and throbbing nature, with intermittent shocking or shooting type that generally starts at the base of the head and goes to the scalp on one or both sides of the head. Patients may have pain behind the eye of the affected side of the head. A movement like brushing hair may trigger pain. Examination include movements of the spine and a neurological examination. CT for structural deformities in vertebrae and MRI for ruling out nerve impingement may be done. A diagnostic occipital nerve block may be performed.

Nonsurgical treatments include hot fomentation, physical therapy, massage, oral nonsteroidal analgesics and local sprays, and occipital nerve blocks with or without steroids.

Occipital nerve stimulation: It is noninvasive stimulation of occipital nerves by placing electrodes on the skin close to occipital nerves. The results are same as DBS, and it uses the same device.

Spinal cord stimulation: This is a surgical procedure where electrodes are surgically placed near spinal cord under the spine. The stimulation results in blocking of pain impulses to spinal cord.

C2,3 ganglionectomy: In this treatment C2-3 dorsal nerve root ganglions are removed surgically. Acar et al. studied the short-term and long-term effects of this procedure. About 95% patients had immediate pain relief and at 1 year postprocedure, 61% patients had continued benefit.

Platelet rich plasma (PRP): This is an emerging biologic treatment. PRP contains high concentrations of platelets, growth factors, and anti-inflammatory molecules. PRP acts to reduce inflammation and encourage tissue repair at the site of injection. PRP is created by collecting a person's own blood, centrifuging it, and extracting the platelet-rich layer of plasma. This platelet rich mixture is then reinjected into the affected area.

OTHER FACIAL PAINS

Persistent idiopathic facial pain (PIFP) is an idiopathic facial pain condition that does not have clinical characteristics of particular neuralgia. Although TN and PIFP are two most common etiologies of paroxysmal pain other red flag conditions (tumors infections, vascular abnormality/dissection, fracture and intracranial bleed) must be excluded. Additionally, other comorbidities like demyelinating, autoimmune or neuromuscular conditions, should be identified. Musculoskeletal conditions like TM disorders may cause dull aching pain or tenderness often worsened by jaw movement, pathology affecting the teeth and gums may result in deep, sharp pain triggered by eating.

CONCLUSION

Neuropathic pain syndromes involving head and neck regions result from unintentional trauma, deafferentation and cephalic neuralgias. Diagnosis is based on clear cut history and detailed investigations. Treatment consists of psychotherapy, pharmacotherapy and if symptoms persist by peripheral interventions or by surgical procedures. RFA and stereotactic surgery are advanced minimally invasive procedures. MVD following craniectomy is the advanced surgical therapy. Rehabilitation of these patients posttherapy is another integral part of treatment in such cases. Establishment of specifically designed exercises, functional restoration programs and restoration of sleep cycle are essential components.

ACKNOWLEDGMENT

I am sincerely grateful to Dr Shweta Gupta CMO in the Department of Anesthesia and Intensive Care for her inputs and preparation of this article.

> **KEY POINTS**
> - Chronic facial pain may result from a diverse assortment of causes including trauma, structural abnormalities, infections, tumors and central nervous system (CNS) disease.
> - Due to complex anatomy and specialized sensory innervation of the head, face, and neck, many of these neuralgias pose diagnostic challenges.
> - Neuropathic pain syndromes result from unintentional trauma, deafferentation and cephalic neuralgia.
> - Common cephalic neuralgias include trigeminal neuralgia, geniculate neuralgia, glossopharyngeal neuralgia, occipital neuralgia and postherpetic neuralgia.
> - Most common cause of trigeminal neuralgia is to vascular compression.
> - Treatment of all neuralgic pains consists of psychological therapy, pharmacotherapy, and when symptoms persists variety of minimally invasive techniques followed by surgery.

REFERENCES

1. Beal MF, Hauser SL. Harrison's Principles of Internal Medicine, 20th edition. New York: Mc Graw-Hill Education; 2018.
2. ICHD-3. (2013). The International Classification of Headache Disorders, 3rd edition. [online] Available from https://ichd-3.org/13-painful-cranial-neuropathies-and-other-facial-pains/13-1-trigeminal-neuralgia/13-1-2-painful-trigeminal-neuropathy/. [Last accessed October, 2020].
3. NICE. (2013). Neuropathic pain in adults: Pharmacological management in non-specialist settings. NICE, Clinical Guideline. 2013. [online] Available from nice.org.uk/guidance/cg173. [Last accessed October, 2020].
4. Dworkin RH, O'Connor AB, Audette J, Baron R, Gourlay GK, Haanpää ML, et al. Recommendations for the pharmacological management of neuropathic pain: an overview and literature update. Mayo Clinic Proc. 2010;85(3 Suppl):S3-14.

5. Cruccu G, Sommer C, Anand P, Attal N, Baron R, Garcia-Larrea L, et al. EFNS guidelines on neuropathic pain assessment: revised 2009. Eur J Neurol. 2010;17(8):1010-8.
6. Zakrzewska JM, Linskey ME. Trigeminal neuralgia. Clin Evid (Online). 2014;10:1207.
7. Campbell FG, Graham JG, Zilkha KJ. Clinical trial of carbamazepine (tegretol) in trigeminal neuralgia. J Neurol Neurosurg Psychiatry. 1966;29(3):265-7.
8. Wiffen PJ, Derry S, Moore RA, Kalso EA. Carbamazepine for chronic neuropathic pain and fibromyalgia in adults. Cochrane Database Syst Rev. 2014;4(4):CD005451.
9. Wiffen P, Collins S, McQuay H, Carroll D, Jadad A, Moore A. Anticonvulsant drugs for acute and chronic pain. Cochrane Database Syst Rev. 2005;(3):CD001133.
10. Nurmikko TJ, Eldridge PR. Trigeminal neuralgia—pathophysiology, diagnosis and current treatment. Br J Anaesth. 2001;87(1):117-132.
11. Beydoun A. Clinical use of tricyclic anticonvulsants in painful neuropathies and bipolar disorders. Epilepsy Behav. 2002;3(3S):S18-22.
12. Beydoun A. Safety and efficacy of oxcarbazepine: results of randomized, double-blind trials. Pharmacotherapy. 2000;20(8 Pt 2):152S-8S.
13. Zakrzewska JM, Linskey ME. Trigeminal neuralgia. BMJ. 2014;348:g474.
14. Hu Y, Guan X, Fan L, Li M, Liao Y, Nie Z, et al. Therapeutic efficacy and safety of botulinum toxin type A in trigeminal neuralgia: a systematic review. J Headache Pain. 2013;14(1):72.
15. Gu W, Zhao W. Microvascular decompression for recurrent trigeminal neuralgia. J Clin Neurosci. 2014;21(9):1549-53.
16. Broggi G, Ferroli P, Franzini A, Servello D, Dones I. Microvascular decompression for trigeminal neuralgia: comments on a series of 250 cases, including 10 patients with multiple sclerosis. J Neurol Neurosurg Psychiatry. 2000;68(1):59-64.
17. Oesman C, Mooij JJ. Long-term follow-up of microvascular decompression for trigeminal neuralgia. Skull Base. 2011;21(5):313-22.
18. Lopez BC, Hamlyn PJ, Zakrzewska JM. Systematic review of ablative neurosurgical techniques for the treatment of trigeminal neuralgia. Neurosurgery. 2004;54(4):973-82.
19. North RB, Kidd DH, Piantadosi S, Carson BS. Percutaneous retrogasserian glycerol rhizotomy: Predictors of success and failure in treatment of trigeminal neuralgia. J Neurosurg. 1990;72(6):851-6.
20. Mullan S, Duda EE, Patronas NJ. Some examples of balloon technology in neurosurgery. J Neurosurg. 1980;52(3):321-9.
21. Mullan S, Lichtor T. Percutaneous microcompression of the trigeminal ganglion for trigeminal neuralgia. J Neurosurg. 1983;59(6):1007-12.
22. Tatli M, Satici O, Kanpolat Y, Sindou M. Various surgical modalities for trigeminal neuralgia: literature study of respective long-term outcomes. Acta Neurochir (Wien). 2008;150(3):243-55.
23. Bergenheim AT, Asplund P, Linderoth B. Percutaneous retrogasserian balloon compression for trigeminal neuralgia: review of critical technical details and outcomes. World Neurosurg. 2013;79(2):359-68.
24. Kondziolka D, Lunsford LD, Flickinger JC, Young RF, Vermeulen S, Duma CM, et al. Stereotactic radiosurgery for trigeminal neuralgia: a multi-institutional study using the gamma unit. J Neurosurg. 1996;84(6):940-94.
25. Skirving DJ, Dan NG. A 20-year review of percutaneous balloon compression of the trigeminal ganglion. J Neurosurg. 2001;94(6):913-7.
26. Maesawa S, Salame C, Flickinger JC, Pirris S, Kondziolka D, Lunsford LD. Clinical outcomes after stereotactic radiosurgery for idiopathic trigeminal neuralgia. J Neurosurg. 2001;94(1):14-20.

27. Murtagh RD, Caracciolo JT, Fernandez G. CT findings associated with Eagle syndrome. Am J Neuroradiol. 2001;22(7):1401-2.
28. Resnick DK, Jannetta PJ, Bissonnette D, Jho HD, Lanzino G. Microvascular decompression for glossopharyngeal neuralgia. Neurosurgery. 1995;36(1):64-8.
29. Dworkin RH, Backonja M, Rowbotham MC, Allen RR, Argoff CR, Bennett GJ, et al. Advances in neuropathic pain: diagnosis, mechanisms, and treatment recommendations. Arch Neurol. 2003;60(11):1524-34.
30. Bean-Lijewski JD. Glossopharyngeal nerve block for pain relief after pediatric tonsillectomy: retrospective analysis and two cases of life-threatening upper airway obstruction from an interrupted trial. Anesth Analg. 1997;84(6):1232-8.
31. Rao S, Rao S. Glossopharyngeal Nerve Block: The Premolar Approach. Craniomaxillofac Trauma Reconstr. 2018;11(4):331-2.
32. Martínez-Álvarez R, Martínez-Moreno N, Kusak ME, Rey-Portolés G. Glossopharyngeal neuralgia and radiosurgery: clinical article. J Neurosurg. 2014;121(Suppl):222-5.
33. Revuelta-Gutiérrez R, Morales-Martínez AH, Mejías-Soto C, Martínez-Anda JJ, Ortega-Porcayo LA. Microvascular decompression for glossopharyngeal neuralgia through a microasterional approach: a case series. Surg Neurol Int. 2016;7:51.
34. Wang X, Tang Y, Zeng Y, Ni J. Long-term outcomes of percutaneous radiofrequency thermocoagulation for glossopharyngeal neuralgia: A retrospective observational study. Medicine (Baltimore). 2016;95(48):e5530.
35. Isamat F, Ferrán E, Acebes JJ. Selective percutaneous thermocoagulation rhizotomy in essential glossopharyngeal neuralgia. J. Neurosurg. 1981;55(4):575-80.
36. Rey-Dios R, Cohen-Gadol AA. Current neurosurgical management of glossopharyngeal neuralgia and technical nuances for microvascular decompression surgery. Neurosurg Focus. 2013;34(3):E8.
37. Mallick-Searle T, Snodgrass B, Brant JM. Postherpetic neuralgia: epidemiology, pathophysiology, and pain management pharmacology. J Multidiscip Healthc. 2016;9:447-54.
38. Werner RN, Nikkels AF, Marinović B, Schäfer M, Czarnecka-Operacz M, Agius AM, et al. European consensus-based (S2k) Guideline on the Management of Herpes Zoster-guided by the European Dermatology Forum (EDF) in cooperation with the European Academy of Dermatology and Venereology (EADV), Part 1: Diagnosis. J Eur Acad Dermatol Venereol. 2017;31(1):9-19.
39. Jeon YH. Herpes Zoster and postherpetic neuralgia: practical consideration for prevention and treatment. Korean J Pain. 2015;28(3):177-84.
40. Bader MS. Herpes zoster: diagnostic, therapeutic, and preventive approaches. Postgrad Med. 2013;125(5):78-91.
41. Johnson RW, Rice AS. Clinical practice. Postherpetic neuralgia. N Engl J Med. 2014;371(16):1526-33.
42. Nalamachu S, Morley-Forster P. Diagnosing and managing postherpetic neuralgia. Drugs Aging. 2012;29(11):863-9.
43. Donahue JG, Choo PW, Manson JE, Platt R. The incidence of herpes zoster. Arch Intern Med. 1995;155(15):1605-9.
44. Galil K, Choo PW, Donahue JG, Platt R. The sequelae of herpes zoster. Arch Intern Med. 1997;157(11):1209-13.
45. Wood MJ, Kay R, Dworkin RH, Soong SJ, Whitley RJ. Oral acyclovir therapy accelerates pain resolution in patients with herpes zoster: a meta-analysis of placebo-controlled trials. Clin Infect Dis. 1996;22(2):341-7.
46. Whitley RJ, Weiss H, Gnann JW Jr, Tyring S, Mertz GJ, Pappas PG, et al. Acyclovir with and without prednisone for the treatment of herpes zoster: A randomized, placebo-controlled trial. The National Institute of Allergy and Infectious Diseases Collaborative Antiviral Study Group. Ann Intern Med. 1996;125(5):376-83.

47. Esmann V, Kroon S, Peterslund NA, Rnne-Rasmussen JO, Geil JP, Fogh H, et al. Prednisolone does not prevent post-herpetic neuralgia. Lancet. 1987;330:126-9.
48. Colding A. Treatment of pain: organization of a pain clinic: treatment of acute herpes zoster. Proc R Soc Med. 1973;66(6):541-3.
49. Chandra K, Shafiq N, Pandhi P, Gupta S, Malhotra S. Gabapentin versus nortriptyline in post-herpetic neuralgia patients: a randomized, double-blind clinical trial—the GONIP trial. Int J Clin Pharmacol Ther. 2006;44(8):358-63.
50. Gilron I, Bailey JM, Tu D, Holden RR, Jackson AC, Houlden RL. Nortriptyline and gabapentin, alone and in combination for neuropathic pain: a double-blind, randomised controlled crossover trial. Lancet. 2009;374(9697):1252-61.
51. Sang CN, Sathyanarayana R, Sweeney M DM-1796 Study Investigators. Gastroretentive gabapentin (G-GR) formulation reduces intensity of pain associated with postherpetic neuralgia (PHN). Clin J Pain. 2013;29(4):281-8.
52. Sharma U, Griesing T, Emir B, Young JP Jr. Time to onset of neuropathic pain reduction: A retrospective analysis of data from nine controlled trials of pregabalin for painful diabetic peripheral neuropathy and postherpetic neuralgia. Am J Ther. 2010;17(6):577-85.
53. Baron R, Mayoral V, Leijon G, Binder A, Steigerwald I, Serpell M. 5% lidocaine medicated plaster versus pregabalin in post-herpetic neuralgia and diabetic polyneuropathy: an open-label, non-inferiority two-stage RCT study. Curr Med Res Opin. 2009;25(7):1663-76.
54. Kanai A, Kumaki C, Niki Y, Suzuki A, Tazawa T, Okamoto H. Efficacy of a metered-dose 8% lidocaine pump spray for patients with post-herpetic neuralgia. Pain Med. 2009;10(5):902-9.
55. Baranidharan G, Das S, Bhaskar A. A review of the high-concentration capsaicin patch and experience in its use in the management of neuropathic pain. Ther Adv Neurol Disord. 2013;6(5):287-97.
56. Irving G, Backonja M, Rauck R, Webster LR, Tobias JK, Vanhove GF. NGX-4010, a capsaicin 8% dermal patch, administered alone or in combination with systemic neuropathic pain medications, reduces pain in patients with postherpetic neuralgia. Clin J Pain. 2012;28(2):101-7.
57. Haanpää M, Rice AS, Rowbotham MC. Treating herpes zoster and postherpetic neuralgia. Pain Clin Updates. 2015;23:1-8.
58. Kumar V, Krone K, Mathieu A. Neuraxial and sympathetic blocks in herpes zoster and postherpetic neuralgia: an appraisal of current evidence. Reg Anesth Pain Med. 2004;29(5):454-61.
59. Opstelten W, van Wijck AJ, Stolker RJ. Interventions to prevent postherpetic neuralgia: cutaneous and percutaneous techniques. Pain. 2004;107(3):202-6.
60. Kuthuru MR, Kabbara AI, Boswell MV. Pulsed radiofrequency ablation of frontal and supraorbital nerves for postherpetic neuralgia: a case report. Reg Anesth Pain Med. 2003;28:A56.
61. Surjya Prasad Upadhyay, Shiv Pratap Rana, Mishra S, Bhatnagar S. Successful treatment of an intractable postherpetic neuralgia (PHN) using peripheral nerve field stimulation (PNFS). Am J Hosp Palliat Care. 2010;27(1):59-62.
62. Vorenkamp Kevin E, Haassett Afton L, Sweet FG, Jonathan M. Trigeminal Neuralgia and other Facial pain conditions. In: Pain Medicine. New York: Oxford University Press; 2015.

CHAPTER 25

Anesthesia Implications in COVID Positive Patients

Anjan Trikha, Venkata Ganesh

INTRODUCTION

The term severe acute respiratory infection (SARI) was instituted by the World Health Organization (WHO) to enable prompt identification of potentially dangerous and possibly novel respiratory infections.[1] The first reporting of the novel pneumonia causing corona virus disease 19 (COVID-19) was from the bronchoalveolar lavage samples of a patient in Wuhan, China in December 2019.[2] This ribonucleic acid (RNA) virus bears phylogenetic similarity with SARS CoV and hence also goes by the moniker SARS-CoV-2.[3] Although estimated mortality rates at the time of this writing range between 0.25 and <6%,[4] lower than the SARS and middle east respiratory syndrome (MERS) cornaviridae, this is probably due to under-reporting and lack of availability widespread testing especially in our country. The hospital fatality rate of such patients, not restricted to those critically ill at presentation, is estimated to near 15% worldover.[5]

The measures advocated for the perioperative as well as critical care management of patients with SARI apply to those infected with SARS-CoV-2 as well. The main mode of transmission is exposure to droplets and surface contact transfer. Coughing and sneezing can usually disperse heavy droplets within a maximum radius of 2 meters. However, aerosol-generating procedures can increase the droplet density and chance of spread to exposed healthcare workers (HCWs). These include procedures such as endotracheal intubation and extubation, noninvasive ventilation, high-flow nasal cannula (HFNC), cardiopulmonary resuscitation, open endotracheal suctioning, bronchoscopy, sputum induction, tracheostomy, nasal endoscopies, colonoscopies, manual bag-mask ventilation and nebulization.[6] All of these procedures come under the purview of the perioperative physician.

Aerosolized SARS-CoV-2 appears to be stable on environmental surfaces, under experimental conditions, lasting up to 72 hours, similar to the original SARS-CoV.[7] In view of the possible earlier and higher accumulation of viral load in the upper respiratory tract of infected individuals[7] combined with patterns of asymptomatic individuals shedding the virus,[8] similar to influenza,[9] implies the need for early case detection and universal respiratory precautions in the operating room (OR).[10] These precautions include appropriate personal protective equipment (PPE), modifications to potentially aerosol-generating procedures, adequate number of disposables and sterilization techniques for reusable equipment.

The estimates for basic reproduction number (R_0) for COVID-19 range from 2.2 to 3.3, higher than SARS and influenza epidemics, is responsible for the rapid progression of this disease to the pandemic stage.[11-13] And this has led to an unprecedented global increase in the demand for PPE, especially N95, filtering face pieces (FFP2/3) respirators and even surgical face masks. Several international organizations and societies have issued recommendations for the perioperative care of COVID-19 patients centering on infection control.[14-17] Many of these are based on continually updated data concerning the evolution of COVID-19 and hence are heavily based on expert recommendations and data from previous experience with SARS and MERS viruses.[18-27]

INFECTION CONTROL FOR ANESTHESIA

The goals of infection control are aimed at prevention of transmission to healthcare providers, prevention of infestation of the anesthesia workstation and other related equipment. These precautions should be the same for all patients, irrespective of the mode of anesthesia, whether suspect or confirmed case. These include strict hand hygiene, contact and droplet precautions especially during aerosol-generating procedures.

Hand Hygiene

Perform standard hand hygiene with soap and water and alcohol-based gel before donning PPE and after removing gloves, after every contact with the patient and before touching anesthesia equipment. Wearing double gloves may offer more safety.

Personal Protective Equipment for Aerosol-generating Procedures

Appropriate PPE includes an N95 mask or the more protective powered air purifying respirator (PAPR), eye protection (face shield, goggles or full face PAPR), gloves, water resistant gown and shoe covers. Disposable OR caps and beard covers should also be donned to prevent droplet inoculation. If available all patients requiring airway management should be approached with airborne precautions (i.e., N95) as there is a risk for asymptomatic or minimally symptomatic SARS-CoV-2 infection.[17,28,29] However, in view of resource limitation and the huge deficit in masks and PPE, a localized risk adaptive approach in the use of PPE may be better.

Personal Protective Equipment for Nonaerosol-generating Procedures

Although similar measures for aerosol-generating procedures would be ideal, recognizing the shortage in respirators affecting even the developed nations, the Centers for Disease Control and Prevention (CDC) and other organizations recommend the use of a surgical mask as a tolerable alternative. However, in the presence of active cough or if the procedure could possibly elicit a cough a respirator or N95 should be mandatory.

Donning and Doffing Personal Protective Equipment

Proper sequence of donning and doffing should be followed to avoid risk of accidental exposure. Even among trained personnel, the varying types or styles of available masks and PPE make this difficult, especially when unmonitored during doffing. There should be cognitive aids such as a legible checklist detailing the steps of donning and doffing in the respective areas. Apart from this there should be real-time direct or indirect observation (for example through a camera and remote monitor) with audio-visual guidance to prevent errors and potential HCW infestation.[30-32] Appropriate disposal measures for PPE should also be in place.

Measures during Patient Transport

Preoperatively the patients should be directly transported to the OR, or to a designated procedure room/airborne infection isolation room (AIIR).[33] These should ideally be negative pressure rooms and should not be used for non-COVID patients. The patient should be wearing at least a surgical mask. If the patient requires oxygen therapy, a surgical mask covering the patient's face, over the oxygen therapy device (i.e., nasal cannula or venturi mask) may limit droplet spread.[34] Using lowest oxygen flows required may minimize aerosol generation. Interestingly, HFNC may generate less aerosol dispersion, in terms of distance, compared to a nonrebreather mask according to some experimental simulator-based studies.[35] A portable tent system with high-efficiency particulate air (HEPA) filtration may be used for additional protection where available.[36] Patients should recover from anesthesia in the OR, or in the isolation room.

For transporting in-hospital, there should be a team consisting of HCW with appropriate PPE, who do not touch environmental surfaces after touching the patient, and a separate person should be assigned to interact with all nonpatient surfaces such as elevator buttons, doors and bystanders and files. If the patient is intubated or requires ventilation during transport, high quality heat and moisture exchanging filter (HMEF) preferably with viral filters should be used between the patient airway and ventilation equipment interface. Use of a transport ventilator is most desired where available. Standard measures and equipment for emergency airway management (such as reintubation) should be available and ready for use.

PROTECTION OF ANESTHESIA EQUIPMENT

In order to avoid unwanted contamination and repeated need for disinfection, only necessary equipment should be kept inside the OR during aerosol-generating procedure. An assistant or "runner" with additional backup equipment can be kept outside the OR.

In brief the best strategy to protect the anesthesia machine from contamination can be summarized as follows:[37]
- Place a "high quality" viral filter between the breathing circuit and the patient's airway with the capability to sample gas from the machine side of the filter.
- Heat and moisture exchanging filter is preferred to preserve humidification. HMEF combine a heat and humidity exchanger with an electrostatic filter in one unit.
- Pleated hydrophobic mechanical filters have the highest viral filtration efficiency (VFE) but they also require a minimum tidal volume of 300 mL and can add a dead-space of 80 mL with increased resistance especially when used in pediatric patients.
- If filter only is used, reducing fresh gas flow is an important strategy for preserving humidity (1–2 L/min or less).
- Place a second filter at the end of the expiratory limb at the connection to the anesthesia machine.
- To provide additional filtration, a 0.22 μ epidural hydrophilic membrane filter can be added to the gas analyzer sampling line. This can, however, affect the quality of the capnogram.
- Breathing circuit and gas-sampling tubing should be discarded after every patient. Water tap may be preserved if sampling was done from HMEF away from the patient.

Surface contamination of the workstation may be prevented by covering the workstation with transparent plastic drapes, especially "high touch" surfaces.[23,38] Such premade covers are also commercially available.[39] However, contamination may still occur during removal of such covers.

Routine cleaning of the anesthesia workstation and reusable equipment should be performed after every case as per manufacturer recommendations.[37] All disposables including breathing circuit, reservoir bag, mask, forced air warming blanket and any others should be considered as contaminated and should be discarded under ideal conditions.[40] However, this may be difficult in resource limited areas and appropriate reusable equipment with adequate sterilization may be considered. There is no evidence to support changing the soda lime CO_2 absorber between cases if it is not depleted as it is highly alkaline and viricidal apart from being protected by filters in the circuit. Sterilizing the internal components of a machine would not be required if appropriate filters have been used. If this is deemed necessary quarantining the machine and following manufacturer's recommendations are the only measures currently available.[37]

OPERATING ROOM DECONTAMINATION

Once the patient has been shifted out of the OR, the room should be sealed and subjected to adequate number of air exchanges to remove aerosolized pathogens, in accordance with standard guidelines.[41] Ultraviolet (UV) light or hydrogen peroxide vapors may be used where available. Appropriate disinfectants should be used on all surfaces (**Table 1**).[42]

TABLE 1: Disinfectants effective against corona virus (1 minute minimum contact time)

Agent	Concentration
Sodium hypochlorite	0.1%
Ethanol	62–71%
Hydrogen peroxide	0.5%
Povidone iodine	0.23–0.75%

MANAGEMENT OF ANESTHESIA

Preoperative Assessment

Standard preoperative assessment should be done for all COVID suspect and positive patients. Performing a regular outpatient preoperative assessment would be challenging as, in the interest of protecting the healthcare workers (HCWs), one would have to do a non-contact or minimal contact clinical examination. This can be achieved by the examiner wearing minimal PPE (in the form of gloves, mask, a gown/apron and face shield) and the patient wearing at minimum a mask and face shield with the examination being conducted across a glass barrier, in a well ventilated or negative pressure room. Pulse, blood pressure and SpO_2 can be recorded for all patients at the entry of the preanesthetic clinic. As auscultation would be difficult with this approach, point-of-care tests such as an ECG, chest X-ray, point-of-care ultrasonography (POCUS) and echocardiography may have to be performed in nearly all patients, however the concerned HCW should be wearing appropriate PPE while performing these. To conserve resources and minimise exposure, making the patients fill a preliminary medical history/questionnaire either online or on paper before entering the clinic may help stratify the need for various blood investigations and the above point-of-care tests, thus minimizing time spent in the clinic as well as overcrowding. An online appointment and record keeping system would be of great use in achieving the above goals. The aims of preoperative assessment should include identification of suspect/high-risk patients **(Table 2)** and high-risk procedures **(Table 3)** as well as optimization of patient condition.[43]

The preoperative assessment should focus on meticulous airway assessment (formulate a patient specific plan), oxygen requirement of the patient (measuring SpO_2) and signs of shock and organ failure (more so in admitted patients). Performing an outpatient airway examination is quite the task one would have to look into the open mouth of the patient. This would be challenging as there is fear of potential aerosolization, exposing the noninfected to the virus. This is further complicated by the fact that the anesthesiologist will have to look through multiple glass barriers and fogging of the goggles, spectacles and face-shield hampers vison further. So, how to perform an airway assessment in such a scenario? One option would be to look at the patient's oral cavity via a video camera/webcam placed across the glass

TABLE 2: Preoperative assessment for identifying high-risk/suspect COVID-19 patients

History
- Fever, dry cough, new onset breathing difficulty
- Travel/contact history with COVID-19 patients
- Workplace exposure such as healthcare workers
- Cluster phenomenon

Physical findings and investigations
- Measure the patient's temperature (noncontact preferable)
- Blood pressure and heart rate for evidence of shock, SpO_2 for desaturation
- Auscultate for wheeze/crepitations
- Leukopenia, lymphopenia, and lymphocytosis on blood counts. Neutrophil/lymphocyte ratio may also be used
- Liver and renal function tests
- Chest X-ray for consolidation
- CT-thorax if available—multilobar ground glass opacities

(CT: computed tomography; COVID: coronavirus disease)

TABLE 3: High-risk and aerosol-generating procedures

Surgical
- Rigid bronchoscopy, fiberoptic bronchoscopy
- Tracheostomy and tracheobronchial surgeries
- Lobectomy and pneumonectomy
- Surgery involving high-speed drilling such as dental and orthopedic surgeries
- Laparoscopic surgeries

Anesthetic
- Awake fiberoptic intubation
- Bag and mask ventilation
- Intubation and extubation
- Suctioning attempts and the use of high-flow oxygen may also aerosolize particles
- High-flow nasal cannula
- Noninvasive ventilation
- Sputum suctioning
- Cardiopulmonary resuscitation (CPR)

barrier. The history taking and inspection part of clinical examination may be done using such a telemedicine approach with the patient and physician in completely different rooms, with patient records being maintained online. This would, however, be difficult in a high-volume center and in over populated countries. Consideration should also include a thorough medication review, especially antivirals and potential drug-drug interaction **(Table 4)**.[44-48]

Due to the lack of consensus guidelines the decision to proceed with a surgical procedure should be keeping in mind the emergent, urgent nature of the procedure and potential hospital facility utilization which may impinge on the availability of resources such as intensive care unit (ICU) beds, trained HCW, blood products and other assets which may be required for the COVID-19 positive cases that are overflowing by the minute.[49-51] Those procedures which are considered nonessential may be deferred and those

TABLE 4: Concerns related to preoperative medications used in the potential treatment of COVID-19

Drug	Concerns
Lopinavir + Ritonavir	Increased plasma concentration of midazolam, fentanyl, erythromycin (prolonged QT), amiodarone, statins, digoxin, warfarin and rivaroxaban
Ribavirin	Hemolysis, anemia and pancytopenia
Remdesivir	May cause hypotension, anemia, AKI, nausea and fever. Limited data on drug interactions, potential interaction with hydroxychloroquine, possible hepatotoxicity with P-glycoprotein inhibitors–amiodarone, PPI, erythromycin, diltiazem, verapamil, etc.
Interferon-1β	Lymphopenia, flu-like symptoms, headache, liver enzyme elevation
Hydroxychloroquine and azithromycin	Arrhythmias, prolonged QT
Low dose dexamethasone, methylprednisolone	Hyperglycemia, increased susceptibility to bacterial and fungal infections
Tocilizumab	Secondary infections
Convalescent plasma	Transfusion reactions, antibody-mediated reactions, although the risk is low
Favipiravir	Limited data. Possible hyperuricemia, transaminitis, diarrhea, leukopenia and neutropenia

(PPI: proton pump inhibitor; AKI: acute kidney injury)

that are essential but, when delayed, do not impart additional morbidity to the patient may be postponed or a conservative route can be considered. This may hold true even in some cases of acute abdomen and local guidelines to triage such patients should be formulated.[52]

Choice of Anesthetic Technique

This should be decided on a case to case basis. However, regional anesthesia as the sole technique may be preferred over general anesthesia.

Regional Anesthesia

Regional anesthesia, where possible, may avoid the need for airway instrumentation, associated aerosolization and contamination of anesthetic equipment when used as the sole technique. There are no specific SARS-CoV-2-related contraindications except may be possible thrombocytopenia. Avoid unplanned conversion to general anesthesia.

The American Society of Regional Anesthesia and Pain Medicine (ASRA) and European Society of Regional Anesthesia and Pain Therapy (ESRA) have issued joint recommendations on the practice of regional anesthesia in COVID-19 cases.[53] A summary is provided here.

- Since it is a nonaerosol-generating procedure surgical mask, eye protection, surgical gown and double gloves may be considered adequate to provide regional anesthesia.[53] Some institutions recommend the use of droplet and contact level precautions at the minimum to account for possible conversion to general anesthesia.[54]
- Perform the procedure in dedicated OR, or procedure room for COVID positive case with routine aseptic precautions. AIIR is preferred but not mandatory.
- Supplemental oxygen can be given where required using lowest possible flows and the patient should wear a surgical mask.
- Periprocedural sedation should be titrated to minimize oxygen requirement.
- The ultrasound equipment, including an ultrasound transducer, should be protected from contamination using plastic covers. Only necessary equipment should be kept near the patient.
- Use disposable paper drapes.

Spinal anesthesia and epidural analgesia:
- Avoid allowing the cerebrospinal fluid (CSF) to drip freely after lumbar puncture as this can cause viral contamination of surfaces.
- No dose adjustment of spinal anesthetic or adjuvant is recommended currently.
- Prophylactic vasopressors should be used to avoid hypotension especially in parturients.
- Epidural infusion is preferred to intermittent boluses.
- Postdural puncture headache (PDPH) should preferably be managed conservatively. Nasal sphenopalatine ganglion block should be avoided. There is no data to absolutely contraindicate use of epidural blood patch.

Peripheral nerve block:
- Choose blocks that least likely interfere with respiration.
- No specific contraindications to the use of adjuvants. Risk of immunosuppression should be weighed when using dexamethasone.
- Catheters may be used based on case by case basis.
- Any additional analgesic block procedures should be avoided if analgesia can be managed systemically.

General Anesthesia

Minimize personnel in the OR, or dedicated AIIR where airway management is to be performed. The most experienced anesthetist in full PPE, one assistant and one "runner" (outside the OR with additional equipment) are required in most instances. Plan the management adequately and also plan the communication strategy, as it is difficult to communicate in full PPE.

Induction
- A rapid sequence induction and intubation, modified according to patient factors, is preferred.[55]
- An HMEF should be preconnected to the circuit and closed suction should be kept at the ready.

- Preoxygenation may be achieved with the patient breathing 100% oxygen spontaneously from the face mask and anesthetic circuit to avoid instituting positive pressure and generating aerosol. A tight seal with a bimanual VE technique is preferred.
- If mask ventilation becomes necessary postinduction use low pressure, small volume 2-person ventilation, maintaining a 2-hand tight mask seal. Placement of wet gauze or towels around the airway and/or nose may be helpful in reducing leaks during mask ventilation.[20]
- For the critically ill patient, etomidate would be ideal, although the effect of single dose steroid suppression on mortality is unknown. Ketamine can also be used. Prophylactic vasopressors may be preferred to overzealous fluid administration which may compromise oxygenation.
- Early paralysis with rocuronium or suxamethonium is advocated.[55]

Airway Management
- Endotracheal intubation with a videolaryngoscope with cricoid pressure is preferred over supraglottic airways (SGAs) to seal the airway and prevent viral spread. A second generation SGA may however be used as a rescue device.[55]
- Intubation may be performed under transparent plastic drapes, clear box (Aerosol box) or other barrier enclosure methods.[56,57] However, these may complicate the difficulty further in untrained hands.
- Avoid aerosol-generating procedures such as high-flow nasal oxygen (HFNO), noninvasive ventilation (NIV), bronchoscopy and tracheal suction without an in-line closed suction system in place.
- Minimize coughing by ensuring deep neuromuscular blockade, additional doses of induction agent or intravenous lignocaine.
- The endotracheal tube is to be place 1–2 cm below the vocal cords to avoid endobronchial intubation. Inflate the cuff before instituting ventilation.
- Auscultation is difficult with PPE and intubation can be confirmed with bilateral chest rise and capnography.
- Avoid disconnections. Clamp endotracheal tube and pause ventilator for airway maneuvers and disconnection.
- Use standard monitors and preplanned failed intubation algorithm with cognitive aid if difficulty arises.
- After induction of anesthesia, clean all equipment and surfaces with antiviral disinfection wipes. Safely place used airway equipment in a dedicated plastic bag.[40]
- In managing an anticipated difficult airway, awake fiberoptic intubation should be avoided.

Tracheal extubation is also at high risk for aerosol generation and precautions similar to intubation should be followed.
- Nonanesthesia personnel should leave the room.
- Full PPE is mandatory.
- Administer prophylaxis for postoperative nausea and vomiting.

- Intravenous lignocaine may be used to minimize cough during extubation.
- Measures should be taken to prevent spread of secretions during extubation. Several experts have suggested different techniques including the use of transparent drapes or clear boxes to cover the patient's face, placement of wet gauze over the patient's mouth and nose just prior to extubation or using a mask over-tube technique.[20,58,59]
- After extubation place an appropriate supplemental oxygen device and cover it with a surgical mask.

OBSTETRIC ANESTHESIA

A team approach takes precedence in managing the obstetric patient for emergency cesarean section. There should be well established lines of communication between the obstetrician and the anesthesia team. Early information about the possibility of a COVID-19 positive or suspect emergency cesarean section will enable OR preparedness and minimize donning time and errors. If the case is a suspect while tests are awaited it is to be managed as a positive case.[60] The increased minute ventilation of pregnancy may increase the chance of aerosol spread and hence all suspect cases should be given a surgical mask.

The Royal College of Obstetricians and Gynecologists (RCOG), Royal College of Anesthetists (RCOA) and the Society for Obstetric Anesthesia and Perinatology (SOAP) support early epidural analgesia which may minimize the need for general anesthesia in case of emergency cesarean section[60] but consideration should also include concurrent prophylactic low-molecular-weight heparin (LMWH). Regional anesthesia is preferred unless contraindicated. Higher morbidity is associated with general anesthesia in an obstetric patient and regional anesthesia is considered safe in COVID-19.[61]

Temporary separation of the mother from the baby may possibly prevent the sharing of respiratory secretions and infecting the baby. There is limited evidence of vertical transmission at the time of this writing, however emerging reports do suggest the possibility[62] and contact precautions (mothers wearing masks and practicing hand hygiene) should be instituted for feeding and care of such babies. Breastfeeding should not be denied as there is no evidence supporting transmission through breast milk.[63] Pasteurized breast milk/human donor milk may be an option as viruses similar to SARS-CoV-2 are destroyed in milk by this process. There is no indication to keep the COVID positive baby isolated from the mother in neonatal intensive care unit (NICU) unless the baby's symptoms warrant NICU admission.[64] The CDC recommends neonatal RT-PCR from upper respiratory swabs at 24 hours of age and if negative a repeat test should be performed at 48 hours of age.[64] An infant being breastfed by a COVID positive mother should be considered as infected when the infants testing results are not available for the duration of the mothers recommended period of home isolation and for 14 days after that.[63] Mothers should be educated to warn the healthcare workers caring for such children, that the infant has had high-risk exposure in the near past.

PEDIATRIC ANESTHESIA

Compared to adults a larger proportion of children infected with SARS-CoV-2 are likely to be asymptomatic or present with only mild disease.[65-68] Hence, it is very important to minimize aerosol-generating procedures. Crying can also be expected to produce aerosol superemission similar to loud speaking in adults[69] and this highlights the importance of adequate premedication and preoperative anxiolysis.

Specific considerations relating to the pediatric population are:
- Nasal premedication should be avoided.
- Intravenous induction is preferred.[28] It may be difficult to secure an intravenous line even in a premedicated child so the care provider may in such cases opt for an inhalational induction with low flow rates, closed circuit and a tight mask seal.
- Parental presence during induction may be avoided to preserve PPE.
- Barrier devices and video laryngoscopy with cuffed endotracheal tube placement is the preferred modality of securing the airway. Rapid sequence induction without cricoid pressure may be used.
- Use in-line closed suction catheters.
- Consider deep extubation and lateral positioning to minimize coughing and bucking during emergence. Other techniques such as the use of total intravenous anesthesia (TIVA) or dexmedetomidine may be used to ensure smooth emergence in the OR. Barrier device during extubation as well is preferred.
- Additional regional analgesia while the child is under general anesthesia may be used to ensure adequate postoperative analgesia to prevent the child from crying.
- Postoperatively the child should be kept in a dedicated unit and caregivers including parents should use droplet and contact precautions in all suspected cases.
- It is a well-known fact that parental presence decreases the anxiety of the child. However, this becomes a problem when the child is COVID positive and the parent has tested negative. In such scenarios we may have to allay anxiety via video calling or in the case of very small children the parent may have to be beside the child with requisite PPE at least for few hours of the day. If the parent is also COVID positive it may not be an issue with allowing them to stay in the same room, albeit with masks, gloves and hand hygiene.

ANESTHESIA AND BRONCHOSCOPY

Bronchoscopy is a high-risk aerosol-generating procedure as the trachea is not secure and the chances of coughing are also very high. It would be prudent to postpone elective bronchoscopies during the COVID-19 pandemic. However, emergent/urgent cases such as massive hemoptysis, severe airway stenosis and foreign body bronchus cannot be postponed.

Bronchoscopies should be conducted in a negative pressure room with only the essential personnel in full PPE and a PAPR especially in confirmed COVID-19 positive cases. Anesthetic concerns include titrating sedation to minimize cough, avoiding atomized or nebulized lidocaine, and instituting paralysis if the procedure is being performed under general anesthesia. Rigid bronchoscopy should be preferably avoided where possible and scope in-out time should be mimimized.[70] Low-flow oxygenation techniques should be used as much as possible and jet ventilation should be avoided. To maintain a constant depth of anesthesia (TIVA) preferably with a target-controlled infusion (TCI) system would be more logical compared to inhalational agents. Creation of a suspended bronchoscopy tent using transparent surgical drapes over the patient's head may facilitate rigid bronchoscopy with some measure of protection to the HCW as demonstrated by Francom et al.[71]

POSTOPERATIVE MANAGEMENT

- Avoid transferring confirmed cases to common postanesthesia care unit (PACU). Have a dedicated PACU to care for suspect as well as confirmed COVID-19 positive cases.
- Apply a surgical mask to all otherwise awake and stable patients in the recovery area.
- Maintain interpatient bed distance of at least 1 meter.
- Avoid giving high-flow oxygen, NIV, or nebulized medications unless absolutely indicated.
- In the event a patient desaturates postoperatively promptly instate rescue measures such as a nonrebreathing mask, helmet NIV and consider early intubation. There might be some merit in self proning or lateral positioning, however, this has not been investigated in the postoperative period.

CONCLUSION

As we know, anesthesia is a balancing act between reversible loss of consciousness, analgesia, maintenance of homeostasis and immobility, the novel coronavirus pandemic has called for maintaining a delicate balance between staff safety and patient safety, especially in terms of infection control. Apart from adapting to the rapidly evolving evidence base surrounding the SARS-CoV-2 pandemic, the principles involved in anesthetic management of such patients include streamlined organizational systems and protocols, rapid patient isolation, appropriate PPE, minimize number of exposed personnel, curtailing aerosol-generating procedures, preferring isolated regional anesthesia over general anesthesia where practicable, and effective decontamination of equipment and hospital environs.

KEY POINTS

- Proper donning and careful doffing of personal protective equipment (PPE) is important to prevent transmission of virus.
- Prioritize and minimize number of personnel and equipment in contact with the patient.
- Limit aerosol-generating procedures (AGPs).
- For AGP wear PPE appropriate for contact, aerosol and airborne precautions which include an N95 respirator or powered air-purifying respirators (PAPR), eye protection (goggles and face shield), double gloves, water resistant gown, head and shoe covers.
- Video-laryngoscopy and barrier precautions during intubation are recommended. Awake fiberoptic should be avoided as far as possible.
- Surgical masks for patients during transport to and from dedicated operating room/postanesthesia care unit (OR/PACU). Facilities should have adequate air exchanges minimum touch points with periodic disinfection. Airborne infection isolation room (AIIR) are preferred.
- Prefer exclusive regional anesthesia where feasible. COVID-19 does not contraindicate regional anesthesia.
- Protect reusable equipment by measures such as using viral filters on all breathing circuits, transparent plastic drapes to cover the workstation and following appropriate decontamination procedures.
- Hand hygiene is paramount.

REFERENCES

1. World Health Organization. Report of the WHO-China Joint Mission on Coronavirus Disease 2019 (COVID-19). [online] Available from https://www.who.int/publications-detail/report-of-the-who-china-joint-mission-on-coronavirus-disease-2019 (COVID-19). [Last accessed November, 2020].
2. Huang C, Wang Y, Li X, Ren L, Zhao J, Hu Y, et al. Clinical features of patients infected with 2019 novel coronavirus in Wuhan, China. Lancet. 2020;395(10223):497-506.
3. Zhu N, Zhang D, Wang W, Li X, Yang B, Song J, et al. A Novel Coronavirus from Patients with Pneumonia in China, 2019. N Engl J Med. 2020;382:727-33.
4. CDC. Case-Fatality Risk Estimates for COVID-19 Calculated by Using a Lag Time for Fatality. (Wilson N, Amanda Kvalsvig A, Barnard LT, Baker MG) Emerging Infectious Disease journal. [online] Available from: https://wwwnc.cdc.gov/eid/article/26/6/20-0320_article. [Last accessed November, 2020].
5. Coronavirus Mortality Rate (COVID-19). Worldometer. [online] Available from https://www.worldometers.info/coronavirus/coronavirus-death-rate. [Last accessed November, 2020].
6. Palmore TN. Coronavirus disease 2019 (COVID-19): Infection control in health care and home settings. UpToDate. [online] Available from https://www.uptodate.com/contents/coronavirus-disease-2019-covid-19-infection-control-in-health-care-and-home-settings?sectionName=Aerosol-generating%20procedures%2Ftreatments&topicRef=127481&anchor=H3802094897&source=see_link#H3802094897. [Last accessed November, 2020].
7. To KK, Tsang OT, Leung WS, Tam AR, Wu TC, Lung DC, et al. Temporal profiles of viral load in posterior oropharyngeal saliva samples and serum antibody responses during infection by SARS-CoV-2: an observational cohort study. Lancet Infect Dis. 2020;20(5):565-74.

8. Rothe C, Schunk M, Sothmann P, Bretzel G, Froeschl G, Wallrauch C, et al. Transmission of 2019-nCoV Infection from an Asymptomatic Contact in Germany. N Engl J Med. 2020;382:970-1.
9. Tsang TK, Cowling BJ, Fang VJ, Chan KH, Ip DK, Leung GM, et al. Influenza A virus shedding and infectivity in households. J Infect Dis. 2015;212(9):1420-8.
10. Livingston EH. Surgery in a time of uncertainty: a need for universal respiratory precautions in the operating room. JAMA. 2020;323(22):2254-55.
11. Zhang S, Diao M, Yu W, Pei L, Lin Z, Chen D. Estimation of the reproductive number of novel coronavirus (COVID-19) and the probable outbreak size on the Diamond Princess cruise ship: a data-driven analysis. Int J Infect Dis. 2020;93:201-4.
12. Liu Y, Gayle AA, Wilder-Smith A, Rocklöv J. The reproductive number of COVID-19 is higher compared to SARS coronavirus. J Travel Med. 2020;27(2).
13. Peak CM, Kahn R, Grad YH, Childs LM, Li R, Lipsitch M, et al. Comparative impact of individual quarantine vs. active monitoring of contacts for the mitigation of COVID-19: a modelling study. medRxiv. 2020;2020.03.05.20031088.
14. Munoz-Price LS, Bowdle A, Johnston BL, Bearman G, Camins BC, Dellinger EP, et al. Infection prevention in the operating room anesthesia work area. Infect Control Hosp Epidemiol. 2019;40(1):1-17.
15. Beers RA. Infectious Disease Risks for Anesthesiologists. ASA Monitor. 2019;83(12):8-10.
16. Anesthesia Patient Safety Foundation. Perioperative Considerations for the 2019 Novel Coronavirus (COVID-19). Anesthesia Patient Safety Foundation. 2020. [online] Available from https://www.apsf.org/news-updates/perioperative-considerations-for-the-2019-novel-coronavirus-covid-19. [Last accessed November, 2020].
17. American Society of Anesthesiologists. General Information about COVID-19. COVID-19 FAQs. [online] Available from https://www.asahq.org/about-asa/governance-and-committees/asa-committees/committee-on-occupational-health/coronavirus/clinical-faqs. [Last accessed November, 2020].
18. Peng PWH, Ho PL, Hota SS. Outbreak of a new coronavirus: what anaesthetists should know. Br J Anaesth. 2020;124(5):497-501.
19. Wax RS, Christian MD. Practical recommendations for critical care and anesthesiology teams caring for novel coronavirus (2019-nCoV) patients. Can J Anaesth. 2020;67(5):568-76.
20. Chen X, Liu Y, Gong Y, Guo X, Zuo M, Li J, et al. Perioperative management of patients infected with the Novel Coronavirus: recommendation from the Joint Task Force of the Chinese Society of Anesthesiology and the Chinese Association of Anesthesiologists. Anesthesiology. 2020;132(6):1307-16.
21. Greenland JR, Michelow MD, Wang L, London MJ. COVID-19 infection: implications for perioperative and critical care physicians. Anesthesiology. 2020;132(6):1346-61.
22. Zhang H-F, Bo L, Lin Y, Li F-X, Sun S, Lin H-B, et al. Response of Chinese Anesthesiologists to the COVID-19 Outbreak. Anesthesiology. 2020;132(6):1333-38.
23. Bowdle A, Munoz-Price LS. Preventing infection of patients and healthcare workers should be the new normal in the era of novel coronavirus epidemics. Anesthesiology. 2020;132(6):1292-95.
24. Chen X, Shang Y, Yao S, Liu R, Liu H. Perioperative care provider's considerations in managing patients with the COVID-19 infections. Transl Perioper Pain Med. 2020;7(2):216-24.
25. Thomas-Rüddel D, Winning J, Dickmann P, Ouart D, Kortgen A, Janssens U, et al. [Coronavirus disease 2019 (COVID-19): update for anesthesiologists and intensivists March 2020]. Anaesthesist. 2020;69(4):225-35.

26. CDC. Donning and doffing personal protective equipment. Centers for Disease Control and Prevention. [online] Available from https://www.cdc.gov/hai/pdfs/ppe/ppe-sequence.pdf. [Last accessed November, 2020].
27. American Society of Anesthesiologists. The use of personal protective equipment by anesthesia professionals during the COVID-19 Pandemic. [online] Available from https://www.asahq.org/about-asa/newsroom/news-releases/2020/03/the-use-of-personal-protective-equipment-by-anesthesia-professionals-during-the-covid-19-pandemic. [Last accessed November, 2020].
28. Matava CT, Kovatsis PG, Lee JK, Castro P, Denning S, Yu J, et al. Pediatric airway management in COVID-19 patients: consensus guidelines from the Society for Pediatric Anesthesia's Pediatric Difficult Intubation Collaborative and the Canadian Pediatric Anesthesia Society. Anesth Analg. 2020;131(1):61-73.
29. American Society of Anesthesiologists. UPDATE: The Use of Personal Protective Equipment by Anesthesia Professionals during the COVID-19 Pandemic. [online] Available from https://www.asahq.org/about-asa/newsroom/news-releases/2020/03/update-the-use-of-personal-protective-equipment-by-anesthesia-professionals-during-the-covid-19-pandemic. [Last accessed November, 2020].
30. Okamoto K, Rhee Y, Schoeny M, Lolans K, Cheng J, Reddy S, et al. Impact of doffing errors on healthcare worker self-contamination when caring for patients on contact precautions. Infect Control Hosp Epidemiol. 2019;40(5):559-65.
31. Tomas ME, Kundrapu S, Thota P, Sunkesula VCK, Cadnum JL, Mana TSC, et al. Contamination of health care personnel during removal of personal protective equipment. JAMA Intern Med. 2015;175(12):1904-10.
32. Singh A, Naik BN, Soni SL, Puri GD. Real-time remote surveillance of doffing during COVID-19 pandemic: enhancing safety of health care workers. Anesthesia & analgesia. [online] Available from https://journals.lww.com/anesthesia-analgesia/fulltext/2020/08000/real_time_remote_surveillance_of_doffing_during.86.aspx. [Last accessed November, 2020].
33. Tuberculosis Infection Control: a practical manual for preventing TB Curry International Tuberculosis Center. [online] Available from https://www.currytbcenter.ucsf.edu/products/tuberculosis-infection-control-practical-manual-preventing-tb. [Last accessed November, 2020].
34. Aerosols CPF of C of D of, Apr 02; DDHVNITU a SSMI for HFNCC 2020, Leonard S, Atwood CW, Walsh BK, DeBellis RJ, Dungan GC, Strasser W, et al. Using a surgical mask to control aerosols and droplets with high-flow nasal cannula. Practice Update. [online] Available from https://www.practiceupdate.com/content/using-a-surgical-mask-to-control-aerosols-and-droplets-with-high-flow-nasal-cannula/98922. [Last accessed November, 2020].
35. Li J, Fink JB, Ehrmann S. High-flow nasal cannula for COVID-19 patients: low risk of bio-aerosol dispersion. European Respiratory Journal. [online] Available from https://erj.ersjournals.com/content/early/2020/04/08/13993003.00892-2020. [Last accessed November, 2020].
36. Wittgen BP, Kunst PW, Perkins WR, Lee JK, Postmus PE. Assessing a system to capture stray aerosol during inhalation of nebulized liposomal cisplatin. J Aerosol Med. 2006;19(3):385-91.
37. Feldman J. FAQ on Anesthesia Machine Use, Protection, and decontamination during the COVID-19 Pandemic Anesthesia Patient Safety Foundation. [online] Available from https://www.apsf.org/faq-on-anesthesia-machine-use-protection-and-decontamination-during-the-covid-19-pandemic. [Last accessed November, 2020].

38. Biddle CJ, George-Gay B, Prasanna P, Hill EM, Davis TC, Verhulst B. Assessing a novel method to reduce anesthesia machine contamination: a prospective, observational trial. Can J Infect Dis Med Microbiol. 2018;2018:1905360.
39. Anesthesia Hygiene Covers. Bell Medical. [online] Available from https://bellmedical.com/anesthesia-hygiene-covers. [Last accessed November, 2020].
40. Dexter F, Parra MC, Brown JR, Loftus RW. Perioperative COVID-19 defense: an evidence-based approach for optimization of infection control and operating room management. Anesth Analg. 2020;131(1):37-42.
41. CDC. Appendix B. Air: Guidelines for Environmental Infection Control in Health-Care Facilities (2003). [online] Available from https://www.cdc.gov/infectioncontrol/guidelines/environmental/appendix/air.html. [Last accessed November, 2020].
42. Kampf G, Todt D, Pfaender S, Steinmann E. Persistence of coronaviruses on inanimate surfaces and their inactivation with biocidal agents. J Hosp Infect. 2020;104(3):246-51.
43. Tang G, Chan AKM. Perioperative management of suspected/confirmed cases of COVID-19. World Fed Soc Anesth; 2020.pp.13.
44. Leegwater E, Strik A, Wilms EB, Bosma LBE, Burger DM, Ottens TH, et al. Drug-induced liver injury in a COVID-19 patient: potential interaction of remdesivir with P-glycoprotein inhibitors. Clin Infect Dis. [online] Available from https://academic.oup.com/cid/advance-article/doi/10.1093/cid/ciaa883/5864408. [Last accessed November, 2020].
45. Beigel JH, Tomashek KM, Dodd LE, Mehta AK, Zingman BS, Kalil AC, et al. Remdesivir for the treatment of Covid-19: preliminary report. N Engl J Med. 2020;383(10):994.
46. Guaraldi G, Meschiari M, Cozzi-Lepri A, Milic J, Tonelli R, Menozzi M, et al. Tocilizumab in patients with severe COVID-19: a retrospective cohort study. Lancet Rheumatol. 2020;2(8):e474-84.
47. Joyner MJ, Bruno KA, Klassen SA, Kunze KL, Johnson PW, Lesser ER, et al. Safety Update: COVID-19 Convalescent Plasma in 20,000 Hospitalized Patients. Mayo Clin Proc. 2020;95(9):1888-97.
48. CDC. Prescribing information: AVIGAN, Influenza antiviral agent. [online] Available from https://www.cdc.gov.tw/Uploads/9401abe5-274f-4090-a67e-70d76d9d425c.pdf#toolbar=0. [Last accessed December, 2020].
49. Stahel PF. How to risk-stratify elective surgery during the COVID-19 pandemic? Patient Saf Surg. [online] Available from https://www.ncbi.nlm.nih.gov/pmc/articles/PMC7107008. [Last accessed December, 2020].
50. Georgia-surgery, invasive-elective-procedure guidelines.pdf. [online] Available from https://www.aaos.org/globalassets/about/covid-19/georgia-surgery--invasive-elective-procedure-guidelines.pdf. [Last accessed December, 2020].
51. Clinical guide to surgical prioritisation during the coronavirus pandemic. [online] Available from https://www.england.nhs.uk/coronavirus/wp-content/uploads/sites/52/2020/03/C0221-specialty-guide-surgical-prioritisation-v1.pdf. [Last accessed December, 2020].
52. March 25 U, 2020. COVID-19 Guidelines for Triage of Emergency General Surgery Patients. American College of Surgeons. [online] Available from https://www.facs.org/covid-19/clinical-guidance/elective-case/emergency-surgery. [Last accessed December, 2020].
53. Medicine AS of RA and P. Practice Recommendations on Neuraxial Anesthesia and Peripheral Nerve Blocks during the COVID-19 Pandemic. [online] Available from https://www.asra.com/page/2905/practice-recommendations-on-neuraxial-anesthesia-and-peripheral-nerve-blocks-dur. [Last accessed December, 2020].

54. World Federation Of Societies of Anaesthesiologists - Coronavirus - guidance for anaesthesia and perioperative care providers. [online] Available from https://www.wfsahq.org/latest-news/latestnews/943-coronavirus-staying-safe. [Last accessed December, 2020].
55. Cook TM, El-Boghdadly K, McGuire B, McNarry AF, Patel A, Higgs A. Consensus guidelines for managing the airway in patients with COVID-19. Anaesthesia. 2020;75(6):785-99.
56. Canelli R, Connor CW, Gonzalez M, Nozari A, Ortega R. Barrier Enclosure during Endotracheal Intubation. Barrier enclosure during endotracheal intubation. N Engl J Med. 2020;382:1957e8.
57. COVID-19 Update: "Aerosol Box" During Intubation/Preventing Outbreaks in Retirement Communities / Guidance on Newborns. [online] Available from https://www.jwatch.org/fw116520/2020/04/05/covid-19-update-aerosol-box-during-intubation-preventing. [Last accessed December, 2020].
58. Zuo M-Z, Huang Y-G, Ma W-H, Xue Z-G, Zhang J-Q, Gong Y-H, et al. Expert recommendations for tracheal intubation in critically ill patients with noval coronavirus disease 2019. Chin Med Sci J; 2020.
59. D'Silva DF, McCulloch TJ, Lim JS, Smith SS, Carayannis D. Extubation of patients with COVID-19. Br J Anaesth. [online] Available from https://bjanaesthesia.org/article/S0007-0912(20)30172-0/abstract. [Last accessed December, 2020].
60. Coronavirus infection and pregnancy. Royal College of Obstetricians & Gynaecologists. [online] Available from https://www.rcog.org.uk/en/guidelines-research-services/guidelines/coronavirus-pregnancy/covid-19-virus-infection-and-pregnancy. [Last accessed December, 2020].
61. Xia H, Zhao S, Wu Z, Luo H, Zhou C, Chen X. Emergency caesarean delivery in a patient with confirmed COVID-19 under spinal anaesthesia. Br J Anaesth. 2020;124(5):e216-8.
62. Dong L, Tian J, He S, Zhu C, Wang J, Liu C, et al. Possible vertical transmission of SARS-CoV-2 from an infected mother to her newborn. JAMA; 2020. [online] Available from https://jamanetwork.com/journals/jama/fullarticle/2763853. [Last accessed December, 2020].
63. CDC. Care for Breastfeeding Women. Interim Guidance on Breastfeeding and Breast Milk Feeds in the Context of COVID-19. Centers for Disease Control and Prevention; 2020. [online] Available from https://www.cdc.gov/coronavirus/2019-ncov/hcp/care-for-breastfeeding-women.html. [Last accessed December, 2020].
64. CDC. Evaluation and Management Considerations for Neonates At Risk for COVID-19. Centers for Disease Control and Prevention; 2020. [online] Available from; https://www.cdc.gov/coronavirus/2019-ncov/hcp/caring-for-newborns.html. [Last accessed December, 2020].
65. Dong Y, Mo X, Hu Y, Qi X, Jiang F, Jiang Z, et al. Epidemiology of COVID-19 Among Children in China. Pediatrics. [online] Available from https://pediatrics.aappublications.org/content/early/2020/03/16/peds.2020-0702. [Last accessed December, 2020].
66. Kelvin AA, Halperin S. COVID-19 in children: the link in the transmission chain. The Lancet Infectious Diseases; 2020. [online] Available from https://www.thelancet.com/journals/laninf/article/PIIS1473-3099(20)30236-X/abstract. [Last accessed December, 2020].
67. Lu X, Zhang L, Du H, Zhang J, Li YY, Qu J, et al. SARS-CoV-2 Infection in children. N Engl J Med. 2020 23;382(17):1663-5.

68. Qiu H, Wu J, Hong L, Luo Y, Song Q, Chen D. Clinical and epidemiological features of 36 children with coronavirus disease 2019 (COVID-19) in Zhejiang, China: an observational cohort study. The Lancet Infectious Diseases. [online] Available from https://www.thelancet.com/journals/laninf/article/PIIS1473-3099(20)30198-5/abstract. [Last accessed December, 2020].
69. Sivabalan S, Srinath M. Does a Crying Child Enhance the Risk for COVID-19 Transmission? Preprint version. Indian Pediatrics. [online] Available from https://indianpediatrics.net/COVID29.03.2020/CORR-00166.pdf. [Last accessed December, 2020].
70. Lentz RJ, Colt H. Summarizing societal guidelines regarding bronchoscopy during the COVID-19 pandemic. Respirology. [online] Available from https://onlinelibrary.wiley.com/doi/abs/10.1111/resp.13824. [Last accessed December, 2020].
71. Francom CR, Javia L, Wolter NE, Lee GS, Wine T, Morrissey T, et al. Pediatric laryngoscopy and bronchoscopy during the COVID-19 pandemic: A four-center collaborative protocol to improve safety with perioperative management strategies and creation of a surgical tent with disposable drapes. Int J Pediatr Otorhinolaryngol. [online] Available from https://www.ncbi.nlm.nih.gov/pmc/articles/PMC7172675. [Last accessed December, 2020].